T0222406

KGMU Book of
Clinical Cases
in Dental Sciences

KGMU Book of
Clinical Cases
in Dental Sciences

The Georgians

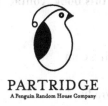

PARTRIDGE
A Penguin Random House Company

To order additional copies of this book, contact
Partridge India
000 800 10062 62
orders.india@partridgepublishing.com

www.partridgepublishing.com/india

Contents

KGMU BOOK OF
CLINICAL CASES IN DENTAL SCIENCES

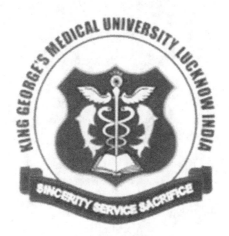

Editor In Chief
Dr. Ravi Kant
Vice Chancellor, KGMU, Lucknow
FRCS (England), FRCS (Ireland), FRCS (Edinburgh),
FRCS (Glasgow), FAMS, MS, DNB, FACS, FAIS

Additional Editor-In Chief
Dr. Shally Awasthi
Head, Department of Medical Education & Prof. of Pediatrics, KGMU, Lucknow
MD, DNB, MMSc, FNAS, FIAS, FIAP, FAMS

Preface

Medical Education is, on the one hand, emphasizing on predefined acquisition of skills and competencies, but on the other hand, is seeing a vast expansion of knowledge and emergence of new specialties and sub-specialties. The students often get caught in the maze of subjects. While competencies are developed in skills laboratories, virtual and real patients, knowledge is acquired, more often than not, by self-directed learning motivated by encounter with facilitators, peers or exposure to assessment.

This Book of Clinical Cases Dental Sciences is a compilation of real life cases seen across 9 Specialties in the dental sciences. Its sister book has done the same across 26 Specialties in the medical sciences. Each clinical vignette is followed by series of related questions or queries which promotes analytic thinking and stimulates linked learning in the reader. Hence this is a text book version of problem bases learning. In this sense the book is unique. Currently the market has many books on multiple choice questions for clearing various examinations. But the this text book transcends above the conventional multiple choice questions books since it will promote learning by reasoning, which will ensure long term of knowledge.

Each vignette is written by the experienced faculty of King George's Medical University, Lucknow, India (www.kgmcindia.edu). They have identified common as well as uncommon presentation of cases seen in medical practice. Since authors are well acquainted with the students' strengthens and weakness in subject specific knowledge, the book will, we are sure, be of great assistance to medical / dental students across all the years of medical and dental education. This book not only prepares a student to clear concepts and examinations but also prepares the practitioners in updating their knowledge in parent as well as allied subjects.

Dr. Ravi Kant
Editor –In Chief
FRCS (Engl). FRCS (Edin), FRCS (Glasg),
FRCS (IREL), MS, DNB
Vice Chancellor,
King George's Medical University,
Lucknow (UP) India

Dr. Shally Awasthi
Additional Editor-In Chief
MD (Pediatrics) DNB (Pediatrics) MMSc
(Clin Epid, USA)
Professor, Department of Pediatrics
Head, Department of Medical Education
King George's Medical University,
Lucknow

Foreword

In his book, "The Structure of Scientific Revolutions", philosopher Thomas Kuhn has argued that paradigm shifts i.e. changes in perspective are a mélange of Sociology, Enthusiasm and Social Promise and are not logically determinate. It has long been a belief with me that paradigm shifts, which are relatively easier during youth can bring about revolutions of positive results provided these are tempered with experience. After all, the human mind which many consider incapable of nothing, is thus also capable of inappropriate shifts in paradigm. It is this reasoning that leads me to believe that it is Medical Education Institutions, where fresh youth meet tempered experience, which are most capable of scientific revolutions in the medical field, several of which I too have witnessed. Thus, it causes me immense pleasure to write a foreword for the multidisciplinary book, KGMU Book of Clinical Cases in Dental Sciences.

Generally, interest in a subject causes it to be discussed and discussion generates new ideas as a result of these paradigm shifts. I think, as a result of being a premier dental education centre and thus fertile meeting ground between the bright young mind and tempered experience, KGMU has, is and will continue to witness such shifts frequently and thus has a social responsibility of sharing such shifts. This book should go a long way towards the fulfillment of this responsibility.

I remember the time when only a few textbooks on Dental Subjects were available to us and were usually written in a European or American setting. It is indeed a welcome move to publish a book of interesting cases of nine dental specialties, which contains 275 clinical situations; each accompanied by 3-5 multiple choice questions, from a local scenario. Not only will this give a better grasp to undergraduates and post graduates but will also be beneficial for faculty members and practitioners alike, thus resulting in an enhanced understanding of disease processes and a more comprehensive approach towards patient care.

Further, multi-specialty information available in a single book is of immense advantage to all practitioners of dentistry and will help dentists and dental specialists to appreciate the difficulties faced by other specialists thus making dental treatment more cohesive. Also, dental surgeons who have left teaching institutions are deprived of the benefits of interdepartmental clinical meetings. This book will be of tremendous help to them in multidisciplinary patient care.

I wish this book great success.

Prof. R. Pradhan
B.Sc.,B.D.S.,M.D.S.,F.I.C.D.,F.I.B.O.M.S.,F.D.S.R.C.P.S (Glasgow)
Former Head, Deptt. of Oral & Maxillofacial Surgery,
Former Dean, Faculty of Dental Sciences
K.G.M.U. Lucknow.
Former Principal & Director P.G. Studies,
Babu Banarsi Das College Of Dental Sciences.

Letter from the Dean's Desk

Dear Friends, I joined Dentistry at King George Medical College in 1978 as a 1st Year BDS Student completing my entire education up to PG here. Today after 37 years it gives me immense pleasure and feeling of pride as I present the KGMU Book of Clinical Cases in Dental Sciences.

Dental Faculty of King George Medical University was born as a section of Department of Surgery in 1949, with 10 Admissions. The Department of Dental Sciences was formed in 1950. It is one of the oldest Dental Educational Facilities in India and Post Graduate courses are running here since 1964. The Dental Department was upgraded to a Dental Faculty in 1980 with 7 Departments. It is considered amongst the top 4 Dental Educational Centre's in the Country.

The Dental Faculty King George Medical University today has 9 Departments, with PG courses running in 7 of them. It has an annual intake of 70 BDS students and 27 MDS students. The Faculty of Dental Sciences, King George Medical University, today treats more than a staggering 100,000 patients in a year. Our Alumni, known all over the World as "Georgians" constitute the who's who of dentistry in India & abroad.

KGMU Book of Clinical Cases in Dental Sciences is a compilation of case scenarios seen in all Dental Departments followed by related close ended questions promoting pertinent learning in the reader. This book is unique as it will ensure long term knowledge. Since authors are well acquainted with the students' problem areas, the book will be of great assistance to dental students across all years. This book will also update the practitioner's knowledge. I am thankful to Hon'ble Vice Chancellor Prof. Ravi Kant for his vision and contribution in enhancing the academic environment of our University.

I wish this book great success.

Prof A.P. Tikku
B.Sc., BDS, MDS, FICD
Dean
Faculty Of Dental Sciences,
King George's Medical University, Lucknow, UP, India.

Vice President, Indian Society of Dental Research
President, Indian Endodontic Society (IES)
President Athletic Association, KGMU
Spokesperson, Faculty of Dental Sciences, KGMU
Ex-Zonal Regent, International College of Dentists
Ex-EC Member, Dental Council of India
Ex- President: Federation of Operative Dentistry, India
Ex- President: India Dental Association, Lucknow Branch
Ex-Dean Student Welfare, KGMU
Ex- Member, State Dental Council, UP.
Ex- President, Kashmiri Association, Lucknow.

2. **Oral & Maxillofacial Surgery**
   Dr. R.K. Singh, *Professor*

3. **Periodontology**
   Dr. Pavitra Kumar Rastogi, *Associate Professor*

4. **Paediatric & Preventive Dentistry**
   Dr. Richa Khanna, *Assistant Professor*

Acknowledgement

We acknowledge the intellectual inputs and time devoted by the faculty of King George's Medical University Lucknow. We are grateful to the patients who formed the basis of case scenarios. We thank Mr. Nikhil Saxena for his tireless efforts in computing and formatting and other staff, Mr. Anand Mohan Singh and Mr. Satyendra Singh for facilitating the logistics and coordination.

Chapter - 1

Conservative Dentistry & Endodontics

Fluorosis Diagnosis and its Management

Dr. Vijay Kumar Shakya, Assistant Professor, Department of Conservative Dentistry & Endodontics

A 20 years old female patient reported to the Department of Conservative Dentistry and Endodontics with the chief complaint of compromised aesthetics due to discoloration of the teeth. These bands become darker from past few months and she wants aesthetic management for the problem. On examination, there was confluent pitting with brown discoloration present on most of the surfaces with some hypoplastic areas on enamel. Oralhygiene was good and the gingival tissue was in healthy state.

1. What would be the most likely clinical diagnosis?

    (A) Dental fluorosis
    (B) Hereditary enamel hypoplasia
    (C) Ectodermal dysplasia
    (D) Incipient dental caries

2. According to Dean's classification, this case is considered as?

    (A) Normal score '0'
    (B) Mild
    (C) Moderate
    (D) Severe

3. What is the most suitable treatment plan for this situation?

    (A) Vital bleaching followed by veneering.
    (B) Veneering only
    (C) Restoration of pitted surface.
    (D) None of the above.

4. Any bonded restoration on bleached surface must be postponed by;

    (A) 7-10 days
    (B) 10-14 days
    (C) 2-7 days
    (D) Does not need any delay

5. Which type of veneer is most suited in this situation?

    (A) Partial
    (B) Full
    (C) Full veneer with incise lapping
    (D) Does not require.

6. According to WHO and Dean's criteria, the optimum level of fluoride in drinking water should be:

   (A) 1.0 mg/l
   (B) 0.1 mg/l
   (C) 0.01 mg/l
   (D) 0.001 mg/l

Answers:

1. (A)

   Dental fluorosis is a type of enamel hypoplasia caused by excessive exposure of fluoride during tooth development usuallylesion are bilaterally symmetrical in nature. It presents as various degree of intermittent white spotting, chalky or opaque areas, yellow or brown discoloration with or without pitting. [1]

2. (D)

   According to Dean's index [2]
   Normal- Smooth, glossy, pale creamy-white translucent surface.
   Questionable- A few white flecks or white spots.
   Very Mild- Small opaque, paper white areas covering less than 25% of the tooth surface.
   Mild- Opaque white areas covering less than 50% of the tooth surface.
   Moderate- All tooth surfaces affected; marked wear on biting surfaces; brown stain may be present.
   Severe- All tooth surfaces affected; discrete or confluent pitting; brown stain present.

3. (A)

   Mild to moderate cases can be treated by bleaching only, however restorative approaches should be considered in severe cases. [1]

4. (A)

   The residual oxygen after bleaching procedure adversely affects polymerization and bonding thus bonded restorations should be avoided up to 7-10 days. [3]

5. (C)

In this case there is generalized defect and intrinsic discoloration present on the most of the facial surface that's why appropriate treatment is full veneer with incisal lapping [4]

6. (A)

Optimum level of fluoride in drinking water is 1.0 mg/l. [5]

References:

1. Ingle JI, Bakland LK, Baumgartner JC, Ingle JI. Ingle's endodontics6th ed. Hamilton, Ontario: BC Decker;2008: 1384.

2. Peter S. Essentials of Preventive and Community Dentistry. 4thed. New Delhi: AryaMedi Publishing House Pvt. Ltd; 2011:352.

3. B. Sureshchandra. V.Gopikrishna. Grossman's Endodontic Practice 10 th ed. New Delhi: Wolters Kluwer Health (India) Pvt. Ltd; 2010: 352,354.

4. Heymann H, Swift EJ, Ritter AV, Sturdevant CM. Non Carious Lesions and their Management. In: Sturdevant's art and science of operative dentistry. South Asian Edition. Haryana (India); EIE Limited-Unit printing press; 2013: 313,324.

5. Peter S. Essentials of Preventive and Community Dentistry 4th ed. New Delhi: Arya Medi Publishing House Pvt.Ltd; 2011:243

Cervical Abrasion Diagnosis and Treatment Planning

Dr. Vijay Kumar Shakya, Assistant Professor, Department
of Conservative Dentistry & Endodontics

A 32 years old male patient reported to the Department of Conservative Dentistry and Endodontics with the complaint of sensitivity in his right maxillary posterior teeth. On examination, tooth no 23 showed slight gingival recession and a 'v' shaped class V lesion on cervical third. Patient also gave the history of using hard tooth brush with a herbal tooth powder in vigorous horizontal motion. The lesion was smooth, shiny in appearance and extended to superficial dentine, incisally on cervical third of enamel and apically on cementum just passing the cervical line.

1. What would be the most likely clinical diagnosis?

    (A) Tooth brush Abrasion
    (B) Erosion
    (C) Abfraction
    (D) Attrition

2. How can we differentiate this lesion from a class V carious lesion?

    (A) Highly polished shiny surface with 'v' shaped defect present on facial surface of tooth.
    (B) Rough margins with soft caries on the lesion
    (C) Most commonly occurs on palatal surface of maxillary anterior
    (D) Catch on proving with soft dentine.

3. Most common cause of this type of lesions is?

    (A) Use of hard tooth brush with abrasive dentifrices.
    (B) Frequent use of acidic beverages.
    (C) Gastro-oesophageal reflex disease.
    (D) High occlusal forces on tooth.

4. Which is the most common site for such lesions?

    (A) Halt or modify the aetiology
    (B) Composite restoration of the lesion
    (C) A and B
    (D) No treatment requires

5. What is the most common site for abrasive lesions caused by faulty tooth brushing?

    (A) Left side teeth of right handed person.
    (B) Left side teeth of left handed person.

(C) Right side teeth of left handed person

(D) A and C

Answers:

1. (A)

   Tooth brush Abrasion is seen as sharp 'v' shaped smooth notch on facial surface of tooth. [1]

2. (A)

   Same as question 1[1]

3. (A)

   Improper tooth brushing habit and high abrasive dentifrices are the most common cause of tooth Abrasion [1]

4. (C)

   Composite restoration are the treatment of choice because of aesthetic consideration [2]

5. (D)

   Tooth brush abrasion are more common on left side of mouth in right handed persons and vice versa. [3]

References:

1. Heymann H, Swift EJ, Ritter AV, Sturdevant CM. Non Carious Lesions and their Management. In: Sturdevant's art and science of operative dentistry. South Asian Edition. Haryana (India);EIE Limited-Unit printing press;2013:293.

2. Heymann H, Swift EJ, Ritter AV, Sturdevant CM. Non Carious Lesions and their Management. In: Sturdevant's art and science of operative dentistry. South Asian Edition. Haryana (India);EIE Limited-Unit printing press;2013: 296-7.

3. R Rajendran. Regressive alteration of the teeth. In: R Rajendran, B Sivapathasundharam, editors. Shafer's textbook of oral pathology. New Delhi; Elsevier publishing Co, Inc; 2012: 573.

Trauma

Dr. Shibha, Junior resident –III, Department of
Conservative Dentistry & Endodontics

A 16 year old girl reported to the Department of Conservative Dentistry and Endodontics with the chief complaint of pain in the right maxillary central incisor due to trauma 3 years back. Endodontic testing revealed tenderness on percussion with negative result for vitality test. Radiographic examination revealed a wide radiolucency along with slight root resorption. Patient was advised apicoectomy followed by retrograde restoration with MTA.

1. In periapical surgery, which of the following flap design limits access to the operative site and often heals with scar formation?

    (A) Envelope
    (B) Rectangular
    (C) Semilunar
    (D) Triangular

2. Which is true about mucogingival flap design?

    (A) Flap should be wider at base
    (B) Flaps should be narrower at the base
    (C) Flaps margins should not rest on the book
    (D) Mucogingival flaps should be avoided

3. Apical surgery is least indicated in

    (A) Maxillary molars
    (B) Maxillary premolars
    (C) Mandibular molars
    (D) Mandibular premolars

4. Draining abscess by cutting a window in the bone is

    (A) Hilton's method
    (B) Trephination
    (C) Marsupialisation
    (D) Odontectomy

Answers:

1. C

   Inaccessibility, excessive haemorrhage, delayed healing, and scarring are the disadvantages of semilunar incision.

2. B

   The base of flap should be wider than the free end to ensure adequate circulation into the flap

3. D

   Apical surgery is done with great caution on mandibular bicuspids because of their proximity to the mental foramen

4. B

   Trephination is a type of artificial fistulation in which, the cortical bone is perforated to release the build up pressure and exudate around root apex to release pain

Reference:

1. B. Sureshchandra, V. Gopikrishna. Grossman's Endodontic Practice, 12th edition, New Delhi; Wolter's-Kluwer (India) Pvt Ltd.;2010:401-405.

Trauma

Dr. Shibha, Junior resident –III, Department of
Conservative Dentistry & Endodontics

A 17 year old girl rushed to the department with swelling of upper lip and avulsion of left central incisors. Tooth re-implantation was carried out by rinsing the avulsed tooth carefully with saline and all the contaminants were removed. After that, splinting of tooth was done.

1. Which medium of storage for avulsed tooth is best for prolonged extra oral periods?
    (A) Hank's balanced salt solution
    (B) Milk
    (C) Distilled water
    (D) Saliva

2. After more than 1 hour of extra oral time, an avulsed tooth is soaked in sodium hypochlorite solution, than it should be soaked in
    (A) 10% NaF for 10 min
    (B) 2% NaF for 10 min
    (C) 8% SnF for 10 min
    (D) 2% SnF for 10 min

3. Stabilisation of avulsed tooth requires
    (A) 1-2weeks
    (B) 2-3weeks
    (C) 4-6weeks
    (D) More than 6 weeks

4. In root fracture of the apical one-third of permanent anterior teeth, the teeth usually
    (A) discolours rapidly
    (B) remains in function and are vital
    (C) undergoes pulpal necrosis and becomes ankylosed
    (D) is indicated for extraction and prosthetic replacement

Answers:

1. A

    If tooth is not reimplanted immediately in dental office HBSS is best storage medium.

2. B

    If more than 1 hour is the extra oral dry time, the avulsed tooth should be immersed in 2 % sodium fluoride solution for 20 minutes.

3. A

    Regardless of the type of splint, splinting should be removed in 7-10 days since prolonged splinting may induce replacement resorption and subsequent ankylosis.

4. B

    In apical root one third root fracture tooth remains vital and resorbs normally.

Reference:

1. B. Sureshchandra, V. Gopikrishna. Grossman's Endodontic Practice, 12th edition, New Delhi; Wolters-Kluwer (India) Pvt Ptd; 2010:380-382.

Extra Oral Sinus

Dr. Ramesh Bharti, Assistant Professor, Department
of Conservative Dentistry & Endodontics

A 30-year-old male patient reported to the Dept. of Conservative Dentistry and Endodontics with chief complaint of pus discharge around the submental region associated with mild pain since last two weeks. Detailed clinical examination revealed grossly carious lower anterior tooth 31. He also presented with deep bite. Extra-oral examination revealed a cutaneous sinus tract near the chin. Radiographic examination revealed that tooth 31 to be the cause. Vitality of mandibular left central incisor and the adjacent teeth was checked using electric pulp tester.

1. What would be the most likely clinical diagnosis?

    (A) Cutaneous abscess
    (B) Cutaneous sinus with periapical abscess
    (C) Furuncle
    (D) all the above

2. Possible differential diagnoses could be

    (A) Tuberculosis
    (B) Impetigo
    (C) Dental sinus
    (D) None

3. Confirmed diagnosis is based on:

    (A) Clinical presentation of the lesion
    (B) Radiographic interpretation
    (C) Clinical and radiographic evaluation of the lesion
    (D) None of the above

4. Condition of the tooth is:

    (A) Vital
    (B) Non-vital
    (C) Partial Non-vital
    (D) Partial Vital

5. What is the etiologic factor of the sinus?

    (A) Periapical infection
    (B) Periodontal
    (C) Both
    (D) None

Answers:

1. B

    It may be due to chronic periapical abscess which leads the resorption of bone and formation of cutaneous sinus.

2. C

    Dental sinus is associated with periapical pathology of the tooth and *Bacteroidesovatus* is detected in the anaerobic culture. Aerobic culture is negative and PCR is negative for Mycobacterium tuberculosis.

3. C

    Radiograph confirmed that the lesion was odontogenic in origin and sinus tract was traced with guttapercha.

4. B

    Non vital

5. C

    Radiograph confirmed that the lesion was odontogenic in origin, traced to 31. So, the diagnosis of pulpal necrosis with suppurativeperiradicular periodontitis with 31 was confirmed.

References:

1. Kaban LB. Draining skin lesions of dental origin: The path of spread of chronic odontogenic infection. PlastReconstrSurg 1980; 66:711-7.

Pulp Polyp

Dr. Ramesh Bharti, Assistant Professor, Department
of Conservative Dentistry & Endodontics

A 30-year-old female patient reported to the Dept. of Conservative Dentistry and
Endodontics with chief complaint of pain and bleeding during chewing since last one
month. Detailed clinical examination revealed grossly carious lower right first molar
tooth and a pinkish red globule of tissue protruding from pulp chamber that was filling
the entire cavity. Vitality of the tooth was checked using electric pulp tester.

1. What would be the most likely diagnosis?

    (A) Acute pulpitis
    (B) Chronic pulpitis
    (C) Chronic hyperplastic pulpitis
    (D) Gingival abscess

2. The confirm diagnosis is based on

    (A) clinical presentation of the lesion
    (B) clinical condition of the patients
    (C) both of the above
    (D) none of the above

3. The above enlargement is

    (A) induced by hormonal change
    (B) induced by inflammation
    (C) due to trauma from occlusion
    (D) chronic inflammation of dental pulp tissue

4. Chronic hyperplastic pulpitis is also known as:

    (A) Gum polyp
    (B) pulp polyp
    (C) Dental polyp
    (D) all of the above

5. Treatment of pulp polyp is

    (A) Root canal treatment with removal of hyperplastic tissue
    (B) direct pulp capping
    (C) indirect pulp capping
    (D) all of the above

Answers:

1. C

    Chronic Hyperplastic pulpitis is essentially an excessive, exuberant proliferation of chronically inflamed dental pulp tissue.

2. A

    Pulp polyp appears as a pinkish-red globule of tissue protruding from pulp chamber and often filling the entire cavity.

3. D

    It occurs because of the unusual proliferation property of pulp tissue due to long standing inflammation of the pulp in young teeth.

4. B

    It appears as a pinkish-red globule of tissue protruding from pulp chamber.

5. A

    Chronic hyperplastic pulpitis may persist as such for long time. This condition is not reversible and may be treated by root canal treatment or some tome extraction of tooth if damage is more.

Reference:

1. William G Shafer. Textbook of oral pathology. 4th edition. Noida: Harcourt Asia PTE Ltd. 1999. 485-86.

Tooth Discoloration

Dr. Jyotsna Singh, Senior Resident, Department of
Conservative Dentistry & Endodontics

A 21 year old male came to the Department of Conservative Dentistry and Endodontics with the chief complaint of discoloured upper front tooth. The tooth was otherwise asymptomatic. He gave history of trauma while playing cricket 10 years back, for which he took no treatment. He wanted the discolouration to be rectified.

1. What could be the reason for discolouration?

    (A) Pulp necrosis
    (B) Fluorosis
    (C) Internal resorption
    (D) External stains

2. What is the treatment that could be done?

    (A) Extraction followed by implant
    (B) Non-vital intracoronal Bleaching/Walking Bleach after root canal treatment.
    (C) Microabrasion
    (D) None of the above

3. What are the agents used for non-vital bleaching?

    (A) Sodium perborate
    (B) Hydrogen peroxide
    (C) Both a and b
    (D) None of the above

4. Complications associated with walking bleach?

    (A) Cervical resorption
    (B) Chemical burns
    (C) Colour could revert back to a darker shade
    (D) All of the above

5. What is the most common age group associated with trauma to anterior teeth?

    (A) 10-12 years old
    (B) 1-2 years old
    (C) Both
    (D) None

Answers:

1. A

    There is decomposition of pulp tissue following trauma which causes discolouration.

2. B

    Walking bleach refers to placement of bleaching agent in the pulp chamber. When sealed into the chamber it oxidises and discolours the stains slowly, continuing its activity over a longer period of time, therefore called walking bleach.

3. C

    Sodium perborate when mixed with water or Hydrogen peroxide decomposes into sodium metaborate and oxygen. This nascent oxygen is responsible for the bleaching effect.

4. D

    To prevent cervical resorption, sealing of the canal orifice with 1mm of cavit over the guttapercha.

5. C

    In toddlers, as they are learning to walk. 10 to 12 yrs old are actively involved in sports activity

Reference:

1. B. Sureshchandra, V. Gopikrishna. Grossman's Endodontic Practice. 12th edition. New Delhi: Wolters-Kluwer (India) Pvt Ltd; 2010. 349-350.

Missed Canal in Maxillary Molar

Dr. Gitika, Junior Resident-III, Department of
Conservative Dentistry & Endodontics

A 32 year old female complained of persistent thermal sensitivity following root canal treatment of upper left 1st molar tooth. There was a composite restoration in access cavity of 26. There were no periodontal probing depths in excess of 4mm & no obvious apical radiolucencies.

1. What could be the most probable cause of this sensitivity?

    (A) Marginal leakage
    (B) ertical root fracture
    (C) Missed canal
    (D) None of above

2. Which canal is most likely to be missed in the maxillary 1st molar?

    (A) mesiobuccal1
    (B) mesiobuccal2
    (C) distobuccal
    (D) palatal

3. What is the frequency of occurrence of 4th canal in maxillary 1st molar?

    (A) 50%
    (B) 65%
    (C) 85%
    (D) 45%

4. Which of the following single rooted tooth has greatest probability of having 2 canals?

    (A) mandibular central incisors
    (B) maxillary central incisors
    (C) maxillary canines
    (D) maxillary lateral incisors

5. Which of the following tooth is an 'enigma to endodontist'?

    (A) maxillary 1st premolar
    (B) mandibular 1st premolar
    (C) maxillary 2nd premolar
    (D) mandibular 2nd premolar

Answers:

1. C

    Missed canal. Causes for "failure" of initial endodontic therapy have been described in the endodontic literature. These include iatrogenic procedural errors, such as poor access cavity design, untreated canals, poorly cleaned and obturated canals, complications of instrumentation and overextensions of root-filling materials [1].

2. C

    Maxillary first molar has four pulp horns (mesiolingual, mesiobuccal, palatal, distobuccal) and almost always has four canals [1].

3. C

    Two separate and distinct mesiobuccal canals occur in 84% of teeth in which two separate orifices are traced [2].

4. A

    Most mandibular incisors have a single root with a dentinal bridge present in the pulp chamber that divides the root into two canals [1].

5. A

    Bifurcations and trifurcations of the roots or root canals are the most common anomalies. They present a challenge during cleaning, shaping and obturation [2].

References:

1. Burn RC, Herbanson EJ. Tooth Morphology and Cavity Preparation. In:Cohen S, Burns RC. Editors; Pathways of the pulp. 9ᵗʰ ed. St. Louis: Mosby, Elsevier; 2006.

2. B. Sureshchandra, V. Gopikrishna. Grossman's Endodontic Practice. 12ᵗʰ edition. New Delhi;Wolter-Kluwer (India) Pvt Ltd; 2010: 472-473.

Vertical Root Fracture

Dr. Gitika, Junior Resident III, Department of
Conservative Dentistry & Endodontics

A 45 year old man reported to the Dept. of Endodontics with the chief complaint of pain on biting in lower right part of jaw. On oral examination, tooth no.46 manifested tenderness on percussion. Radiographic and periodontal evaluation was carried out which revealed isolated bone loss.

1. What is the probable diagnosis?

    (A) Acute irreversible pulpitis
    (B) Acute reversible pulpitis
    (C) Vertical root fracture
    (D) Periodontitis

2. What is the etiology of this condition?

    (A) Parafunctional habits
    (B) Iatrogenic dental treatment
    (C) Poor oral hygiene
    (D) Both A and B

3. Endodontically treated teeth are prone to this as

    (A) Such teeth have decreased hydration.
    (B) Excessive compaction pressure during obturation.
    (C) No correlation to endodontic treatment.
    (D) Teeth are heavily restored.

4. Radiographic evaluation is critical in this condition as

    (A) Isolated bone loss in the absence of advanced periodontal disease is unusual.
    (B) A "halo-like" appearance, traversing circumferentially around the root will be seen.
    (C) Sometimes "cement trail" can be seen across the root.
    (D) All of the above.

Answers:

1. C

   A tooth with vertical root fracture is typically painful with selective sensitivity on percussion. A vertical root fracture left undetected, creates a dehiscence in the bone and an isolated, deep and narrow bone loss (1).

2. D

   Vertical root fractures may arise from a physical trauma, repetitive parafunctional habits, resorption induced pathologic root fractures and iatrogenic dental treatment (1).

3. C

   Intracanal forces from excessive compaction pressure during obturation may also contribute to an increased incidence of vertical root fractures (1).

4. D

   Isolated bone loss to just one tooth in the absence of advanced periodontal disease is suggestive of vertical root fracture. The bone loss has a tendency to give a "halo-like" appearance. Split root with fracture extending from the mesial to the distal of the tooth can be interpretated after endodontic treatment by a "cement trail" seen up or across the root (1).

Reference:

1. B. Sureshchandra, V. Gopikrishna. Grossman's Endodontic Practice. 12th edition. New Delhi; Wolter-Kluwer (India) Pvt Ltd; 2010: 372-375.

Amelogenesis Imperfecta

Dr.Gunjan Garg, Senior Resident –III, Department of
Conservative Dentistry & Endodontics

A 13 year old male reported to the Department of Conservative Dentistry and Endodontics with chief complaint of sensitivity to cold and unesthetic smile. On clinical examination, enamel surface of all teeth was found to be yellow, soft, thin and pitted. There was no carious exposure or periodontal involvement of any tooth.

1. What is the most likelydiagnosis?

   (A) Hypocalcificamelogenesis imperfecta
   (B) Hypoplasticamelogenesis imperfecta
   (C) Hypomaturativeamelogenesis imperfecta
   (D) None of the above

2. What should be the treatment?

   (A) Full prosthetic coverage
   (B) Vital bleaching
   (C) Direct composite restoration
   (D) none of the above

3. Which esthetic treatment is contraindicated in such type of situation?

   (A) Full prosthetic coverage
   (B) Vital bleaching
   (C) Direct composite restoration
   (D) none of the above

4. Amelogenesis imperfecta affects

   (A) Only primary dentition
   (B) Only permanent dentition
   (C) Both
   (D) None of the above

Answers:

1. B

   Enamel found in this group is quite thin, often to the point of eliminating interproximal contacts. They usually have smooth hair, yellow appearance, although some pitting found on occasion

2. A

   The more common, as well as more predictable treatment is to provide full prosthetic coverage for affected teeth.

3. B

   Any vital bleaching is contraindicated because teeth exhibit insufficient, weak or abraded enamel

4. C

   Generally it is considered as genetic defect which affect both primary and permanent dentition.

Reference:

1. G. *Mclaughlin* and G.A. Freedman. *Color atlas of tooth whitening*, Ishiyaku Euro America Publishing, Missouri; *1991*: 17-18.

Replantation

Dr. Harsh Bhoot, Junior resident –II, Department of
Conservative Dentistry & Endodontics

A 15 year old patient reported to the Department of Conservative Dentistry & Endodontics with a chief complaint of injury about 1 hour back, by a swing that had backed up prematurely when she was not looking, knocking out the maxillary central incisor.

1. What would be the most likely clinical diagnosis?

    (A) Avulsion
    (B) Subluxation
    (C) Extrusion
    (D) Concussion

2. Ideal medium to carry the tooth is:

    (A) Saliva
    (B) HBSS
    (C) Water
    (D) Viaspan

3. Treatment of choice will be:

    (A) Replantation
    (B) Curettage of socket
    (C) Both a & b
    (D) None of the above

4. Ellis classification for this condition is:

    (A) IV
    (B) V
    (C) III
    (D) VI

Answers:

1. A

   Complete displacement of tooth out of socket is called avulsion

2. D

   Viaspan has been shown to decrease resorption and maintain fibroblast vitality, better than HBSS.

3. A

   The replacement of a tooth that has been removed from the alveolar socket, either intentionally or by trauma is called, replantation.

4. B

   that is tooth loss due to trauma.

Reference:

1. Weine FS. Endodontic therapy. 6th ed. St. Louis: Mosby; 2004: 88-89.

Condensing Osteitis

Dr. Harsh Bhoot, Junior resident –II, Department of
Conservative Dentistry & Endodontics

A 35 year old patient reported to the Department of Conservative Dentistry and Endodontics with an asymptomatic deeply carious tooth. Radiographic examination revealed a radiopaque mass attached to the apex of tooth.

1. The mass is most likely to be:

   (A) Cementoma
   (B) Condensing Osteitis
   (C) Rarefying osteitis
   (D) acute apical periodontitis

2. Which of the following differentiates between condensing ostietis and benign cementoblastoma?

   (A) Condensing osteitis is associated with vital teeth and benign cementoblastoma with non-vital tooth.
   (B) In condensing osteitis radio opacity is attached to the tooth, whereas in benign cementoblastoma, it is not.
   (C) Cementoblastoma is associated with vital tooth whereas condensing ostietis with non-vital tooth.
   (D) In cementoblastoma radio opacity is attached to the tooth whereas in condensing osteitis it is not.

3. Tooth most commonly involved in condensing osteitis is:

   (A) Maxillary 2nd molar
   (B) Maxillary 3rd molar
   (C) Maxillary 1st molar
   (D) Mandibular 1st molar

4. The clinical situation described above is also known as

   (A) Garre's disease
   (B) Chronic focal sclerosing osteomyelitis
   (C) Both a and b
   (D) None of the above

Answers:

1. B

   In condensing osteitis, the periodontal ligament space is widened and this is an important feature in distinguishing it from benign cementoblastoma.

2. D

   In condensing osteitis, radiographs demonstrate radiopacity which is not attached to tooth, entire root outline is visible, lamina dura intact and periodontal ligament is widened. These features differentiate it from cementoblastoma.

3. D

   Most commonly involved teeth are premolars and molars.

4. C

   It was described by Dr. Carl Garre in 1893.The sclerotic reaction results from good patient immunity and a low degree of virulence of the offending bacteria.

Reference:

1. William G Shafer. Textbook of oral pathology. 4th edition. Noida: Harcourt Asia PTE Ltd. 1999. 502-503

Chronic Apical Periodontitis

Dr. Isha, Junior resident –II, Department of
Conservative Dentistry & Endodontics

Michael, a 35 year old male patient reported with the chief complaint of pain in his lower right back tooth region since 2 days. On examination, a large carious lesion in the right mandibular first molar along with tenderness on percussionwas found. Radiograph of the particular tooth revealed widening of PDL space.

1.   What is the most likely diagnosis for the problem?

    (A) Reversible pulpitis.

    (B) Acute irreversible pulpitis.

    (C) Acute periapical abscess.

    (D) Periapical periodontitis.

2.   Which tests is not required to be included in routine clinical examination for confirmation of the endodontic diagnosis?

    (A) Cold test

    (B) Radiograpgh

    (C) Mobility

    (D) Electric pulp test.

3.   What is the treatment of choice in such cases?

    (A) Pulpotomy

    (B) Root canal treatment

    (C) Apicoetomy

    (D) Root amputation

4.   Which instrument is used to enlarge and smooth the root canals?

    (A) Barbed broach

    (B) Endodontic files

    (C) Endodontic reamer

    (D) Pesos reamer

5.   What is the most commonly used material to fill the root canal space after root canal treatment?

    (A) Silver points.

    (B) Guttapercha cones

    (C) Calcium hydroxide paste

    (D) Glass ionomer cement

Answers:

1. D

   The tooth is tender on percussion.

2. C

   Mobility determines the periodontal status of the tooth.

3. B

   Root canal treatment is the treatment of choice

4. B

   Endodontic K files are the commonly used instruments for enlargement and smoothening of root canals

5. B

   Guttapercha is the most commonly used obturating material

Reference:

1. B. Sureshchandra, V. Gopikrishna. Grossman's Endodontic Practice. 12th edition. New Delhi: Wolters-Kluwer (India) Pvt. Ltd; 2010:106-108.

Periapical Abscess

Dr. Isha, Junior resident –II, Department of
Conservative Dentistry & Endodontics

A 55 year old male patient reported with the chief complaint of pain and pus discharge in the upper front tooth region since 5 days. Patient gave history of root canal treatment followed by restoration in the front tooth 5 years back. On examination, a restoration was found in right upper lateral incisor and a draining sinus in its periapical region. Radiographic examination showed presence of a periapical radiolucency involving the root apex of the right lateral with well defined borders.

1. What is the likely diagnosis?

    (A) Chronic periapical abscess
    (B) Acute reversible pulpitis
    (C) Apical periodontitis
    (D) Irreversible pulpitis

2. What is the status of pulp vitality in such cases?

    (A) Vital
    (B) Non vital
    (C) Hyperresponsive
    (D) Hyporesponsive

3. What is the treatment of choice in such case?

    (A) Non surgical retreatment
    (B) Periapical surgery
    (C) Extraction
    (D) No treatment.

4. The type of restoration most commonly advocated for badly broken anterior teeth is

    (A) Composite restoration.
    (B) Post and core followed by crown.
    (C) Cast gold restoration
    (D) Glass ionomer filling

5. In case of persistence of pathosis even after retreatment, the next choice of treatment?

    (A) Extraction
    (B) No treatment
    (C) Periradicular surgery
    (D) Any of the above

Answers:

1. A

    A large periapical lesion with a draining sinus indicates periapical abscess.

2. B

    A root canal treated tooth becomes non vital.

3. A

    Non surgical retreatment is the most appropriate treatment option.

4. B

    Badly broken tooth is has to be restored using post core and crown.

5. C

    In case the retreatment fails, the next most appropriate treatment of choice is periapical surgery.

Reference:

1. B. Sureshchandra, V. Gopikrishna. Grossman's Endodontic Practice. 12th edition. New Delhi: Wolters-Kluwer (India) Pvt Ltd; 2010: 108-109.

Discoluration of Teeth due to Trauma

Dr Nidhi Bharti, Junior resident –III, Department of
Conservative Dentistry & Endodontics

A 20 year old patient reported to the OPD of Dept. of Conservative Dentistry and Endodontics with chief complaint of discolouration of upper front tooth. He gave historyof road side accident 10 years back, due to which his upper front tooth got fractured. He did not visit any dentist that time and took analgesics. The tooth was left unattended once pain was relieved. He noticed discolouration around 6-7 years back along with occasional pain. He found the discolouration to be increasing in intensity in the last few years leading to his present condition. On investigation, tooth was found to be non vital with cold test and radiograph showed a well defined radiolucency in the periapical region and incomplete apex.

1. What is the present pulp condition of the tooth?

    (A) Acute irreversible pulpitis.
    (B) Acute reversible pulpitis
    (C) Chronic irreversible pulpitis with apical periodontitis
    (D) Normal vital pulp.

2. What is the reason behind discolouration?

    (A) External staining
    (B) Intrinsic developmental staining
    (C) Intrinsic staining due to pulpal haemorrhage
    (D) Intrinsic staining due to fluorosis.

3. What is the cause of incomplete apex?

    (A) External root resorption due to trauma
    (B) Internal root resorption due to trauma
    (C) Incomplete apex formation due to trauma before root completion
    (D) None of the above.

4. Choose the Elle's classification for trauma to tooth

    (A) Class I
    (B) Class II
    (C) Class III
    (D) Class IV

5. What is the cause of radiolucency seen on radiograph?

    (A) Decrease in density of bone in periapical region
    (B) Localised destruction of periodontium due to inflammatory products.

(C) Incomplete apex

(D) Radiographic artifact.

Answers:

1. C

   The patient in question has a long back history of trauma which had irreversibly affected the pulp. Since he did not attend to the condition at that time the condition became chronic leading to the apical periodontitis.

2. C

   The physical impact on the pulp lead to the haemorrhage in the blood vessels supplying the pulpal tissue, leading to extravasation of red blood cells. These gradually broke down with time producing heam containing iron and other products that occluded the deninal tubules and hence the colour change.

3. C

   The tooth got traumatized at the age of 11. The normal chronological time for root completion of upper central incisor is 13. Due to trauma the normal root formation was disturbed as the pulp was insulted and devitalized, so completion of root apex did not take place.

4. D

   According to the classification given by Elle. Type IV fracture stands for fracture tooth in which the devitalisation of pulp occur due to trauma which may or may not involve the tooth structure. This stands true for the present case.

5. B

   Trauma to the pulp lead to inflammatory response forming products that in this case had easy access to the periodontium due to incomplete apex formation. they caused activation of osteoclasts in the periapical bone region and hence localized destruction of bone occurred.

Reference:

1. B. Sureshchandra, V. Gopikrishna. Grossman's Endodontic Practice. 12th edition. New Delhi; Wolters-Kluwer (India) Pvt Ltd. 2010: 330-335.

Dentine Hypersensitivity

Dr. Rakesh Yadav, Associate Professor,
Department of Conservative Dentistry & Endodontics

A 64 year male came to department of Conservative Dentistry with the chief complaint of hypersensitivity to cold in his lower teeth. On clinical examination, extensive loss of incisal andocclusal tooth structure of anterior teeth and premolars, root canal treatment with crown fabrication in molars due to same problem was found. There was no tenderness on palpation and no periapical radiolucency. Patient had history of supari and gutukha chewing along with use of gull powder since last 20 years.

1. What is the most likely diagnosis?

    (A) abrasion
    (B) attrition
    (C) erosion
    (D) abfraction

2. Most commonly accepted theory of hypersensitivity is

    (A) hydrodynamic theory
    (B) neural theory
    (C) odontoblastic transduction theory
    (D) none of the above

3. Treatment of hypersensitivity includes

    (A) occluding dentinal tubule
    (B) desensitize the nerve
    (C) both
    (D) none

4. The mechanism of action of Nd: YAG laser is by

    (A) occluding dentinal tubule
    (B) desensitizing the nerve
    (C) decreasing blood flow
    (D) none

5. Helium-Neon low output power laser used in hypersensitivity

    (A) affects electric activity (action potential)
    (B) affects A delta fibers
    (C) affects C fiber nociceptors
    (D) occludes dentinal tubules

Answers:

1. B

   As teeth exhibit extensive loss of incisal & occlusal tooth structure. [1].

2. A

   Brannstromproposed that nerve endings in the dentin–pulp border area are activated by hydrodynamic fluid flow in response to dentinal stimulation (the hydrodynamic mechanism). According to the hydrodynamic theory, rapid dentinal fluid flow serves as the final stimulus in activating intradentalnociceptors for many different types of stimuli[1].

3. C

   The rationale for laser-induced reduction in dentinal hypersensitivity is based on two possible mechanisms that differ greatly from each other. The first mechanism implies the direct effect of laser irradiation on the electric activity of nerve fibers within the dental pulp, whereas the second involves modification of the tubular structure of the dentin by melting and fusing of the hard tissue or smear layer and subsequent sealing of the dentinal tubules[1].

4. A

   Nd:YAG laser effect on dentin hypersensitivity is related to the laser-induced occlusion or narrowing of the dentinal tubules[1].

5. A

   Helium-Neon laser irradiation affects electric activity (action potential) rather than Ad- or C-fiber nociceptors.[2]

References:

1. Burn RC, Herbanson EJ. Tooth Morphology and Cavity Preparation. In: Cohen S, Burns RC. Editors; Pathways of the pulp. 9th ed. St. Louis: Mosby, Elsevier; 2006:434-435.

2. Stabholz A, Sahar-Helft S, Moshonov J. Lasers in endodontics. 2004;48:809-832.

Crown Lengthening

Dr. Rakesh Yadav, Associate Professor Department
of Conservative Dentistry & Endodontics

A 12 year old girl undergoing orthodontic treatment for malocclusion complained of unesthetic smile. On examination, protruded incisors and impacted canine was found. So, it was planned to manage the case by multidisciplinary approach involving orthodontic extrusion followed by crown lengthening.

1. Method used for surgical crown lengthening

    (A) Gingivectomy
    (B) Apically positioned flap
    (C) Apically positioned flapwith bone reduction
    (D) all of the above

2. Average biological width is

    (A) 3mm
    (B) 2mm
    (C) 3.5 mm
    (D) 1mm

3. The greatest advantage of the laser is

    (A) lack of local anesthesia injection
    (B) associated pre- and postoperative discomfort
    (C) enhances epithelization and improves wound healing after gingivectomy and gingivoplasty operations
    (D) all of the above

4. Crown lengthening with monopolarelectrosurgery is

    (A) painless
    (B) better than laser
    (C) produces pain and smoke thus necessitating the use of local anesthetics.
    (D) none of the above

Answers:

1. D

    Surgical crown lengthening procedure is done to increase the clinical crown length without violating the biologic width. Several techniques have been proposed for clinical crown lengthening which includes gingivectomy, apically displaced flap with or without resective osseous surgery, and surgical extrusion using periotome. [1]

2. B

Biologic width is composed of junctional epithelium and supracrestal connective tissues both acting as a biologic seal surrounding the teeth to protect subgingival connective tissue from microorganisms' actions and their products and support alveolar bone simultaneously. Width of each two sections is about 1mm while the biologic width has been reported to be about 2m. [1]

3. D

Laser is the least-invasive and predictable method of performing crown lengthening procedure. It has a high level of precision, requires minimal anesthesia and causes very low collateral tissue damage. [2]

4. C

There are two basic types of ES, monopolar and bipolar units. In monopolar ES units, the current begins with the ES device and travels along a wire to the oral site, then to an indifferent plate placed behind the patient's back. As the surgical electrode contacts the patient's oral soft tissues, heat is produced and controlled cutting is achieved. Bipolar ES devices have two electrodes on the cutting tip. The current flows from one electrode to the other, making a broader cut than does the monopolar unit, but eliminating the need for the indifferent plate. [3]

References:

1. Huynh-ba G. e ss e n z i Surgical lengthening of the clinical crown : a periodontal concept for reconstructive dentistry. 2007;4(3):193-201.

2. Agrawal AA. Esthetic crown lengthening with depigmentation using an 810 nm GaAlAs diode laser. Indian J. Dent. 2014;5(4):222-4.

3. Bashetty K, Nadig G, Kapoor S. Electrosurgery in aesthetic and restorative dentistry: A literature review and case reports. J. Conserv. Dent. 2009;12(4):139-44.

Trauma

Dr. Rhythm, Assistant Professor, Department of
Conservative Dentistry & Endodontics

A 22 year old, male patient reported to the department of conservative dentistry with the chief complaint of pain and mobility in his upper front teeth since few months. Clinical examination showed fractured maxillary central incisors with grade I mobility in the right central incisor. Intra-oral periapical radiograph revealed a horizontal fracture in the middle third of the root.

1. The IOPA X-ray depicts:
   (A) Vertical fracture of root
   (B) Horizontal fracture of root
   (C) Root resorption
   (D) Internal Resorption

2. What should be the immediate treatment given to this patient?
   (A) Root canal treatment
   (B) Extraction
   (C) Splinting of teeth
   (D) Post and core treatment

3. Which of the following is one of the healing patterns for this type of condition?
   (A) callus formation
   (B) celoid formation
   (C) keratin formation
   (D) scar formation

4. What type of intraradicular splint is used for such cases?
   (A) flexible
   (B) plastic
   (C) rigid
   (D) soft

Answers:

1. B

   The IOPA shows a horizontal break in continuity in the mid root region suggestive of horizontal root fracture [1].

2. C

The immediate treatment involves splinting and stabilization of the fractured root and is successful in approximately 80% cases with middle and apical root fractures [2].

3. A

Various types of histological responses seen at the fracture line in the roots can be categorised into four types: type I, interposition of calcified tissue (callus formation, radiographically fractured fragments appear in close contact); type II, interposition of connective tissue, (peripheral rounding of the fracture's ends visible); type III, interposition of bone and connective tissue, (appears on a radiograph as a clear separation between fractured ends); and type IV, the interposition of granulation tissue, caused by an infected or necrotic pulp [3].

4. C

Reinforcement of the tooth is desirable in such cases, and use of stainless steel files, metal posts and fibre posts has been documented to stabilise the fractured root[4].

References:

1. Andreasen F M, Andreasen J O, Cvek M (2007) Root fractures. In: Andreasen J O, Andreasen F M,Andersson L (Ed.): Textbook and color atlas of traumatic injuries to the teeth. Munksgaard, Kopenhagen, 337–371.

2. Oikarinen K, AndreasenJO, AndreasenFM Rigidity of various fixation methods used as dental splints. Dental Traumatol1992 8(3), 113–119.

3. B. Sureshchandra, V. Gopikrishna. Grossman's Endodontic Practice. 12th edition. New Delhi: Wolters-Kluwer; 2010: 371-372.

4. Subay RK, Subay MO, Yilmaz B, Kayatas M. Intraradicular splinting of a horizontally fractured central incisor: a case report. Dent Traumatol 2008;24(6): 680-84.

Complication of Local Anaesthesia – Soft Tissue Injury

Dr.Sakshma, Junior resident –II, Department of
Conservative Dentistry & Endodontics

A 22-yr-old female reported with swollen lower lip. She gave history of ongoing endodontic treatment and sudden appearance of the swelling in her lower lip. Oral examination revealed access cavity preparation with respect to tooth number 46.

1. This condition is

    (A) Frequent in younger children and mentally disabled adults
    (B) Painless
    (C) Self-inflicted trauma
    (D) Both A and C

2. What is the cause of this condition?

    (A) Itching in soft tissue due to intracanal irrigation
    (B) Allergic reaction to local anaesthesia
    (C) Soft-tissue anaesthesia lasts significantly longer than pulpal anaesthesia
    (D) Habitual, unrelated to endodontic treatment.

3. Management of the patient includes

    (A) Cold sponging
    (B) Antibiotics are unnecessary
    (C) Lukewarm saline rinses and analgesics
    (D) All of the above

4. This condition could be avoided by

    (A) Intradermal patch test before anaesthetizing the patient
    (B) Use of vasoconstrictor-free anaesthetic
    (C) Placement of cotton roll between the lips and teeth at the time of discharge
    (D) None of the above. Condition is a chance phenomenon.

Answers:

1. D

    Self-inflicted trauma occurs most frequently in younger children and in mentally or physically disabled children or adults. [1]

2. C

    Soft-tissue anaesthesia lasts significantly longer than pulpal anaesthesia. The primary cause is the fact that soft-tissue anaesthesia lasts significantly longer than does pulpal anaesthesia. A local anesthetic of appropriate duration should be selected if dental appointments are brief. [1]

3. C

    Management is symptomatic with analgesics for pain, antibiotics as necessary in the unlikely situation that infection results and lukewarm saline rinses to decrease swelling present. [1]

4. C

    A cotton roll can be placed between the lips and teeth if they are still anesthetized at the time of discharge. [1]

References:

1. Malamed SF. Handbook of local anesthesia. 6th ed. St. Louis: Elsevier Mosby; 2013: 292-309.

Complication of Local Anaesthesia-Facial Nerve Paralysis

Dr.Sakshma, Junior resident II, Department of
Conservative Dentistry & Endodontics

A 17 year old female patient reported with chief complaint of pain in lower right side of face. Her medical history was insignificant with no history of drug allergies. After examination and diagnosis, endodontic treatment was planned for the patient. But her face appeared lopsided after administration of local anaesthetic. She was also unable to wink her right eye.

1. This situation suggests

   (A) Contaminated local anaesthetic solution was used.
   (B) Needle has been broken and retained within tissues.
   (C) Tetanic spasm of the jaw muscles.
   (D) Introduction of local anaesthetic into the parotid gland.

2. This situation is

   (A) Transitory and will be resolved within hours.
   (B) Transitory and will be resolved within days.
   (C) Transitory but may progress to chronic hypomobility.
   (D) Permanent.

3. It could have been prevented by

   (A) A needle tip contact with medial aspect of ramus before L.A. deposition during IAN block.
   (B) Use of larger-gauge needles.
   (C) Use of aseptic technique.
   (D) Both A and B.

4. Management includes

   (A) Reassure the patient and advise use of eye patch on the affected eye until muscle tone returns.
   (B) Prescribe analgesics and muscle relaxants.
   (C) Immediate removal of the broken needle if visible.
   (D) All of the above

Answers:

1. D

   Facial muscle droop is observed when motor fibres are anesthetized by inadvertent deposition of local anesthetic into deep lobe of parotid gland, through which terminal portions of the facial nerve extend. [1]

2. A

   This loss is transitory and lasts no more than several hours. [1]

3. A

   It is preventable by adhering to protocol with IAN block correct positioning of needle tip in contact with bone. [1]

4. A

   There is no treatment other than waiting until the action of the drug resolves. Reassure the patient. Remove contact lenses and apply eye patch to the affected eye until muscle tone returns. [1]

References:

1. Malamed SF. Handbook of local anesthesia. 6th ed. St. Louis: Elsevier Mosby; 2013:292-309.

Vitality Test

Dr. Sanghamitra Suman, Junior resident – II, Department
of Conservative Dentistry & Endodontics

A 19 year old boy reported with chief complaint of slight discolouration of her right front tooth. Patient gave history of trauma 4 years back. On examination, 11 was found to be discoloured, so vitality test was carried out.

1. The preferred temperature to perform a heat test is

    (A) 55 degree Celsius
    (B) 65.5 degree Celsius
    (C) 77 degree Celsius
    (D) 63.5 degree Celsius

2. Laser Doppler Flowmetry is a method used to assess blood flow to

    (A) microvascular systems
    (B) microlymphatics
    (C) microvesicles
    (D) microspaces

3. Electric pulp tester detects pain by stimulating which nerve fibres

    (A) A alpha
    (B) A beta
    (C) A delta
    (D) C fibres

4. Testing with cold is carried out best

    (A) to localize pulpal pain
    (B) to localize periodontal pain
    (C) to localize referred pain
    (D) to test pulp necrosis

5. The most reliable among vitality test is

    (A) heat test
    (B) cold test
    (C) electric pulp test
    (D) test cavity

Answers:

1. B

   The preferred temperature for performing a heat test is 65.5 degree Celsius or 150 degree Fahrenheit.

2. A

   Laser Doppler Flowmetry is a non- invasive, better and more reliable method for determining the pulp vitality by measuring the blood flow.

3. C

   In Electric pulp testing, A delta fibres are stimulated directly.

4. A

   Cold test is a more accurate method than heat test to localize pulpal pain.

5. D

   When the sensitivity tests (thermal and electric pulp test) give inconclusive results, it will most often be possible to determine whether the pulp is vital or not by the preparation of a test cavity.

Reference:

1. B. Sureshchandra, V. Gopikrishna. Grossman's Endodontic Practice. 12th edition. New Delhi: Wolters-Kluwer; 2010: 67-70.

Bleaching

Dr. Sanghamitra Suman, Junior resident II, Department
of Conservative Dentistry & Endodontics

A 20 year old female reported with history of long term use of tetracycline. The anterior teeth had mild yellowish brown discolouration. The patient wanted to get the discolouration rectified.

1. Minimum dose of tetracycline which will show tooth discoloration is

    (A) 5mg/kg body weight
    (B) 20mg/kg body weight
    (C) 50mg/kg body weight
    (D) 80mg/kg body weight

2. Dentist prescribed home applied bleaching technique uses

    (A) 35%hydrogen peroxide
    (B) 10%carbamide peroxide
    (C) 18%hydrochloric acid
    (D) sodium perborate

3. Carbamide solution used for bleaching degrades into

    (A) 0.3% sodium perborate
    (B) 30%hydrogen peroxide
    (C) 3% hydrogen peroxide
    (D) 30% sodium perborate

4. the most common consequence of bleaching non vital teeth is

    (A) discoloration
    (B) Cervical resorption
    (C) Apical periodontitis
    (D) root resorption

5. Following intra-coronal bleaching, immediate composite restoration was required, so pretreatment with which of the following is required?

    (A) treat with catalase
    (B) wait for 7 days is mandatory
    (C) treat with hydrogen peroxide for 3 minutes
    (D) not possible

Answers:

1. B

    20 mg/kg of body weight is the minimum dose of tetracycline that may cause tooth discolouration.

2. B

    Night guard bleach or home technique uses 10% carbamide peroxide that degrades into 3% hydrogen peroxide and 7 % urea.

3. C

    10% carbamide peroxide used in night guard bleaching breaks into 3% hydrogen peroxide and 7%urea.

4. B

    Cervical resorption is a common consequence of bleaching of non vital teeth whereas apical periodontitis is a common sequel of bleaching vital teeth.

5. A

    Composite should be delayed for 2-3 weeks after bleaching, catalase treatment at the final visit may enhance removal of residual peroxides allowing for immediate composite restorations.

Reference:

1. B. Sureshchandra, V. Gopikrishna. Grossman's Endodontic Practice. 12th edition. New Delhi: Wolters-Kluwer; 2010: 359-360.

Endodontic Flare Up

Dr. Simith Yadav, Junior resident –II, Department of
Conservative Dentistry & Endodontics

A 27 year old female reported to the department of Conservative Dentistry & Endodontics with the chief complaint of food lodgement in upper left maxillary 1st molar area. On clinical examination, a class II caries approximating pulp was seen. Maxillary 1st molar had been asymptomatic before treatment but large periapical radiolucency was present. Canal had been enlarged to a size 40 at previous appointment but patient returned next day with severe swelling and pain.

1. What is the probable diagnosis?

    (A) Endodontic Flare up
    (B) acute exacerbation of chronic periapical abscess.
    (C) Necrotic pulp
    (D) none of the above

2. What precaution is advisable to prevent above situation?

    (A) No instrumentation beyond CEJ
    (B) Antibiotic prophylaxis
    (C) Irrigation between instrumentation
    (D) none of the above

3. This condition most commonly affects

    (A) Women
    (B) Men
    (C) Children
    (D) Elderly males

4. Most appropriate treatment will be

    (A) Completion of RCT
    (B) Corticosteroid antibiotic prophylaxis
    (C) No instrumentation and relief of occlusion
    (D) all of the above

Answers:

1. A

    The tooth is tender to percussion and palapation and area may be swollen and tense.

2. A

    The desire to remove unwanted tissue from the canal is most commendable, but if carried to any extreme, it may lead to the undesirable acute secondary apical periodontitis.

3. A

    Instrumentation beyond CEJ leads to the irritation of periapical tissue and exacerbation of existing chronic condition.

4. C

    Instrumentation beyond CEJ leads to the irritation of periapical tissue which in case of chronic pulp necrosis might exacerbate the chronic condition, manifesting as severe pain and swelling.

Reference:

1. Weine FS. Endodontic therapy. 6ᵗʰ ed. St. Louis: Mosby; 2004: 73.

Acute Alveolar Abscess

Dr.Simith Yadav, Junior resident –II, Department of
Conservative Dentistry & Endodontics

A 34 years old male reported to the Department of Endodontics with pain and swelling in the upper right back tooth region with an associated pus discharge. On taking history, patient revealed that swelling occurred 1 day back and patient was on self-medication for past 1 week for the pain associated with the tooth. On clinical examination, deep occlusal caries approximating the pulp was seen. Radiographic examination also revealed radiolucent lesion on the occlusal surface approximating the pulp.

1. What can be the probable diagnosis of this clinical situation?

    (A) Acute alveolar abscess
    (B) pulp necrosis
    (C) Apical periodontitis
    (D) none of the above

2. Most appropriate treatment plan:

    (A) Immediate access opening and drainage
    (B) antibiotic regime
    (C) Analgesics & wait and watch
    (D) none of the above

3. The confirmation of diagnosis is based on

    (A) Only clinical examination
    (B) clinical & radio graphical examination
    (C) Only radio graphical examination
    (D) none of the above

4. Most appropriate irrigant for this condition will be

    (A) Saline
    (B) NaOCl
    (C) H2O2
    (D) All of the above

Answers:

1. A

    Diagnosis of acute periapical abscess ranges from large diffuse swelling, targeted tooth being tender to percussion, mobile and lacking vitality. Radiograph ranges from no periapical change to definite radiolucency.

2. A

    Whenever possible, the acute periapical abscess should be incised and drained though root canal space, even if it requires damage to existing restoration.

3. A

    Swelling, tenderness to percussion and presence or absence of associated pus discharge in the form of sinus are all indication of acute periapical abscess.

4. A

    At the emergency appointment the preferred irrigant in the initial stages of inducing drainage should be warm sterile water or saline. The NaOCl has a tendency to clump the exudate, which might cause plugging of the apical constriction and halt the drainage.

Reference:

1. Weine FS. Endodontic therapy. 6th ed. St. Louis: Mosby; 2004: 77-78.

In Office Vital Bleaching

Dr. Umesh Kumar Yadav, Junior resident –III, Department
of Conservative Dentistry & Endodontics

A 29 years old female reported to the department of Conservative Dentistry & Endodontics with a chief complaint of discoloured anterior teeth. On taking history, she revealed that she was a heavy tea drinker.

1. What exactly is this clinical situation?

    (A) extrinsic discoloration
    (B) intrinsic discoloration
    (C) abrasion
    (D) erosion

2. Most appropriate treatment plan for this condition:

    (A) In office vital bleaching
    (B) non vital bleaching
    (C) night guard bleaching
    (D) walking bleach

3. Most common problem of sensitivity associated with bleaching is due to:

    (A) H2O2
    (B) NaOCl
    (C) Carbamide peroxide
    (D) Superoxol

4. Normal bleaching appointment is for:

    (A) 30-45mins
    (B) 20-20mins
    (C) 10-15mins
    (D) 60-90mins.

Answers:

1. A

   Stains on the external surface of teeth due to poor oral hygiene and habit like heavy coffee, tea and tobacco consumption.

2. A

   Vital bleaching procedure is indicated in various situations like discoloured teeth due to aging, trauma, drug ingestion or habits like heavy tea and coffee drinking.

3. A

   Small molecular size of Hydrogen peroxide enables it to penetrate enamel and dentin and thereby leading to temporary sensitivity.

4. A

   Normal bleaching time should be 30-45mins.

Reference:

1. B. Sureshchandra, V. Gopikrishna. Grossman's Endodontic Practice. 12th edition. New Delhi: Wolters-Kluwer (India) Pvt Ltd; 2010: 352-355.

Replantation

Dr. Umesh Kumar Yadav, Junior resident –II, Department
of Conservative Dentistry & Endodontics

A 35 years old male reported to the Department of Conservative Dentistry & Endodontics with a complaint of increase sensitivity to percussion and biting after non-surgical re treatment. Radiograph revealed periapical radiolucent lesion. But the tooth had a thick buccal bone, shallow vestibular depth and close proximity to the mandibular canal.

1. Treatment of choice for above mentioned situation is:
    (A) replantation
    (B) apicoectomy
    (C) extraction
    (D) hemisection

2. Which of the following is a contraindication to replantation?
    (A) vertical root fracture
    (B) periapical pathology
    (C) apical periodontitis
    (D) thick overlying buccal bone

3. QAfter replantation, sutures should ideally be removed by:
    (A) 1-2 day's
    (B) 2-4days
    (C) 4-5 days
    (D) 5-7 days

4. Ideal extra oral time for completing replantation procedure should be?
    (A) 7-8 mins
    (B) 10-12mins
    (C) 9-8mins
    (D) 3-4mins

Answers:

1. A

    Intentional replantation may be a treatment of choice when surgical access is very limited or presents unacceptable risks. Such as thick overlying buccal bone, close proximity to mandibular canal.

2. A

    Contraindication to replantation includes vertical root fracture, moderately curved roots and periodontal disease.

3. A

    Sutures should ideally be removed within 2-4 days to remove any potential irritant.

4. A

    Extra oral dry time should not be more then 7-8mins.

Reference:

1. B. Sureshchandra, V. Gopikrishna. Grossman's Endodontic Practice. 12th edition. New Delhi: Wolters-Kluwer (India) Pvt Ltd; 2010: 419-420.

Chapter - 2

Oral & Maxillofacial Surgery

Temporo-Mandibular Joint

Dr. Divya Mehrotra, Professor, Dr. Nitin Mahajan, Senior
Resident, Department of Oral & Maxillofacial Surgery

A ten year boy presented with chief complaint of inability to open mouth for past four years. He had history of fall from height five years back. On extra-oral examination, scar was present over the chin, and the chin was shifted towards the left side with prominent left antegonial notch. TMJ movements were not palpable on left side with almost nil mouth opening. OPG was advised and is shown below:

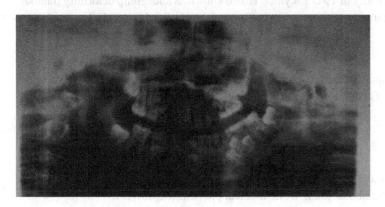

1. What is the most probable diagnosis?

   (A) Left hemifacialmicrosomia
   (B) Right TMJ ankylosis
   (C) Left TMJ ankylosis
   (D) Right mandibular hypertrophy

2. Facial deformity in TMJ ankylosisis represented as **EXCEPT**:-

   (A) Fullness on the affected side, flatness on unaffected side
   (B) Ande Gump deformity
   (C) Vogelgesicht deformity
   (D) Fullness on unaffected side

3. What is the treatment of choice in this case?

   (A) Gap arthroplasty
   (B) Gap arthroplasty with genioplasty
   (C) TMJ osteoarthrectomy, reconstruction of condyle with costochondral graft
   (D) TMJ ostearthrectomy with reconstruction of condyle with TMJ prosthesis.

Answers:

1. C

In TMJ Ankylosis, there is fullness on the affected sideand chin is shifted on ipsilateral side, flatness of mandible on contralateral side, and prominent antegonial notch with retruded mandible.[1]

2. D

Facial deformity in TMJ ankylosis is also known as andegump deformity (famous cartoon character without lower jaw), vogelgesicht (bird facies).[1,]

3. C

Gap arthroplasty leads to reankylosis. TMJ prosthesis are not advised in growing patient, CCG can be considered due to its growth potential.[2]

References:

1. Norman JE,deBurgh,Bramley P. Ankylosis: A textbook and color atlas of the temporomandibular joint: Wolfe medical publication;p151-171.

2. Fonseca RJ. Oral & Maxillofacial Surgery. 1st edition. Vol 4, TMJ Disorders. WB Saunders Company, Philadelphia. p 125-144.

Oral Tumours

Dr.DivyaMehrotra, Professor, Dr.NitinMahajan, SeniorResident,
Department of Oral & Maxillofacial Surgery

A 15 year old girl presented with chief complaint of painful bony swelling of lower jaw for past 1 year. On examination swelling was firm; temperature and color of overlying skin was normal. Orthopantomogram showed multilocular radiolucent lesion crossing the midline present. CT face was advised and a axial section through the mandible is shown below.

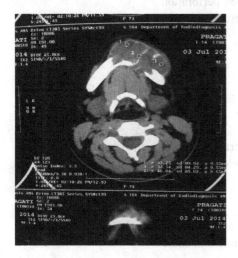

1. All these lesions have similar histopathologic findings EXCEPT:

   (A) Brown tumor of hyperparathyroidism
   (B) Cherubism
   (C) Central giant cell granuloma.
   (D) Odontogenicmyxoma

2. What is the treatment of choice for non aggressive type of central giant cell reparative granuloma?

   (A) Wide surgical resection
   (B) Composite excision of lesion with removal of next uninvolved barrier
   (C) Aggressive curettage
   (D) Resection of lesion without continuity defect.

3. What are the different non surgical treatments used in its management?

    (A) Weekly intralesionalinj. Triamcinolol for 6 weeks
    (B) Human Calcitonin inj subcutaneously
    (C) Interferon alpha
    (D) All of above

4. What are criteria behind the classification into aggressive and non aggressive type?

    (A) Lesion size and root resorption
    (B) Root displacement and cortical bone perforation
    (C) Growth rate, recurrence after curettage
    (D) All of the above

Answers:

1. D

    Central giant cell granuloma, hyperparathyroid tumor and cherubism are giant cell lesions and have similar histopathologic findings

2. C

    For non aggressive lesion –curettage and for aggressive lesion resection with histologically clear margins is the treatment of choice.

3. D

    Non surgical interventions used are weekly intalesionalinj triamcinolone for six weeks, 0.5mg (100 IU) S.C and interferon alpha 2a/2b

4. D

    Chuong R classified central giant cell granuloma as aggressive and non aggressive criteria for being graded as aggressive as size>5cm, rapid growth, root resorption, root displacement, cortical bone perforation and recurrence after curettage.

References:

1. Schmidt Brian L. Benign NonodontogenicTumors.in:MarcianiRobertD,voleditor. Oral and Maxillofacial surgery 2ndEd.VolII. Saunders Elsevier;2009.p.592-593.

Oral Tumours

Dr. Divya Mehrotra, Professor, Dr. Nitin Mahajan, Senior
Resident, Department of Oral & Maxillofacial Surgery

A patient comes with a history of pain and gradual increase in the size of swelling over the past few years and his orthopantomogram presents a picture like this, and there is no fluid on aspiration

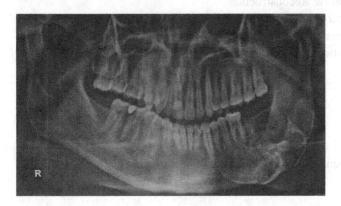

1. What does this radiographic picture show:

    (A) radio-opaque lesion in left body of mandible

    (B) mixed radiolucent-opaque lesion in left body of mandible

    (C) multicystic lesion in left body of mandible

    (D) fracture of body of mandible

2. What is the most probable diagnosis?

    (A) Dentigerous cyst

    (B) Amoeloblastoma

    (C) Ossifying fibroma

    (D) Odontogenicmyxoma

3. Which investigations would you require to confirm the lesion?

    (A) CT scan

    (B) Immunohistochemistry

    (C) Biopsy

    (D) MRI

4. What is the fate of inferior alveolar Nerve

    (A) is pushed inferiorly by the lesion
    (B) is pushed laterally by the lesion
    (C) is passing through the lesion
    (D) is involved with the lesion

5. What is the best management option

    (A) Surgical excision & Reconstruction
    (B) En Bloc Resection & Reconstruction
    (C) Segmental resection with continuity defect & Reconstruction
    (D) Marginal resection & Reconstruction

Answers:

1. B

    A mixed radio-opaque and radiolucent type of radiographic picture.

2. C

    Ossifying fibroma is a mixed radiolucent and radio opaque lesion

    Amelobastoma, dentigerouscyst, odontogenicmyxoma- radiolucent lesion.

3. C

    Histopathological examination is done to confirm the diagnosis of disease.

4. C

    Inferior alveolar nerve is pushed inferiorly as seen in OPG

5. C

    Segmental resection with continuity defect & Reconstruction is the standard treatment for Odontogenic Fibroma.

References:

1. Schmidt Brian L. Benign NonodontogenicTumors.in:MarcianiRobertD, voleditor. Oral and Maxillofacial surgery 2ⁿᵈEd.VolII. Saunders Elsevier;2009 .p.598.

Oral Tumours

Dr. Divya Mehrotra, Professor, Dr. Nitin Mahajan, Senior
Resident, Department of Oral & Maxillofacial Surgery

A young female patient presents with a swelling in anterior mandible, enlarging slowly over the past few years, crossing midline and presents a picture like this. On aspiration, there comes straw coloured fluid.

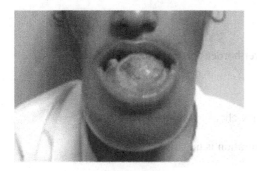

1. What clinical features does the picture show?

   (A) Incompetent lips
   (B) lesion in tongue
   (C) lesion in mandible expanding buccal cortex, lower border
   (D) peripheral lesion in mandible expanding buccal, lingual & lower border

2. What is the most probable diagnosis?

   (A) Odontogenickeratocyst
   (B) Amoeloblastoma
   (C) Ossifying fibroma
   (D) Odontogenicmyxoma

3. Straw coloured fluid is present in?

   (A) Dentigerous cysts
   (B) OdontogenicKeratocyst
   (C) Dermal cyst
   (D) Epidermal cyst

4. What should be the treatment plan

   (A) Resection till next anatomic barrier along with 1 cm of normal bone
   (B) Resection with 1 cm of normal bone
   (C) Curettage
   (D) Enucleation

5. What is the best reconstructive option
   (A) Reconstruction plate and iliac crest graft
   (B) Vascularized bone graft
   (C) Reconstruction plate
   (D) Reconstruction plate with cortico-cancellous chips in titanium mesh

Answers:

1. C

   Lesion of mandible buccal and lower border cortical expansion.

2. B

   Odontogenic cyst-cystic fluid is dirty cheesy in appearance

   Ossifying fibroma-solid tumor, aspiration is negative

   Odontogenicmyxoma-rare lesion

   Most probable diagnosis is ameloblastoma, cystic ameloblastoma shows straw coloured fluid on aspiration.

3. A

   Cystic fluid of dentigerous cyst is straw colored

4. A

   Treatment advised for large ameloblastoma is composite resection till next uninvolved anatomic barrier along with 1 cm of normal bone.

5. A

   Best reconstruction option is with load bearing plate and iliac crest bone graft.

References:

1. Schmidt Brian L. Odontogenic Tumors.in:MarcianiRobertD, voleditor.Oral and Maxillofacial surgery 2ndEd.VolII. Saunders Elsevier;2009 .p.476-502

Dental Implantology

Dr. Divya Mehrotra, Professor, Dr. Nitin Mahajan, Senior
Resident, Department of Oral & Maxillofacial Surgery

An adult male visits us for dental rehabilitation. His orthopantomogram shows a picture like this:

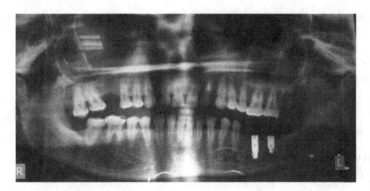

1. What does this radiographic picture show:

    (A) two submerged intra-osseous screws in left body mandible
    (B) two dental implants in left body mandible
    (C) odontome in anterior mandible
    (D) bilateral parasymphyseal fracture mandible

2. What is the best management option for right maxillary edentulous site

    (A) Fixed Bridge
    (B) Partial denture
    (C) Sinus lift & dental implant
    (D) Dental implant

3. What is the fate of inferior alveolar Nerve if dental implant impinges on it,

    (A) It is pushed inferiorly
    (B) It recovers within a month
    (C) It may recover within 6 months
    (D) It does not recover

4. When should rehabilitation routinely be done after implant placement

    (A) immediately
    (B) after 1 month
    (C) after 3 months
    (D) after 6 months

Answers:

1. B

    OPG shows two dental implants inserted w.r.t left body of mandible

2. D

    Dental implant is the best restorative procedure.

3. D

    Whenever a dental implant impinges over the canal, it should be removed and re implanted.

4. D

    Rehabilitation should be done after 6 months of implant placement.

References:

1. Malik N A. Dental Imlants an overview in: textbook of Oral and Maxillofacial surgery 3rd Ed..jaypee bros medical publisher, New Delhi.; 2011 .p.843-854.

Facial Deformity

Dr. Divya Mehrotra, Professor, Dr.Nitin Mahajan, Senior
Resident, Department of Oral & Maxillofacial Surgery

A 21 years old male presented with a prognathic mandible. His CT scan profile picture is seen below:

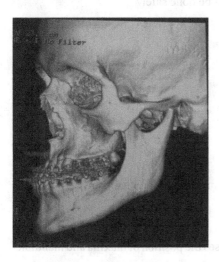

1. What does this radiographic picture show:

    (A) Midface hypoplasia

    (B) Zygomatic hypoplasia

    (C) Mandibular prognathism with maxillary hypoplasia

    (D) Mandibular prognathism

2. What Cephalometric measurements are NOT required?

    (A) SNA

    (B) SNB

    (C) Gonial angle

    (D) Nasion to Pogonion

3. What is the best management option

    (A) Lefort I osteotomy for maxillary advancement and Vertical Sub sigmoid osteotomy for mandibular set back

    (B) Lefort II osteotomy for maxillary advancement, and Bilateral sagittal split osteotomy for mandibular set back

    (C) Lefort I osteotomy for maxillary advancement and unilateral sagittal split osteotomy for mandibular set back

    (D) Bilateral sagittal split osteotomy for mandibular set back

4. Why is BSSO preferred osteotomy for advancement

   (A) Provides good bony overlap
   (B) Can be fixed with bone plates and screws
   (C) It is a versatile procedure
   (D) All of the above

5. How much of setback or advancement can be done safely

   (A) 1 cm
   (B) 0.5 cm
   (C) 0.8 cm
   (D) 1.5 cm

Answers:

1. C

CT scan shows maxillary hypoplasia and mandibular prognathism

2. D

SNA, SNB, Gonial angle all required to asses the position of maxilla and mandible to cranium and growth pattern of patient.

3. B

Excessive setback is not stable and is more prone to relapse, so both jaw surgery is advised to get a stable relation.

4. D

BSSO is considered as most stable orthognathic surgery as there is good bony overlap, stable fixation can be achieved and it's a versatile procedure.

5. A

Reference:

1. Fonseca RJ, voleditor. Oral and Maxillofacial surgery, Vol II. Saunders Elsevier; 2000:24-56.

Hemifacial Microsomia

Dr. Divya Mehrotra, Professor, Dr.Nitin Mahajan, Senior
Resident, Department of Oral & Maxillofacial Surgery

A 16 years old male presents with gross facial deformity. His picture is as below:

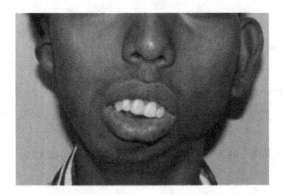

1. Which clinical features are NOT in the picture:

    (A) Midline shift in mandible

    (B) Canting of occlusion

    (C) Retrognathic chin

    (D) Extreme Overjet

2. What is the most probable diagnosis?

    (A) Treacher Collins Syndrome

    (B) HemifacialMicrosomia

    (C) TMJankylosis

    (D) Sleepapnoea

3. Treacher Collins Syndromepresents with

    (A) blue sclera

    (B) multiple jaw cysts

    (C) retrognathic mandible

    (D) frontal bossing

4. TMJ ankylosis presents with all EXCEPT

    (A) Ipsilateral chin shift

    (B) Contralateral chin shift

    (C) Retrognathic mandible

    (D) Reduced mouth opening

5. What should NOT be included in the treatment plan

    (A) Distraction osteogenesis
    (B) Genioplasty
    (C) Le Fort I osteotomy
    (D) Verticalsubsigmoid osteotomy

Answers:

1. D

    Extremeoverjet cannot be assessed in this picture

2. B

    Facial deformity on right half along with ear deformity points to hemifacialmicrosomia.

3. C

    Treachercollins syndrome presents with retrudedmandible, zygomatichypoplasia, ear deformity and orbital deformity.

4. B

    TMJ ankylosis presents with ipsilateral chin shift, retrognathic mandible and reduced mouth opening.

5. D

    For correction of facial deformity, distraction osteogenesis can be used to lengthen the mandible, genioplasty is to correct the shifted chin, while lefortI osteotomy is done to correct the occlusal cant.

References:

1. Fonseca RJ, vol editor. Oral and Maxillofacial surgery, Vol II. Saunders Elsevier; 2000 .p.24-56.

Maxillofacial Trauma

Dr. R. K. Singh, Professor, Oral & Maxillofacial Surgery

A 30 years female reported to the Oral & Maxillofacial Surgery Clinic at trauma centre, KG Medical University with chief complaint of pain and inability to close jaw since four day following road traffic accident. Her clinical examination revealed swelling and ecchymosis at mandibular angle region, disturbed occlusion, paresthesia on the lower lip right side with blood stained saliva dribbling from the corner of the mouth. Intra oral examination revealed the presence of lingual hematoma in right side third molar region. Buccal mucosa was lacerated between mandibular second and third molar region.

1. What is the most probable diagnosis?

   (A) Mandibular Symphysis fracture
   (B) Mandibular right angle fracture.
   (C) Mandibular Ramus fracture right side
   (D) Mandibular right body fracture

2. Inferior Alveolar nerve paresthesia is present in

   (A) Mandibular parasymphysis fracture
   (B) Mandibular Body fracture
   (C) Mandibular angle fracture
   (D) Mandibular Body& Angle fracture

3. Mandibular fracture are usually

   (A) Simple fracture
   (B) Compound fracture
   (C) Comminuted type fracture
   (D) Impacted type fracture

4. What is the most appropriate treatment for undisplaced Mandibular angle fracture?

   (A) Open reduction and single miniplatefixation at superior border.
   (B) Open reduction and reconstruction plate at the lower border.
   (C) Open reduction and two miniplate at upper and lower border of the mandible.
   (D) External pin fixation at angle of mandible.

5. Mandibular angle fracture are usually displaced due to muscles action of

   (A) Medial pterygoid and lateral pterygoid muscle
   (B) Lateral pterygoid and temporalis muscle pull
   (C) Medial Pterygoid and Masseter muscle pull
   (D) Masseter, Medialpterygoid and Temporalis muscles pull.

Answers:

1. B

   Lingual hematoma in 3rd molar region, buccal mucosa laceration b/w 2nd and 3rd molar and paresthesia points toward Rt angle Fracture is the most probable diagnosis.[1]

2. D

   Inferior alveolar paresthesia may be present in body as well as angle fracture of mandible.[1]

3. B

   Mandibular fractures are usually compound as fracture communicates through the lamina dura.[2]

4. A

   Open reduction and single miniplate fixation over superior border is most appropriate. [3]

5. C

   Mandibular angle fractures are displaced due to muscle pull of medial pterygoid and masseter.[3]

References:

1. Peter Banks. Killy's Fractures of the Mandible. 4th ed. Glasgow (UK):Wright Publishers 1991.

2. Malik NA editor. Text book of Oral & Maxillofacial Surgery. 3[rd]ed. New Delhi (India): Jaypee Publications 2012.

3. Balaji SM. The CompleteText book on Oral & Maxillofacial Surgery. 1st ed. Elsevier 2007.

Maxillofacial Trauma

Dr. R. K. Singh, Professor, Oral & Maxillofacial Surgery

A 22 year old male patient of road traffic accident, reported to department of oral & Maxillofacial Surgery with complaint of pain and difficulty in chewing for past two days. His chief complaint was pain in jaw since day of trauma. Clinical examination revealed swelling in the submental region, blood stained saliva and disturbed dental occlusion with mandibular arch collapsed anteriorly. CT scan showed fracture in the parasymphysis with overlapping of the fractured fragments. Intraorallyopen reduction and two miniplate fixation was done under local anaesthesia.

1. Mandibular symphysis fracture dislpaced due to pull of

    (A) Geniohyoid and genioglossus muscle pull
    (B) Geniohyoid, Genioglossus and Mylohyoid muscles pull
    (C) Geniohyoid, genioglossus, anterior belly of digastric muscle and mylohyoid muscle pull.
    (D) Geniohyoid, Genioglossus and anterior belly of digastric muscles pull.

2. Mandibular parasymphysis fracture results from

    (A) Direct violence
    (B) Indirect Violence
    (C) Direct and indirect violence.
    (D) Sudden excessive muscle contraction.

3. In mandibular Symphysis fracture maxillomandibular fixation (MMF)as treatment method is contraindicated in:

    (A) Pregnant patient
    (B) Head injury patient
    (C) Compound mandibular fracture
    (D) Mandibular condylar fracture.

4. Displaced Mandibular bilateral parasymphysis can cause:

    (A) Reduced tongue space
    (B) Reduce tongue space and airway problem
    (C) Reduce tongue space and difficulty in Maxillomandibular fixation.
    (D) Airway problem may not allow intraorally open reduction and internal fixation.

5. Mandibular angle fracture is usually associated with

    (A) ContralateralBody fracture
    (B) Ipsilateralsubcondylar fracture
    (C) Contralateralsubcondylar fracture.
    (D) Contralateral canine region or subcondylar fracture.

Answers:

1. B

    Muscle pull of geniohyoid, genioglossus, andmylohyoid makes the symphysis fracture displaced.[1]

2. A

    Mandibular parasymphysis fracture is usually due to direct violence.[1]

3. B

    IMF should not be done unless head injury is ruled out.[2]

4. B

    Displaced bilateral parasymphysis fracture displaces fracture fragment downwards and backwards reducing the tongue space and impinges over the airway.[3]

5. D

    Mandibular angle fracture is usually fractured with associated contralateral canine region or sub condylar fracture.[2]

References:

1. Malik NA editor. Text book of Oral & Maxillofacial Surgery. 3rded. New Delhi (India): Jaypee Publications 2012.

2. Peter Banks. Killy's Fractures of the Mandible. 4th ed. Glasgow (UK):Wright Publishers 1991.

3. Balaji SM. The CompleteText book on Oral & Maxillofacial Surgery. 1st ed. Elsevier 2007.

Maxillary Sinus Afflictions

Dr. R. K. Singh, Professor, Oral & Maxillofacial Surgery

A 45 years old patient reported to department of Oral &Maxillofacial surgery with the complaint of nasal fluid regurgitation following extraction of upper right first molar one month previously. Patient had nasal voice and intra oral examination revealed a small opening at tooth extraction side. Further examinations confirmed abnormal communication opens into maxillary sinus. Nose blowing sign was positive. On drinking water, fluid was regurgitated and escape from nose.

1. What is your diagnosis:
    (A) Acute Maxillary Sinusitis
    (B) Oro-antral Communication
    (C) Oro-antral fistula
    (D) Le forte I Fracture.

2. What is difference between Oro-antral communication (OAC) and oral antral fistula (OAF)
    (A) OAC and OAF are lined by epithelium
    (B) OAC is lined by epithelium.
    (C) OAF is lined by epithelium
    (D) Fresh antral opening is lined by epithelium.

3. Maxillary sinus opens into
    (A) Inferior meatus
    (B) Middle meatus
    (C) Superior Meatus
    (D) Ostium Maxillae.

4. The average volume of Maxillary sinus is
    (A) 10 to 15 ml
    (B) 15 to 30 ml
    (C) 10 to 25 ml
    (D) 20 to 35 ml

5. Fresh accidental opening during dental extraction can be treated by
    (A) Primary Wound closure and antibiotic therapy
    (B) Tongue flap only
    (C) Palatal flap only
    (D) Saline irrigation of wound and antibiotic therapy.

Answers:

1. C

   Whena oral antral communication tract gets epithelialized, it become oroantral fistula.

2. C [1]

3. B

   Maxillary sinus opens into middle meatus.

4. B

   Volume of maxillary sinus is 15- 30ml.

5. A

   Fresh accidental openings during extraction can be treated by primary wound closure and antibiotic therapy.

References:

1. Malik NA editor. Text book of Oral & Maxillofacial Surgery. 3rded. New Delhi (India): Jaypee Publications 2012.

Trigeminal Neuralgia

Dr. R.K. Singh, Professor, Department of Oral & Maxillofacial Surgery

A 55 years female presented with history of sharp stabbing pain of right side of face since past 4 years. Pain was triggered by eating, talking and touching in affected area. Her pain was sharp, shooting, intermittent type which lasted for few seconds to minutes. Pain was of unilateral type and never crossed midline or involved whole face. All teeth were healthy, without any symptoms. Diagnostic nerve block confirmed the involvement of inferior alveolar nerve.

1. What is most likely diagnosis?
   (A) Paroxysmal trigeminal neuralgia
   (B) Facial palsy
   (C) Phantom pain
   (D) Post trauma neuritis.

2. Post traumatic neuritis can be caused by
   (A) Nerve injury due to its exposure
   (B) Nerve injury during trans alveolar tooth extraction
   (C) Nerve stretching during osteotomy.
   (D) Transalveolar extraction & osteotomy procedures

3. In sweet diagnostic criteria for trigeminal neuralgia pain is of
   (A) The Pain is paroxysmal, unilateral
   (B) The pain is paroxysmal, unilateral and may be provoked by light touch to the face.
   (C) The pain is paroxysmal, bilateral and may be provoked by light touch to the face.
   (D) The pain is paroxysmal and can be provoked by light touch to the face.

4. The side effects of Carbamazepine therapy are all except -
   (A) Visual blurring, Dizziness, Somnolence
   (B) Hepatic dysfunction
   (C) Bone marrow suppression
   (D) Gingival hyperplasia

5. Repeated injection of 95% absolute alcohol should be avoided because
   (A) Causes local tissue toxicity and fibrosis
   (B) Causes local tissue toxicity, fibrosis and inflammation.
   (C) Causes fibrosis and inflammation
   (D) Causes fibrosis

Answers:

1. A

    White & Sweets diagnostic criteria for trigeminal neuralgia:
    *   Pain is paroxysmal.
    *   Pain may provoked by light touch to face(trigger zones).
    *   Confined to trigeminal distribution.
    *   Unilateral
    *   Clinical sensory examination normal

2. D

    Nerve injury while doing Tranalveolar extraction and osteotomy procedure may cause post traumatic neuritis

3. B

4. D

    Side effects of carbamazepine therapy are visual blurring, dizziness, somnolence, skin rashes and ataxia and in rare cases hepatic dysfunction, leucopenia, thrombocytopenia.

5. B

    Repated absolute alcohol injections causes local tissue toxicity, fibrosis and inflammation.

References:

1. Malik NA editor. Text book of Oral & Maxillofacial Surgery. 3rded. New Delhi (India): Jaypee Publications 2012.

Maxillofacial Trauma

Dr. R. K. Singh, Professor, Oral & Maxillofacial Surgery

A 26 years male presented with pain in the right side Tempero Mandibular Joint following assault that took place two days earlier. The extra oral examinations showed facial asymmetry and shifting of the chin towards injured side (right side). Sutured lacerated wound and edema was present on the chin. Intra oral examination revealed a malocclusion and shift in midline towards right side. Interincisal mouth opening was 20mm. Extra oral palpation showed diminishedcondylarmovements on right side and tenderness in the Subcondylar region.

1. What is most probable diagnosis:

    (A) Extracapsular mandibularSubcondylar fracture right side.
    (B) Intracapsular mandibular Subcondylar fracture right side.
    (C) Bilateral mandibular Subcondylar fracture
    (D) Condylar dislocation right side.

2. Mandibular condylar fractures are usually result of

    (A) Direct violence
    (B) Indirect violence
    (C) Direct or indirect violence
    (D) Excessive muscular contraction

3. Which radiograph is advised to visualize mandibularcondylar fracture

    (A) PA view of Mandible
    (B) Sub mento vertex view of skull.
    (C) Orthopentogram
    (D) CT Scan

4. The displacement of Fractured condylar fragment is due to

    (A) Lateral pterygoid muscle pull
    (B) Lateral pterygoid and Temporalis muscle pull
    (C) TMJ ligament and stylomandibular ligament pull
    (D) Sphenomandibular ligament pull

5. Complication of untreated Intracapsular fracture in children

    (A) Infection to middle ear
    (B) TMJ ankylosis
    (C) Condylar Hyperplasia
    (D) Internal derangement of TMJoint.

Answers:

1. A

    Swelling and laceration over chin, shifting of chin to right side, diminished condylar movement palpated on Rt side and tenderness over sub condyle region all pertains to extracapsular sub condylar fracture on right side.[1]

2. B

    Mandibular condylar fracture are usually result of indirect violence.[1]

3. D

    CT Scan is the gold standard to study the condylar fracture and interrelation and position of fracture fragments.[1]

4. A

    Lateral pterygoid muscle pull over condylar fracture fragment antero-medially causes displacement of fracture fragment.[1]

5. B

    Intra capsular fracture in children may leads to TMJ ankylosis. [1]

References:

1. Malik NA editor. Text book of Oral & Maxillofacial Surgery. 3rded. New Delhi (India): Jaypee Publications; 2012.

2. Peter Banks. Killy's Fractures of the Mandible. 4th ed. Glasgow (UK):Wright Publishers; 1991.

3. Ehrenfield M, Manson P, PrienJ.Principles of Internal fixation of the Craniomaxillofacial Skeleton: Trauma and Orthognathic Surgery. Dubendorf (Switzerland): AO Education- Publishing; 2012.

Maxillofacial Trauma

Dr. Vibha Singh, Professor, Department of Oral & Maxillofacial Surgery

A 21 years old female patient reported to the outpatient department of oral and maxillofacial surgery with the complain of restricted mouth opening, pain swelling and double vision. Patient was apparently normal 3 days back when she met with road traffic accident. There was no history of loss of conciousness, vomiting.

1. What will be the most likely diagnosis.

   (A) Left zygomatic complex feacture.
   (B) Left zygomatic complex fracture with lefort 2 fracture.
   (C) Bilateral zygomatic complex fracture.
   (D) Left zygomatic complex fracture with nasal bone fracture.

2. Diplopia may be because of

   (A) Alteration in globe level.
   (B) Muscle entrapment with fractured segments.
   (C) Paralysis of nerve.
   (D) All of the above.

3. In Force ductiontest with the tissue holding forceps we should hold the tendon of
   (A) Inferior rectus muscle
   (B) Inferior oblique muscle
   (C) Superior oblique muscle
   (D) Superior rectus muscle.

4. Treatment modality for above case will be
   (A) Open reduction with fixation
   (B) Close reduction
   (C) Transosseouswiring.
   (D) Open reduction fixation with reconstruction of orbital floor.

Answers:

1. B

   Frontal view NCCT Face shows a line of discontinuity from medial orbital wall, involving the infraorbital rim and passing downwards and laterally medial to infra orbital foramen till zygomatic buttress, breach in contiuity of body of zygoma and frontozygomatic suture region, with inward rotation of zygoma along the vertical axis. Most probable diagnosis is #Lt. LF II,Lt. ZMC.

2. D

   Alteration in globe level, muscle entrapment with in fractured segments, paralysis of nerve all leads to diplopia.

3. A

   Tendon of Inferior Rectus Muscle is holded in forced duction test to check the entrapment of muscle with in fracture fragment leading to inability to upward movement of eyeball.

4. D

   Open reduction and internal fixation along with reconstruction of orbital floor is the best option among all the options provided

Reference:

1. Malik N A, Injuries to the maxillofacial skeleton, Text book of Oral and Maxillofacial Surgery. Jaypee Brothers Medical Publisher New Delhi. 2005;p-301

Fractures

Dr. Vibha Singh, Professor, Department of Oral & Maxillofacial Surgery

A 25 years old male reported to the department of oral and maxillofacial surgery with the complaint of restricted mouth opening, inability to chew for 5 days. Patient was apparently asymptomatic 5 days back when he met with road traffic accident on clinical examination there was step and tenderness on both fronto- zygomatic region, at frontonasal region, tenderness over right zygomatic buttress, occlusion was deranged, step and tendeness on the lower border of mandible in the symphysis region.

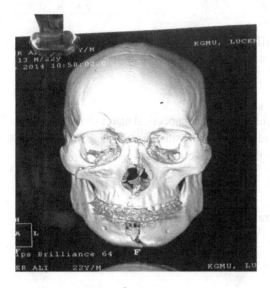

1. What will be the most probable diagnosis.

   (A) Bilateral lefort 3 fracture with right zygomatic complex fracture.
   (B) Bilateral lefor 3 with right zygomatic complex fracture with fracture mandible parasymphysis with dentoalveolar fracture mandible.
   (C) Right zygomatic complex fracture with fracture mandible parasymphysis.
   (D) All of the above are correct.

2. Management of mandibular fracture in the above case ideally how many plates should be placed?

   (A) One bicortical plate
   (B) Two monocortical plate
   (C) One monocortical and one bicortical plate
   (D) Two bicortical plate

3. Champys line of osteosynthesis are for fracture anterior to the mental foramina
   (A) Two plates are necessary to neutralize the torsional forces.
   (B) One plate is sufficient to neutralize the torsional forces.
   (C) Onemonocorical and one bicortical plates is sufficient to neutralize the torsional forces.
   (D) all of the above are correct

Answers:

1. B

   Complete diagnosis is #B/L LF-III, Rt.ZMC,Rt. Parasymphysis, dentoalveolar # of mandible.

2. B

   Acc to champy's principle of osteosynthesis, 2monocotical plates should be fixed in inter-foraminal region of mandible one below the apex of teeth and other at lower border. Both the plates should be atleast 5mm apart.

3. A

   Two plates are necessary to neutralize the tortional forces.

Reference:

1. Malik N A, Injuries to the maxillofacial skeleton, Text book of Oral and Maxillofacial Surgery. Jaypee Brothers Medical Publisher New Delhi. 2005;p-301

Trauma

Dr. Vibha Singh, Associate Professor, Department of Oral & Maxillofacial Surgery

Looking at the radiograph, the case may be assessed as:

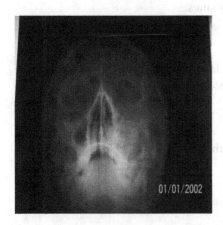

1.   What will be the most probable diagnosis.

    (A) Left zygomatic complex fracture.
    (B) Left Lefort 2 fracture., with zygomatic complex fracture
    (C) Right zygomatic complex fracture.
    (D) All of the above.

2.   Treatment modality for above case will be

    (A) Close reduction
    (B) Open reduction and fixation.
    (C) Open reduction and fixation at 3 places.
    (D) Open reduction and fixation at two places.

3.   In the above case these clinical findings will be present **EXCEPT**

    (A) Circumoribitalecchymosis.
    (B) Circumorbitaledema.
    (C) Diplopia.
    (D) CSF Rhinorrhea.

Answers:

1. B

    OMV view shows breach in continuity over Lt F-Z region, Lt.infraorbital rim, Lt zygomatic buttress and hazy Lt maxillary sinus.

2. C

    Open reduction and internal fixation should be done at Lt F-Z region, infraorbital rim and zygomatic buttress to get the stable fixation.

3. D

    All the options are correct but CSF rhinorrhea less likely to occur until cribriform plate of ethmoid bone has been fractured.

Reference:

1. Malik N A, Injuries to the maxillofacial skeleton, Text book of Oral and Maxillofacial Surgery. Jaypee Brothers Medical Publisher New Delhi. 2005;p-301

Cysts and Tumours

Dr. Vibha Singh, Professor, Department of Oral & Maxillofacial Surgery

A 18 years old girl reported to the department of oral and maxillofacial surgery with the complaint of swelling on right side of face for one year. Radiograph of the patient showing a large radiolucent lesion with a radio opaque mass and a tooth like structure on the lower border of the mandible. On aspiration clear straw color fluid was aspirated which shows total protein content -6.4g/dl, and albumin 3.8g/dl.

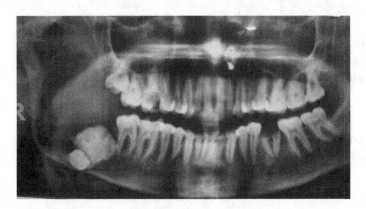

1. What will be the most probable diagnosis.

   (A) Dentigerouscyst.
   (B) Keratocysticodontogenictumor.
   (C) Priapicalcyst.
   (D) Dermoid cyst

2. Treatment of choice for above case will be

   (A) Marsupialization.
   (B) Marsupialization +enucleation
   (C) Enucleation
   (D) All of the above.

3. The complications of the cystic lesion are

   (A) Fracture of jaw
   (B) Infection prior to surgery
   (C) Dysplastic, or neoplastic changes
   (D) All of the above are correct.

4. Marsupialization is indicated in

   (A) Younger age group of patient
   (B) Proximity to vital structure
   (C) In very large cyst
   (D) All of the above

Answers:

1. A

   Points in favour of dentigerous cyst-Radiolucent lesion in relation to impacted tooth in molar-angle –ramus region of mandible with straw colored clear cystic fluid with protein content >4gm/dl

2. B

   Marsupialization and then enucleation is done if there is size of cyst is large, proximity to a vital structure, or risk of pathological fracture.

3. D

   All options are correct

4. D

References:

1. Malik N A,Cyst of the jaws oral and facial soft tissues, Text book of Oral and Maxillofacial Surgery. Jaypee Brothers Medical Publisher New Delhi .2005;p-401

Swelling

Dr. Vibha Singh, Professor, Department of Oral & Maxillofacial Surgery

55 years old male reported to the department of oral and maxillofacial surgery with the complaint of swelling on right lower jaw for 6 months. Patient was advised for radiograph OPG which was showing a radiolucent lesion involving right body of the mandible crossing midline..On aspiration there was thick cheesy material was found.

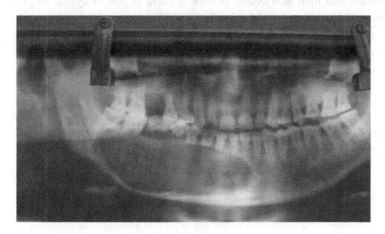

1. What will be the most probable diagnosis.

    (A) Dentigerouscyst.
    (B) Keratocysticodontogenictumor.
    (C) Priapicalcyst.
    (D) Dermoid cyst

2. Treatment of choice for above case will be

    (A) Marsupialization.
    (B) Marsupialization +enucleation
    (C) Enucleation
    (D) All of the above.

3. The complications of the cystic lesion are

    (A) Fracture of jaw
    (B) Infection prior to surgery
    (C) Dysplastic, or neoplastic changes
    (D) All of the above are correct.

Answers:

1. B

   KCOT has thick cheesy cystic fluid with protein content <4gm/dl.

2. B

   Marsupialization and then enucleation is done if there is size of cyst is large, proximity to a vital structure, or risk of pathological fracture.

3. D

References:

1. Malik N A,Cyst of the jaws oral and facial soft tissues, Text book of Oral and Maxillofacial Surgery. Jaypee Brothers Medical Publisher New Delhi .2005;p-401

White Lesions

Dr. Geeta Singh, Assistant Professor, Dr. Dichen Palmo Bhutia,
Resident, Department of Oral and Maxillofacial Surgery

A 45 yrs old male patient, with history of chronic smoking reported to dept of OMFS with chief complaint of white unscrappable lesion on his right buccal mucosa and adjoining gingival mucosa of mandibular posterior teeth of same side. The lesion appeared exophytic and non homogenous in texture.

1. Diagnosis on basic of clinical examination can be

    (A) Proliferative verrucous leukoplakia
    (B) Leukoplakia erosive
    (C) Nodular leukoplakia
    (D) Erythroleukoplakia

2. Moderate epithelial dysplasia refers to

    (A) Alteration limited to basal and parabasal layer
    (B) Alteration of basal to mid portion of spinous layer
    (C) Alteration from basal layer to level above epithelium
    (D) Alteration from subbasal layer to spinous layer.

3. Type of leukoplakia with high risk of converting to malignancy is

    (A) Prolferativeverrucous leukoplakia
    (B) Nodular leukoplakia
    (C) Leukoplakia simplex
    (D) Erythroplakia

4. Which among the following is not a hisopathological feature of leukoplakia

    (A) enlarged nuclei and cells
    (B) absence of rete pegs
    (C) increased nuclear to cytoplasmic ratio
    (D) pleomorphic nuclei and cells.

5. Leukoplakia can be most commonly superinfected with

    (A) Strepcococcal species
    (B) Candidal species
    (C) Gram negative rods
    (D) Staphylococcal species.

Answers:

1. A

PVL is characterized by multiple keratotic plaques with roughened surface projection.[1,2]

2. B

Option A is mild, option C is severe and option D is carcinoma in situ.[1,2]

3. D

PVL exhibit persistent growth becoming exophytic and verrucous in nature which can further progress into a stage indistinguishable from veruccous carcinoma. [1,2]

4. B

Leukoplakia exhibits bulbous and tear drop shaped rete pegs.[1,2]

5. B

Candida hyphae are found to isolated from the lesion. [1,2]

References:

1. Neville BW, Damm DD, Allen CM, Bouquot JE. Oral and maxillofacial pathology. 2nd ed. Pennsylvania: Saunders 2002.

2. Neelima AN. Oral and maxillofacial surgery. 3rded. New Delhi:Jaypee Brothers 2012.

Reduced Mouth Opening

Dr.Geeta Singh, Assistant Professor, Dr.Dichen Palmo Bhutia,
Resident, Department of Oral and Maxillofacial Surgery

A young male 24 yrs old presented to our Out Door Patient Department with complain of reduced mouth opening since 3 months. He has a habit of chewing 5 – 6 pouches of pan masala daily with the duration of 10 yrs. On palpation dense fibrous bands were palpated on bilateral buccal mucosa and also in retromolar region extending uptotonsillar pillars.

1. The condition is

   (A) Oral sub mucous fibrosis
   (B) leukoplakia
   (C) nicotine stomatitis
   (D) actinic chelosis

2. Malignant transformation rate of oral submucous fibrosis is

   (A) 7-13%
   (B) 20-25%
   (C) 5-10%
   (D) 25-50%

3. Grade III OSMF have interincisal distance

   (A) 15-25mm
   (B) 26-35mm
   (C) Less than 15mm
   (D) Less than 10mm

4. Prodromal symptoms in oral submucous fibrosis include all, EXCEPT

   (A) Blister apperance.
   (B) Dry mouth
   (C) Ulceration of oral mucosa.
   (D) Burning sensation

5. Pathogenesis of **oral submucous fibrosis** may be all except

   (A) Clonal secretion of fibroblast
   (B) Increased secretion of collagenase
   (C) Deficiency in collagen phagocytosis
   (D) Increased collagen cross linking

Answers:

1. A

OSMF is characterized by mucosal rigidity of varied intensity with chronic progressive scarring caused due to release of an alkaloid (arecaidine) from areca nuts.[1,2]

2. A

OSMF is chronic, progressive, scarring, high risk precancerous condition of the oral mucosa caused by fibroelastic hyperplasia and modification of superficial connective tissue..[1,2]

3. A

Grade I is earliest stage with interincisal distance greater than 35mm. grade II interincisal distance 26-35mm, gradeIII advanced stage eith IID less than 15mm, grade IV extensive fibrosis of all oral mucosa.[1,2]

4. B

Prodromal symptoms in OSMF exhibits excessive salivation with defective gustatory sensation. [1,2]

5. B

Stimulation of fibroblast proliferation and collagen synthesis with decreased secretion of collagenase.[1,2]

References:

1. Neville BW, Damm DD, Allen CM, Bouquot JE. Oral and maxillofacial pathology. 2nd ed. Pennsylvania: Saunders 2002.

2. Neelima AN. Oral and maxillofacial surgery. 3rded. New Delhi: Jaypee Brothers 2012.

Sublingual Hematoma

Dr. Geeta Singh, Assistant Professor, Dr. Dichen Palmo Bhutia,
Resident, Department of Oral and Maxillofacial Surgery

A 30 years male reported to our trauma centre unit with history of Road traffic accident few hours ago. On examination there was tenderness over right preauricular region with deviation of mouth to the left side. Intraoral examination revealed sublingual hematoma.

1. Sublingual haematoma is pathognomic of
    (A) symphyseal fracture
    (B) body of mandible fracture
    (C) Angular fracture
    (D) condylar fracture

2. Highest incidence of mandibular fracture site is

    (A) body
    (B) angle
    (C) symphysis
    (D) condyle

3. According to Kazanjian and Converse classification of fracture of mandible class III is
    (A) teeth present on both sides of fracture line
    (B) teeth present only on one side of fracture line
    (C) edentulous arches
    (D) fracture behind third molar

4. Group of muscles responsible for inward and inferior displacement of bilateralparasymphyseal fracture

    (A) Mylohyoid, geniohyoid, digrastic
    (B) Diagastric, gehiohyoid and genioglossus
    (C) Mylohyoid, geniohyoid and genioglossus
    (D) Mylohyoid, genioglossus and diagrastic

5. Overbending of plates during ORIF of mandibular fracture is done primarily for
    (A) Avoiding splaying of lingual cortices
    (B) Immediate pain relief and functional stability
    (C) Augmentation of tension band
    (D) Overcoming concentrated tensile forces

Answers:

1. A

    Extravasation of blood in the subcutenous or submucosal space in the floor of the mouth or sublingually refered *as Cormans sign* is pathognomic of symphyseal fracture. [1,2,3,&4]

2. D

    According to Dingman and Natvig incidence of mandibular site fracture is condylar process> angle>body>symphysis>ramus>dento alveolar> coronoid.. [1,2,3,&4]

3. C

    ClassIII when both the fragments on each side of fracture line is edentulous. [1,2,3,&4]

4. B

    If the bilateral fracture line in symphysis fracture runs obliquely forward and medially from the inner to outer cortical plate than due to pull of geniohyoid, genioglossus and anterior belly of diagrastic the entire anterior segment is displaced posteriorly eading to tongue fall..[1,2,3,&4]

5. A

    During Screw tighting achieve compression of fracture fragments avoid lingual spaying. [1,2,3,&4]

References:

1. Michael M, Ghali GE, Larsen P, Waite P. Peterson's principles of oral and maxillofacial surgery. 3rd ed. USA: People's Medical Publishing House 2011.

2. Fonseca RJ, Walker RV, Betts NJ, Barber HD, Powers MP. Oral and maxillofacial trauma. 4th ed. USA: Saunders; 2012.

3. Spiessel B, Rahn BA. Internal fixation of the mandible: a manual of AO/ASIF principles. Berlin: Springer; 1989.

4. Neelima AN. Oral and maxillofacial surgery. 3rd ed. New Delhi: Jaypee Brothers; 2012

Maxillofacial Trauma

Dr.Geeta Singh, Assistant Professor, Dr. Dichen Palmo Bhutia,
Resident, Department of Oral and Maxillofacial Surgery

A patient of road traffic accident was brought to our trauma centre unit with frank epistaxis from right side, bilateral circumorbital edema and ecchymosis and flattened nasal bridge. On examination there was enblock mobility of maxilla, step over bilateral infraorbital rim region, with pain and difficulty in opening of mouth.

1. Ptosis of uppereyelid is caused by damage to

    (A) Oculomotor nerve
    (B) Abducent nerve
    (C) Supra orbital nerve
    (D) facial nerve

2. Intercanthal distance in normal adult male measures

    (A) 28-35 mm
    (B) 30-35 mm
    (C) 32-38 mm
    (D) 32- 36 mm

3. Horizontal buttresses of midface are all except

    (A) Zygomaticomaxillary
    (B) Supraorbital
    (C) Infraorbital
    (D) Zygomatic arches

4. Dish- face deformity is pathognomic of

    (A) ZMC fracture
    (B) LF-I
    (C) LF-II.
    (D) F-III

5. According to Hendrickson classification of palatal fracture sagittal palatal split of median palatal fissure is seen in

    (A) type II
    (B) type IA
    (C) TYPE III
    (D) TYPE I B.

6. According to Gruss et al order of midfacial trauma reconstruction begin as
   (A) Zygomatico frontal, zygomatico temporal and thannasofrontal
   (B) Nasofrontal, zygomatico temporal and zygomaticofrontal
   (C) Zygomatico frontal, nasofrontal, andzygomaticotemporal.
   (D) None of the above.

Answers:

1. A

   Levatorpalpebraesuperiosis maintains level of eyelid when eyelids are open which is innervated by CN III.[1,2,&3]

2. A

   The average intercanthal distance in male is 33-34mm and in female 32-34mm. [1,2,&3]

3. A

   Zygomatico maxillary, pterygomaxillary and nasomaxillary buttresses are the vertical buttresses of midface.[1,2,&3]

4. D

   Craniofacial dysjunction with NOE fracture gives a characteristic dish-face deformatiy in LFIII fracture.[1,2,&3]

5. A

   Type I is alveolar fracture, type II sagittal fracture in the midline and type III para sagittal fracture.[1,2,&3]

6. A[1,2&3]

References:

1. Michael M, Ghali GE, Larsen P, Waite P. Peterson's principles of oral and maxillofacial surgery. 3rd ed. USA: People's Medical Publishing House 2011.

2. Fonseca RJ, Walker RV, Betts NJ, Barber HD, Powers MP. Oral and maxillofacial trauma. 4th ed. USA: Saunders; 2012.

3. Spiessel B, Rahn BA. Internal fixation of the mandible: a manual of AO/ASIF principles. Berlin: Springer; 1989.

Extraoral Sinus

Dr. Geeta Singh, Assistant Professor, Dr. DichenPalmoBhutia,
Resident, Department of Oral and Maxillofacial Surgery

A lady of 55 yrs presented to our OPD with pus discharge and difficulty in opening of mouth since 20 days associated with fever. On examination an extraoral sinus over the left body region with active discharge of pus was present. She gave a history of extraction of left 2nd molar 22 days ago. OPG revealed a typical "moth –eaten appearance"

1. The condition is

    (A) Fibrousdyslplasia
    (B) Osteoradionecrosis
    (C) Osteomylites
    (D) Paget's disease

2. Saucerization involves-

    (A) Removing infected and avascular pieces of bone
    (B) Removal of adjacent cortices and open packing to permit healing by secondary intension
    (C) Removal of infected bone and placement of vascular periosteum to medullary bone.
    (D) Removal of bone 1-2 cm beyond area of involvement.

3. "Onion skin" appearance in Garresosteomylities is due to

    (A) Subperiosteal bone formation
    (B) Due to granulomatous and suppurutive reaction
    (C) Due to cortical hyperostosis
    (D) Dense mass of bone trabuclae.

4. Hudson classified osteomylities as

    (A) Suppurutive and non suppurutive
    (B) Haematogenous and contigeous
    (C) Acute and chronic
    (D) Scleorising and recurrent.

5. True about osteomylities are all EXCEPT

    (A) Prime organisms are streptococci and aerobic bacteria
    (B) Infections are often mixed
    (C) Pus can travel via haversian and volksmann channels
    (D) Pain are described as deep and boring.

Answers:

1. C

   Granulation tissue between living and dead bone produces irregular lines and zones of radiolucency resulting in moth eaten appearance. [1,2,&3]

2. B

   Saucerization involves removal of formed and forming sequestrum eliminating dead space:[1,2,&3]

3. A

   Garre's osteomyelitis is chronic non supurrativesclerosing OML with proliferative periostitis and periostitisossificans.[1,2,&3]

4. C

   Patient history and clinical sign& symptom classify acute and chronic osteomyelitis.[1,2,&3]

5. A

   Prime organisms are streptococci and *anaerobic* bacteria.[1,2,&3]

References:

1. Michael M, Ghali GE, Larsen P, Waite P. Peterson's principles of oral and maxillofacial surgery. 3rd ed. USA: People's Medical Publishing House 2011.

2. Neville BW, Damm DD, Allen CM, Bouquot JE. Oral and maxillofacial pathology. 2nd ed. Pennsylvania: Saunders; 2002.

3. Wood NK, Goaz PW. Differential diagnosis of oral and maxillofacial lesions. 5th ed. Missouri: Mosby; 1997.

Chapter - 3

Orthodontics & Dentofacial Orthopaedics

Mouth Breathing

Dr. Alka Singh, Associate Professor; Dr Pradeep Tandon,
Professor & Head and Dr. Gulshan K. Singh, Professor,
Department of Orthodontics & Dentofacial Orthopaedics

A 12 year old male patient presented to the outpatient Department of Orthodontics with the chief complaint of forward placement of anterior teeth. On taking history he reported repeated cold and cough, with adenoidectomy by ENT surgeon one year back. On extraoral examination convex profile, increased lower face height & incompetent lips were present. Intraorally generalized gingival inflammation, proclination of maxillary anterior teeth, constricted upper arch with a high narrow palatal vault was observed.

1. The most likely cause of generalized gingival inflammation in this case may be?

    (A) Allergy

    (B) Constant wetting and drying of gingiva

    (C) Juvenile periodontitis

    (D) None

2. What would be the cause for increased facial height?

    (A) Supraeruption of posterior teeth only

    (B) Alteration in head posture alone

    (C) Altered respiratory pattern, change in head posture & supraeruption of posterior teeth

    (D) Altered respiratory pattern and supraeruption of posterior teeth

3. Which is not the commonly used test for mouth breathing?

    (A) Water holding test

    (B) Cotton wisp test

    (C) Blanch test

    (D) Mirror condensation test

4. What will be the ideal treatment plan for this patient?

    (A) A habit breaking appliance should be given to the patient immediately

    (B) Patient should be referred to ENT for further treatment

    (C) Patient should be given appliance for maxillary expansion to reduce nasal resistance after consultation with the otolaryngologist

    (D) None of the above

5. What would be the cause for maxillary constriction in this patient?

(A) Lowered tongue posture & incompetent lip posture
(B) Protruded anterior teeth& hyperactive mentalis muscle
(C) Lowered tongue posture & active buccinator mechanism
(D) Lowered tongue posture & hyperactive mentalis muscle

6. "Adenoid Facies" term was coined by?

(A) Norland (1918)
(B) Tomes (1872)
(C) Linder-Aronsen (1970)
(D) Solow and Krugburgh (1977)

Answer:

1. B

When the patient breathes through the mouth instead of nose, oral mucosa becomes dry leading to the cycle of constant wetting and drying of gingiva which causes irritation, saliva about the exposed gingival tend to accumulate debris resulting in an increase in bacterial population. [1]

2. C

Altered respiratory pattern would cause lower tongue and mandibular postural along with increase in craniovertebral angle, that will lead to supraeruption of posterior teeth & increase in lower face height. [2]

3. C

Blanch test is used to diagnose high labial frenum, all other test are used for mouth breathing. [3]

4. C

Patient had already taken treatment from the ENT surgeon and passed the stage of early intervention to prevent the adverse effect of mouth breathing. Now the treatment should be corrective that is RME appliance without extrusive mechanics (to control vertical) to reduce nasal resistance and promote nasal breathing along with the maxillary expansion [4]

5. C

Lowered tongue is less capable of balancing the lateral pressure of the cheek on the maxillary arch. This pressure differential across the hard palate in the absence of nasal airflow contributes to narrow high arch palate.[5]

6. B

Tomes (1872) [6]

References:

1. Kapoor TJ, Singh G. Oral Habits and their Management. In: Singh G, Textbook of orthodontics. 3rd edition. Jaypee, 2015: 607

2. Proffit WR, Fields HW. Etiology of Orthodontic Problems. Contemporary Orthodontics. 3th edition. Mosby, Inc, 2000: 137

3. Kapoor TJ, Singh G. Oral Habits and their Management. In: Singh G, Textbook of orthodontics. 3rd edition, Jaypee, 2015: 608

4. Kharbanda OP, Gupta A. Altered orofacial functions on development of face and occlusion. Orthodontics, Diagnosis and management of Malocclusion and Dentofacial Deformities. 1st edition. Mosby, Elsevier, 2009: 80

5. Proffit WR, Fields HW. Etiology of Orthodontic Problems. Contemporary Orthodontics. 3th edition. Mosby, Inc, 2000: 137

6. Kharbanda OP, Gupta A. Altered orofacial functions on development of face and occlusion: Orthodontics, Diagnosis and management of Malocclusion and Dentofacial Deformities, 1st edition, Mosby, Elsevier; 2009: 79

Tongue Thrusting

Dr. Sudhir Sharma, Senior Resident; Dr Pradeep Tandon,
Professor and Head and Dr Alka Singh, Associate Professor,
Department of Orthodontics & Dentofacial Orthopaedics

A boy aged 15 years came to the department with a chief complaint of spacing in upper front teeth. Medical and Dental history were irrelevant. On extra-oral examination patient was having apparently bilateral symmetrical face and convex Profile. Intraoral examination showed the patient in permanent dentition having proclined maxillary and mandibular incisors with spacing and Angle's Class I relationship. Drooling out of saliva through the spaced dentition was observed during swallowing. Cephalometric finding showed class I skeletal bases with average growth pattern.

1. What would be other procedure we can use for assessing this case?

    (A) Grummon's Analysis
    (B) Moyers Analysis
    (C) Assessing Oral Habits
    (D) Technitium Scan

2. What would be the probable diagnosis for this case?

    (A) Angle's class II div 1 malocclusion
    (B) Angle's class III Malocclusion
    (C) Angle's class I malocclusion with tongue thrusting habit
    (D) Angle's class I type 1 malocclusion

3. All Anatomic factors causes tongue thrusting habit except?

    (A) Prognathic Maxilla
    (B) Macroglossia
    (C) Enlarged Adenoids
    (D) Retruded Mandible

4. Interception and treatment of tongue thrust habit is commonly done with?

    (A) Headgear
    (B) Rapid maxillary expansion
    (C) Palatal cribs and spurs
    (D) Twin block

5. Tongue exercises, a treatment modalities in tongue thrust habit are all except?

    (A) Elastic band swallow
    (B) Speech exercises
    (C) Water swallow
    (D) Water holding test

Answer:

1. C

   The Tongue thrusting or abnormal swallowing pattern can be responsible for protrusion, spacing in the dentition or bidental protrusion. Grummons analysis is a comparative and quantitative. PA cephalometric analysis assesses transverse discrepancy. Moyers is a mixed dentition model analysis used for tooth material arch length discrepancy. Technitium scan involves imaging the skeleton using gamma emitting isotopes and can detect trabecular bone destruction before any radiographic abnormality is visible.[1]

2. C

   Molar relationship is Class I and patient is having Tongue thrusting habit so the malocclusion is Angle's class I with tongue thrusting habit.[2]

3. A

   Causes of tongue thrusting are Maturational, Anatomic and Neurogenic factors. In Anatomic factors macroglossia is overgrowth of the tongue, enlarged adenoids causes the tongue to be positioned anteriorly and retruded mandible also developed tongue thrusting habit. [3]

4. C

   Treatment modalities are reminder therapy and corrective therapy. In reminder therapy palatal crib, spurs, palatal rolling ball are given. In corrective therapy removal of obstruction, tongue exercises and lip exercises have been used.[4]

5. D

   Tongue exercises used to break the habit are elastic band swallow, water swallow, candy swallow and speech exercises. Water holding test is for diagnosis of mouth breathing habit. [5]

References:

1. Kharbanda OP. Diagnostic records. In: Kharbanda OP, Orthodontics: Diagnosis and Management of Malocclusion and Dentofacial Deformities. 2nd Edition. Elsevier, 2013: 188

2. Kharbanda OP, Gupta A. Altered orofacial functions and development of face and occlusion. In:Kharbanda OP, Orthodontics: Diagnosis and Management of Malocclusion and Dentofacial Deformities. 2nd Edition. Elsevier, 2013: 138

3. Kharbanda OP, Gupta A. Altered orofacial functions and development of face and occlusion. In:Kharbanda OP, Orthodontics: Diagnosis and Management of Malocclusion and Dentofacial Deformities. 2nd Edition. Elsevier, 2013: 138

4. Kharbanda OP, Gupta A. Altered orofacial functions and development of face and occlusion. In:Kharbanda OP, Orthodontics: Diagnosis and Management of Malocclusion and Dentofacial Deformities. 2nd Edition. Elsevier, 2013: 139

5. Kharbanda OP, Gupta A. Altered orofacial functions and development of face and occlusion. In:Kharbanda OP, Orthodontics: Diagnosis and Management of Malocclusion and Dentofacial Deformities. 2nd Edition. Elsevier, 2013: 141

Oligodontia

Dr. Gyan P.Singh, Associate Professor; Dr Pradeep
Tandon, Professor & Head and Dr. Alka Singh, Associate Professor,
Department of Orthodontics and Dentofacial Orthopaedics

A 20 years old female of normal mental and physical status has the complaint of multiple missing teeth in both the arches. Oral examination reveals multiple retained deciduous teeth, poor oral hygiene, end-on molar relationship on both side, overjet-2mm and overbite-2mm. Her upper lateral incisors, second premolars and lower second premolars are bilaterally missing. All the third molars are also missing. Patient's father is also having a similar problem.

1. What is the above mentioned condition called?

   (A) Anodontia
   (B) Oligodontia
   (C) Microdontia
   (D) Macrodontia

2. The main etiology behind this condition is?

   (A) Environmental
   (B) Genetic
   (C) Both A and B
   (D) Psychological

3. The term used to refer to the condition of second deciduous molar in this case is?

   (A) Ankylosed teeth
   (B) Fused tooth
   (C) Submerged tooth
   (D) Dentin dysplasia

4. The best approach to treat this type of malocclusion is?

   (A) Unidisciplinary approach
   (B) Multidisciplinary approach
   (C) Orthodontic approach
   (D) Prosthodontic approach

5. What is the best treatment strategy for the above patient problem?

   (A) Extraction of retained tooth
   (B) Move nearby tooth partially into edentulous space, then prosthetic management
   (C) Canine Space maintenance is recommended
   (D) Over denture placement

Answer:

1. B

    Oligodontia refers to congenital missing of many but not all teeth [1]

2. B

    It appears that a polygenetic multifactorial model is the best explanation of etiology [2]

3. C

    Submerged deciduous tooth - most commonly mandibular second molars undergo a variable degree of root resorption. [3]

4. B

    Oligodontia, often erroneously called partial anodontia, presents some of the most demanding problems in adult orthodontics and collaboration with other branches of dentistry is required to provide long term stable and functional occlusion. [4]

5. B

    It is best to move the tooth at least partially into the edentulous space so that new bone is formed and then the final prosthesis can be planned. [5]

References:

1. Proffit WR. The Etiology Orthodontic Problems. In: Proffit WR, Fields FW, Sarver DM. Contemporary Orthodontics. 5th edition. Mosby, St Louis, 2013: 128

2. Proffit WR. The Etiology Orthodontic Problems (Chapter 5). In: Proffit WR, Fields FW, Sarver DM. Contemporary Orthodontics. 5th edition. Mosby, St Louis, 2013: 128

3. Shafer WG, Hine MK, Levy BM. Developmental disturbances of oral and paraoral structures.. A textbook of Oral Pathology. 4th edition. W.B. Saunders Company, 1997: 69

4. Moyers RE, DrylandVig KWL,Fonseca RJ. Adult treatment. Handbook of Orthodontics for the student and general practitioner. 4ᵗʰedition. Year Book Publisher, 1988: 485

5. Proffit WR, Fields F W. Special considerations in comprehensive treatment of adults. Contemporary Orthodontics. 3ʳᵈ edition. Mosby, St Louis, 2000: 660

Cephalometrics

Dr.Gyan P.Singh, Associate Professor; Dr Pradeep Tandon, Professor & Head and Dr Alka Singh, Associate Professor, Department of Orthodontics and Dentofacial Orthopaedics

Lateral cephalogram is a supplemental diagnostic aid, use to diagnose the sketetal, dental and soft-tissue problems in the sagittal and vertical dimensions of the patient. It also uses to observe the treatment changes and the growth status of the individuals. There are various cephalometric analysis used to evaluate the skeletal, dental and soft-tissue structures like Down's, Steiner's and Tweed's etc. In these analysis there are anatomic landmarks, derived landmarks and reference planes which are used to draw the required information.

1. The analysis which uses the S-N plane as cranial reference plane?

   (A) Down's analysis
   (B) Steiner's analysis
   (C) COGS analysis
   (D) Tweed's analysis

2. The value of SNA=90^0 indicates?

   (A) Prognathic Maxilla
   (B) Retrognathic Maxilla
   (C) Prognathic Mandible
   (D) Retrognathic Mandible

3. Lateral cephalogram helps in the evaluation of various structures except?

   (A) Sagittal position of the jaws
   (B) Soft-tissue profile
   (C) Antero-posterior facial height
   (D) Transverse relation of the jaws

4. The additional information we can also get from the lateral cephalogram is?

   (A) Accurate age of the patient
   (B) Sex of the patient
   (C) Asymmetry of the jaws
   (D) Growth status (CVMI)

5. Frankfort horizontal is a reference plane constructed by joining?

    (A) Porion & Orbitale
    (B) Nasion & Sella
    (C) Porion & Sella
    (D) Porion & Nasion

Answer:

1. B

    The S (sella) and N (nasion) are easily discernible in a lateral cephalogram and can be located with relatively higher accuracy. Another advantage is their being located in the mid-sagittal plane of the head, they therefore move minimally with any deviation of head from true profile position. [1]

2. A

    Point A (anterior limit of the maxilla) reveals the position of the maxilla in relation to the cranium. [2]

3. D

    The PA cephalogram offers an effective tool in evaluating the craniofacial structures in transverse and vertical dimensions. [3]

4. B

    The size and shape changes in the bodies of five cervical vertebrae are good indicators of skeletal maturity. [4]

5. A

    Another stable reference plane used in Down's cephalometric analysis is the Frankfort horizontal plane. [5]

References:

1. Kharbanda OP. Steiner analysis. In: Kharbanda OP. Orthodontics: Diagnosis and Management of Malocclusion and Dentofacial Deformities.,2nd Edition. Elsevier, 2013: 231

2. Kharbanda OP. Steiner analysis. In: Kharbanda OP. Orthodontics: Diagnosis and Management of Malocclusion and Dentofacial Deformities.,2nd Edition. Elsevier, 2013: 232

3. Kharbanda OP. PA Cephalometric Analysis. In:Kharbanda OP, Orthodontics: Diagnosis and Management of Malocclusion and Dentofacial Deformities. 2nd Edition. Elsevier, 2013: 255

4. Kharbanda OP. Diagnostic records. In: Kharbanda OP, Orthodontics: Diagnosis and Management of Malocclusion and Dentofacial Deformities. 2nd Edition. Elsevier, 2013: 187

5. Kharbanda OP. Down's Analysis. In: Kharbanda OP.Orthodontics: Diagnosis and Management of Malocclusion and Dentofacial Deformities. 2nd Edition. Elsevier, 2013: 223

Mesiodens

Dr. Gyan P. Singh, Associate Professor, Dr. Pradeep Tandon,
Professor & Head; Dr Gulshan K. Singh, Professor, Department
of Orthodontics and Dentofacial Orthopaedics

A female patient aged 13 years presented with the chief complaint of proclined anterior tooth and an extra tooth present in between two upper central incisors. The patient had Angle's Class I molar relationship, overjet 4 mm and overbite 3 mm. The oral hygiene of patient was poor and patient had a family history of this presentation.

1. Tooth that lies in between the maxillary central incisors is known as?

    (A) Mesiodens
    (B) Peg lateral
    (C) Supplemental tooth
    (D) Dilacerated tooth

2. This kind of tooth is most commonly found in which region of mouth in maxillary arch?

    (A) Anterior region
    (B) First molar region
    (C) Premolar region
    (D) Third molar region

3. The presence of extra tooth is most commonly due to which factor?

    (A) Genetic
    (B) Developmental
    (C) Functional
    (D) Infection

4. All are commonly seen supernumerary teeth, except?

    (A) Paramolar
    (B) Parapremolar
    (C) Distomolar
    (D) Canine

5. Treatment of the supernumerary tooth preferably should be?

    (A) Extraction without space closure
    (B) Extraction with space closure
    (C) Observation only
    (D) Extraction and placement of implant

Answers:

1. A

    The most common supernumerary tooth that appears in maxillary midline is called a mesiodens. [1]

2. A

    Maxillary midline is the most common location for a supernumerary tooth.[2]

3. A

    Sedano and Gorlin have stated that the "mesiodens" is transmitted as an autosomal dominant trait, with lack of penetrance in some generations.[3]

4. D

    Supernumerary lateral incisors, extra premolars, and 4th molars occassionally occur. [4]

5. B

    Supernumerary teeth can disrupt the normal eruption of other teeth and cause crowding. Treatment is aimed at extracting the extra tooth and consolidating the available space.[5]

References:

1. Proffit WR. The Etiology Orthodontic Problems. In: Proffit WR, Fields FW, Sarver DM. Contemporary Orthodontics. 5th edition. Mosby, St Louis, 2013: 129

2. Proffit WR. The Etiology Orthodontic Problems. In: Proffit WR, Fields FW, Sarver DM. Contemporary Orthodontics. 5th edition. Mosby, St Louis, 2013: 129

3. Shafer WG, Hine MK, Levy BM. Developmental disturbances of oral and paraoral structures. A textbook of Oral Pathology. 4th edition. W.B. Saunders Company, 1997: 49

4. Proffit WR. The Etiology Orthodontic Problems. In: Proffit WR, Fields FW, Sarver DM. Contemporary Orthodontics. 5th edition. Mosby, St Louis, 2013: 129

5. Fields F W, Proffit WR. Moderate Nonskeletal Problems in Preadolescent Children. In: Proffit WR, Fields FW, Sarver DM. Contemporary Orthodontics. 5thedition. Mosby, St Louis,2013:424

Physiological Spacing

Dr. Amit Nagar, Professor; Dr Gulshan K. Singh, Professor and Dr Alka Singh, Associate Professor, Department of Orthodontics and Dentofacial Orthopaedics

Parents of a 5 year old child reports to a dental surgeon with the chief complaint of spacing in the dentition. The child has a normal growth pattern with no caries in any of the teeth, and the eruption schedule of deciduous teeth was normal. There was no habit of mouth breathing, tongue thrusting or thumb sucking. None of the permanent teeth have erupted in the oral cavity. Jaws show a normal growth pattern.

1. What could be the possible cause of spacing in this child?

    (A) Tooth size arch length discrepancy
    (B) Rampant caries.
    (C) Tongue thrusting habit.
    (D) Presence of spacing at this age is normal.

2. Second deciduous molar relationship (terminal plane relationship) in this patient is likely to be?

    (A) Mesial step
    (B) Distal step
    (C) Flush terminal plane
    (D) None of the above.

3. Primate spaces are present in deciduous dentition between?

    (A) Mesial to Maxillary and mandibular canines
    (B) Distal to maxillary and mandibular canines.
    (C) Distal to maxillary and mesial to mandibular canines.
    (D) Mesial to maxillary and distal to mandibular canines.

4. Leeway space of Nance is?

    (A) 3.4mm in mandibular and 1.8 mm in maxillary arch.
    (B) 1.8mm in mandibular and 3.6 mm in maxillary arch.
    (C) It is equal in both the arches.
    (D) Is present in permanent dentition only.

5. The spacing present in the above case?

    (A) Should be treated immediately with removable orthodontic appliance.
    (B) Should be treated after 1 year with removable or fixed orthodontic appliance.
    (C) Should be treated with functional appliance.
    (D) Should not be treated.

Answers:

1. D

   In deciduous dentition the presence of spacing is a normal occurrence. Various spaces present are physiologic spaces, primate spaces and leeway spaces.[1]

2. C

   In normally growing child, the deciduous molar relationship is flush terminal plane relationship. In this relationship, distal surfaces of both maxillary and mandibular second molars are in a straight line.[2]

3. D

   Primate spaces are present in majority of deciduous dentition between lateral incisor and canines in maxillary arch and distal to canine in mandibular arch.[3]

4. A

   Leeway space is greater in mandibular arch ie.3.4 mm in mandibular arch and 1.8mm in maxillary arch.[4]

5. D

   Since the spaces present in deciduous dentition are considered normal, they do not require any treatment.[5]

<u>Reference:</u>

1. Samir EB. Development of Dental Occlusion. Text Book Of Orthodontics. 1stedition. W.B. Saunders Company, 2001: 56.

2. Samir EB. Development of Dental Occlusion. Text Book Of Orthodontics. 1stedition. W.B.Saunders Company, 2001: 57.

3. Samir EB. Development of Dental Occlusion. Text Book Of Orthodontics. 1stedition. W.B.Saunders Company, 2001: 54.

4. Samir EB. Development of Dental Occlusion. Text Book Of Orthodontics. 1st edition. W.B.Saunders Company, 2001: 57.

5. Samir EB. Development of Dental Occlusion. Text Book Of Orthodontics. 1st edition. W.B.Saunders Company, 2001: 54.

Severe Crowding

Dr. Gyan P. Singh, Associate Professor; Dr. Pradeep Tandon,
Professor and Head and Dr. Amit Nagar, Professor, Department
of Orthodontics and Dentofacial Orthopaedics

A 13 year old female patient presented with unpleasant smile and irregularity of teeth, Molar relationship was Angle's Class I with crowding of 9 mm in both upper and lower arches. Extraction treatment was planned and fixed 022 slot edgewise appliance was selected.

1. Which is the commonest malocclusion normally found in population?

    (A) Angle's Class I
    (B) Angle's Class II Div.1
    (C) Angle's Class II Div.2
    (D) Angle's Class III

2. The commonest tooth extracted for orthodontic purpose is?

    (A) Canine
    (B) Incisor
    (C) Molar
    (D) First Premolar

3. The most common reason of seeking orthodontic treatment?

    (A) Functional concern
    (B) Esthetic concern
    (C) Stability concern
    (D) Status concern

4. Exraction cases can be best treated by the use of?

    (A) Functional appliance
    (B) Fixed appliance
    (C) Semifixed appliance
    (D) Removable appliance

5. Exraction of premolars is helpful in resolving all problems **except**?

    (A) Relieve crowding
    (B) Overjet correction
    (C) Levelling of curve of spee
    (D) Reduced anchorage requirement

Answers:

1. A

    A normal relationship of primary molar teeth is flush terminal plane. Mandibular molar normally moves mesially more than its maxillary counterpart. This differential movement contributes to the normal transition from a flush terminal plane relationship in the mixed dentition to a Class I relationship in the permanent dentition.[1]

2. D

    The Extraction of first premolar provides the greater range of differential movements as per individual need to protract the posterior, or retract anterior teeth as well.[2]

3. B

    A major motivation for seeking orthodontic treatment is to enhance dental and facial aesthetics, besides improvement of function and status of oral health.[3]

4. B

    The fixed appliance is able to better control tooth movement in all the three dimensions.[4]

5. D

    Retraction of the anterior segment is required to close the space created by extraction of first premolars. The premolar extraction spaces are closed using buccal segments as anchor teeth.[5]

References:

1. Proffit WR, Fields FW. Early stages of development. Contemporary Orthodontics. 3rd edition. Mosby, St Louis, 2000: 90

2. Proffit WR, Fields FW. Complex Nonskeletal problems in preadolescent children. Contemporary Orthodontics. 3rd edition. Mosby, St Louis, 2000: 458

3. Kharbanda OP. Psychological implications of malocclusions and orthodontic treatment. In: Kharbanda OP, Orthodontics: Diagnosis and Management of Malocclusion and Dentofacial Deformities. 2nd edition. Elsevier,2013: 57

4. Kharbanda OP. Components of fixed orthodontic appliance. In: Kharbanda OP, Orthodontics: Diagnosis and Management of Malocclusion and Dentofacial Deformities. 2nd Edition. Elsevier, 2013: 317

5. Kharbanda OP. Anchorage in orthodontic practice. In: Kharbanda OP, Orthodontics: Diagnosis and Management of Malocclusion and Dentofacial Deformities. 2nd Edition. Mosby Elsevier, 2013: 371

Anterior Cross Bite

Dr. Sanjeev Sharma, Junior Resident, Dr. Pradeep Tandon, Professor & Head and
Dr. Alka Singh, Associate Professor, Department of
Orthodontics and Dentofacial Orthopaedics

A 22 year old female reported to the Department of Orthodontics and Dentofacial Orthopaedics with the chief complaint of irregular placement of her front teeth. Clinical Examination revealed molars in Angle's Class I relationship with crossbite in maxillary right central and lateral incisor.

1. Angle's class I molar relation with anterior crossbite is classified as?

    (A) Dewey modification type 1
    (B) Dewey modification type 2
    (C) Dewey modification type 3
    (D) Dewey modification type 4

2. Which of the following is the treatment of anterior cross bite?

    (A) Maxillary removable appliance with z-spring
    (B) Maxillary removable appliance with expansion screw in anterior region
    (C) Maxillary lingual arch with finger spring
    (D) All of the above with occlusal extensions

3. Early correction of anterior crossbite is indicated because?

    (A) Lingually positioned incisor limit lateral jaw movement
    (B) Lingually positioned incisor or their mandibular counterpart sometimes suffer significant incisal abrasion
    (C) In crossbite, lower incisors are likely to have gingival recession.
    (D) All of the above

4. What is whip spring?

    (A) Maxillary removable appliance with z-spring
    (B) Maxillary removable appliance with expansion screw in anterior region
    (C) Maxillary lingual arch with finger spring
    (D) Maxillary removable appliance with finger springs

5. Which of the following is the disadvantage of lower anterior inclined plane used for correction of anterior crossbite?

    (A) Creation of temporary speech defect
    (B) Anterior open bite if the appliance is left in place too long
    (C) Dietary restriction
    (D) All of the above

Answers:

1. C

    Dewey's modification of Angle's Class I malocclusion [1]
    Type 1: Crowded anterior teeth
    Type 2: maxillary incisors in labioversion
    Type 3: Anterior crossbite
    Type 4: Posterior crossbite
    Type 5: Molars are in mesioversion due to shifting after loss of tooth mesial to first molars

2. D

    All the appliances are used for correction of crossbite along with the occlusal extensions to relieve the occlusion [2]

3. D

    Anterior crossbite can lead to limited jaw movement, incisal abrasion and gingival recession, so early correction is indicated. [3]

4. C

    Whip spring is maxillary lingual arch with finger spring. [4]

5. D

    All are the disadvantages of anterior inclined plane.[5]

References:

1. Kharbanda OP. Classification and methods of recording malocclusion. In: Kharbanda OP, Orthodontics: Diagnosis and Management of Malocclusion and Dentofacial Deformities. 2nd Edition. Mosby Elsevier, 2013: 50.

2. Proffit WR, Fields FW, Sarver DM. Moderate Nonskeletal Problems In Preadolescent Children: Preventive And Interceptive Treatment In Family Practice, Henry W. Fields. Contemporary Orthodontics. 5th edition. Mosby Elsevier, St Louis, 2000:: 410

3. Proffit WR, Fields FW, Sarver DM. Moderate Nonskeletal Problems In Preadolescent Children: Preventive And Interceptive Treatment In Family

Practice, Henry W. Fields. Contemporary Orthodontics. 5ᵗʰ edition. Mosby Elsevier, St Louis, 2000:: 409

4. Proffit WR, Fields FW, Sarver DM. Moderate Nonskeletal Problems In Preadolescent Children: Preventive And Interceptive Treatment In Family Practice, Henry W. Fields. Contemporary Orthodontics. 5ᵗʰ edition. Mosby Elsevier, St Louis, 2000:: 410

5. Graber T M, Classification of malocclusion. Orthodontics- Principles and Practice; 3ʳᵈ edition,W.B. Saunders company;1992: 840

Class I Malocclusion With Posterior Cross-Bite

Dr. Jitesh K. Haryani, Junior Resident; Dr. Pradeep Tandon, Professor & Head and Dr. Gyan P. Singh, Associate Professor, Department of Orthodontics and Dentofacial Orthopaedics

An 11 year 8 month old boy complains of irregular upper teeth. He has straight profile with incompetent lips. TMJ examination reveals that he has a centric relation/centric occlusion discrepancy and the path of closure is deflected to left side. He has overjet of 5 mm, overbite 4 mm, and molar relation is Class I on both sides with a bilateral posterior crossbite at CR and unilateral posterior crossbite on the left side at CO. His upper arch is constricted, and lower arch is U shaped. There is 5 mm of arch length discrepancy in upper arch. Treatment plan included an occlusal splint for 1 month to deprogramme the muscles followed by upper arch expansion.

1. What is the diagnosis in accordance to Dewey's modification?
   (A) Type 1
   (B) Type 2
   (C) Type 3
   (D) Type 4

2. On an average, a 1 mm increase in interpremolar width increases arch perimeter values by?
   (A) 0.4 mm
   (B) 0.7 mm
   (C) 1.2 mm
   (D) 1.5 mm

3. Method of arch expantion includes all **except**?
   (A) Quad helix
   (B) Coffin spring
   (C) Removable appliance with jack screw
   (D) Nance palatal arch

4. Quad helix is made of?
   (A) 38 mil SS
   (B) 36 mil NiTi
   (C) 28 mil SS
   (D) 32 mil TMA

5. Expansion rate of quad helix is?

   (A) 0.5 mm/day
   (B) 0.25 mm/day
   (C) 1 mm/week
   (D) None

Answers:

1. D

   Dewey's modification of Angle's Class I malocclusion [1]
   Type 1: Crowded anterior teeth
   Type 2: maxillary incisors in labioversion
   Type 3: Anterior crossbite
   Type 4: Posterior crossbite
   Type 5: Molars are in mesioversion due to shifting following loss of tooth anterior to first molars

2. B

   Correction of posterior crossbite increases arch circumference. on an average, a 1 mm increase in interpremolar width increases arch perimeter values by 0.7 mm. [2]

3. D

   Nance palatal appliance is used to augment the anchorage. All other appliances are used for maxillary expansion.[3]

4. A

   The quad helix is used to correct maxillary constriction. It is made of 38 mil SS wire soldered to the molar bands.[4]

5. C

   Fixed expanders can be activated for either Rapid (0.5 mm/day), semi rapid (0.25 mm/day) or slow (1 mm/week). Quad helix is a type of slow expansion appliance.[5]

References:

1. Kharbanda OP. Classification and methods of recording malocclusion. In: Kharbanda OP. Orthodontics: Diagnosis and Management of Malocclusion and Dentofacial Deformities; 2nd ed. Mosby Elsevier, 2013: 49

2. Proffit WR, Fields F W, Sarver D M; Moderate nonskeletal problems in preadolescent children: preventive and interceptive treatment in family practice; Contemporary orthodontics, 5th ed. Mosby Elsevier, 2013: Page 403 – 408

3. Kharbanda OP. Anchorage in orthodontic practice. In: Kharbanda OP.Orthodontics: Diagnosis and Management of Malocclusion and Dentofacial Deformities. 2nd ed. Mosby Elsevier, 2013: 373

4. Proffit WR, Fields F W, Sarver D M. Moderate non skeletal problems in preadolescent children, Contemporary orthodontics. 5thed 201Mosby Elsevier, 2013: 404

5. Proffit WR, Fields F W, Sarver D M. Treatment of skeletal problem in children and preadolescent, Contemporary orthodontics, 5thed, Mosby Elsevier, 2013: 476

Bilateral Maxillary Canine Impactions

Dr. Gyan P. Singh, Associate Professor; Dr. Pradeep Tandon, Professor & Head and Dr. Gulshan K. Singh, Professor, Department of
Orthodontics and Dentofacial Orthopaedics

A 16 years old female reported to the department with the complaint of unpleasant smile. The clinical examination showed that she had Angle's Class I Molar relationship, overjet of 3 mm, overbite of 4 mm, with retained deciduous maxillary cuspids.

1. Which diagnostic aid will provide most useful information on the long axis and the inclination of the impacted tooth?

    (A) Study models
    (B) IOPA X-Ray
    (C) Orthopantomogram
    (D) Posterio-anterior cephalogram

2. Orthopantomogram is helpful in the diagnosis and treatment planning **except**?

    (A) Soft-tissue profile analysis
    (B) Angulation of the roots of the teeth
    (C) Missing or impacted tooth
    (D) Mandibular asymmetry

3. In this patient the maxillary canines are normal but not erupted in the oral cavity. This condition is called?

    (A) Impaction
    (B) Transmigration
    (C) Transposition
    (D) Transillumination

4. The best treatment planning of the case should be?

    (A) Extraction of the impacted canines
    (B) Observation
    (C) Orthodontic guidance to eruption and alignment of canines
    (D) Autologous transplantation of teeth

5. Teeth in order of frequency of occurrence of impaction?

    (A) Mandibular 3rd molar, Mandibular cuspids, 2nd premolar and 1st premolar
    (B) Max. cuspids, Mandibular 3rd molar, 2nd premolar and 1st premolar
    (C) Mandibular 3rd molar, Max. cuspids, 1st Premolar and 2nd premolar
    (D) Mandibular 3rd molar, Max. cuspids, 2nd premolar and 1st premolar

Answers:

1. D

    Posterio-anterior cephalogram provide most useful information on the long axis and the inclination of the impacted tooth. [1]

2. A

    The soft-tissue profile can be best analysed with the help of lateral cephalogram. [2]

3. A

    In current perspective, an impacted tooth is one "Whose eruption is considerably delayed and for which there is clinical or radiographic evidence that further eruption may not take place".[3]

4. C

    Orthodontic guidance/intervention for the relocation of the impacted tooth involves one or more methods like extraction of the retained deciduous canine, removal of physical barrier, creation of the sufficient space and orthodontic guidance.[4]

5. D

    Third molars are commonest tooth to be impacted. Maxillary canines has the longest path to travel before eruption in to oral cavity and the last tooth to erupt in the anterior region, therefore it has more chances of impaction.[5]

References:

1. Kharbanda OP.Orthodontic aspects of impacted teeth. In: Kharbanda OP. Orthodontics: Diagnosis and Management of Malocclusion and Dentofacial Deformities;2nd edition, Mosby Elsevier; 2013: 629

2. Kharbanda OP.Diagnostic records. In Kharbanda OP.Orthodontics: Diagnosis and Management of Malocclusion and Dentofacial Deformities; 2nd edition, Mosby Elsevier; 2013: 185.

3. Kharbanda OP.Orthodontic aspects of impacted teeth. In: Kharbanda OP, Orthodontics: Diagnosis and Management of Malocclusion and Dentofacial Deformities;2nd edition, Mosby Elsevier; 2013: 621.

4. Kharbanda OP.Orthodontic aspects of impacted teeth. In: Kharbanda OP. Orthodontics: Diagnosis and Management of Malocclusion and Dentofacial Deformities;2nd edition, Mosby Elsevier; 2013: 630

5. Kharbanda OP.Orthodontic aspects of impacted teeth. In: Kharbanda OP. Orthodontics: Diagnosis and Management of Malocclusion and Dentofacial Deformities;2nd edition, Mosby Elsevier; 2013:622

Unilateral Canine Impaction

Dr. Dipti Shastri, Senior Resident; Dr. Pradeep Tandon, Professor
& Head and Dr. Alka Singh, Associate Professor, Department
of Orthodontics and Dentofacial Orthopaedics

An 18 year old female presented with missing maxillary left canine. Patient had a pleasing profile. Study cast analysis shows 6 mm discrepancy in maxillary arch and 5mm in mandibular arch. Intraoral examination revealed Angle's Class I molar relationship on both side with 2 mm overjet and deep overbite. Occlusal X-ray revealed palatally impacted maxillary left canine. Analysis of orthopantomogram showed impacted maxillary left canine in Sector II, angulation of maxillary canine in relation to midline of 21^0 and linear distance of 19 mm from the occlusal plane.

1. Sector classification was given by?

   (A) Ericson and Kurol

   (B) Power and Short

   (C) Adams and Vohris

   (D) Nanda and Burstone

2. Impacted canine are commonly found in?

   (A) Female and mandibular arch

   (B) Female, and maxillary arch

   (C) Male and maxillary arch

   (D) d. Male and mandibular arch

3. 'SLOB' rule is?

   (A) Same buccal opposite lingual

   (B) Some light orthodontic base

   (C) Some local occlusal barrier

   (D) Same side lingual opposite side buccal

4. Sector IV includes?

   (A) All area mesial to sector III

   (B) All area distal to sector III

   (C) Mesial to sector I, but distal to sector II

   (D) Mesial to sector II, but distal to sector I

5. A detailed clinical examination of the...............is important when looking for signs of canine impaction?
   (A) Deciduous central incisor
   (B) Permanent premolar
   (C) Permanent lateral incisor
   (D) Permanent maxillary molar

Answers:

1. A

   Sector classification was given by Ericson and Kurol in 1987, and later modified by Lindauer in 1994.[1]

2. B

   Gender may play a role because maxillary canine impactions occur twice as often in female than in males in ratio 2.3:Majority of the canine impaction occur in maxilla as compared to mandible and the ratio is 8:1.[2]

3. D

   'SLOB' rule = Same lingual opposite buccal[3]

4. A

   Sector I – Area distal to line tangent to distal heights of contour of lateral incisor crown and root
   Sector II – Is mesial to sector I, but distal to bisector of lateral incisor's long axis
   Sector III – Is mesial to sector II, but distal to mesial heights of contour of lateral incisor crown and root
   Sector IV – Includes all area mesial to sector III[4]

5. C

   Permanent lateral incisor should be evaluated in canine impaction like missing lateral incisor, small size, unusual rotation etc.[5]

References:

1. Ericson S. and Kurol, J.Radiographic examination of ectopically erupting maxillary canines. Am J Orthod. 1987; 91: 483-492.

2. Kharbanda OP. Orthodontic aspects of impacted teeth. In: Orthodontics: Diagnosis and Management of Malocclusion and Dentofacial Deformities; 2nd Edition, Elsevier; 2013: 631

3. Kharbanda OP. Orthodontic aspects of impacted teeth. In: Orthodontics: Diagnosis and Management of Malocclusion and Dentofacial Deformities; 2nd Edition, Elsevier; 2013: 626

4. Kharbanda OP. Orthodontic aspects of impacted teeth. In: Orthodontics: Diagnosis and Management of Malocclusion and Dentofacial Deformities; 2nd Edition, Elsevier; 2013: 630

5. Kharbanda OP. Orthodontic aspects of impacted teeth. In: Orthodontics: Diagnosis and Management of Malocclusion and Dentofacial Deformities; 2nd Edition, Elsevier;2013: 630

Class II Div 1 Malocclusion

Dr. Alka Singh, Associate Professor; Dr. Pradeep Tandon, Professor & Head and Dr. Amit Nagar, Professor, Department of Orthodontics and Dentofacial Orthopaedics

A 12 year old male reported to the department with forward placement of anterior teeth. Extra-oral examination showed that patient had convex profile, retruded mandible, 10 mm overjet, 7mm overbite with class II molar relationship. His cephalometrc readings were: SNA-82°, SNB-75°, IMPA-102° and FMA-26°

1. What was the growth pattern of the patient's mandible?

    (A) Mandible was growing downward and forward
    (B) Mandible was growing upward and forward
    (C) Mandible was growing downward and backward
    (D) Mandible was growing upward and backward

2. What is the diagnosis of the patient?

    (A) Class II div 1 with increased maxillary growth and normal mandible
    (B) Class II div 1 with increased maxillary and mandibular growth
    (C) Class II div 1 with normal maxilla and deficient mandible
    (D) Class II div 1 with increased maxillary growth and deficient mandible

3. What was the CVMI stage?

    (A) CVMI- IV
    (B) CVMI- II
    (C) CVMI- III
    (D) CVMI-V

4. What should be the suitable treatment plan for the patient?

    (A) Extraction of upper first premolars and anterior retraction with no treatment in mandible
    (B) Extraction of first premolars in maxilla and second premolars in mandible with anchorage loss in mandible to correct molar relationship
    (C) Functional appliance to modulate the growth of mandible
    (D) Extraction of upper first premolars and anterior retraction with fixed functional appliance

5. What will be the **ideal** functional appliance for this patient in present scenario?

    (A) Activator
    (B) Frankel
    (C) Twinblock
    (D) Bionator

Answers:

1. A

    Patient's FMA was 26^0 so patient was having a normal growth pattern that is downward and forward. [1]

2. C

    Patient's SNA was 82^0 and SNB 75^0 so the growth of maxilla was normal but the mandibular growth was deficient.[2]

3. B

    Distinct concavities are present at the lower border of C-2, C-3 and C-The bodies of both C-3, C-4 are rectangular horizontal in shape, so the patient is in the CVMI-III stage.[3]

4. C

    Patient is at the peak of mandibular skeletal growth so the functional orthopaedic appliance should be given to the patient to enhance the growth of the lower jaw[4]

5. C

    Twin block is the only two piece functional appliance which does not obstruct speech or other oral functions, instead, it takes advantage of forces of mastication when compared with one piece functional appliances.[5]

References:

1. Kharbanda OP. Tweed's analysis. In: Orthodontics: Diagnosis and Management of Malocclusion and Dentofacial Deformities; 2nd Edition, Elsevier; 2013: 228

2. Kharbanda OP. Features and early intervention of growing maxillary excess. In: Orthodontics: Diagnosis and Management of Malocclusion and Dentofacial Deformities; 2nd Edition, Elsevier; 2013: 461

3. Kharbanda OP, Nanda RS, Wadhawan N. Concepts of growth and development. In: Kharbanda OP (ed): Orthodontics: Diagnosis and Management of Malocclusion and Dentofacial Deformities; 2nd Edition, Elsevier; 2013: 110

4. Kharbanda OP. Fundamentals of functional appliance therapy. In: Orthodontics: Diagnosis and Management of Malocclusion and Dentofacial Deformities; 5th Edition, Elsevier;2013: 475

5. Kharbanda OP. Interception and treatment of mandibular retrusion.: functional appliance. In: Orthodontics: Diagnosis and Management of Malocclusion and Dentofacial Deformities; 2nd Edition, Elsevier;2013: 492

Class II DIV1 Camouflage Treatment

Dr. Noshi, Junior Resident, Department of Orthodontics; Dr. Pradeep Tandon, Professor & Head and Dr. Alka Singh, Associate Professor, Department of Orthodontics and Dentofacial Orthopaedics

A 16 year old female patient came to the department with chief complaint of forwardly placed front teeth. Clinical examination revealed convex facial profile, acute nasolabial angle and incompetent lips. Intraoral examination revealed class II molar relation on both sides, overjet of 10mm and overbite of 6mm. Cephalometric values are: ANB=6^0,$\underline{1}$ to NA=10mm/42^0, $\overline{1}$ to NB= 7mm/38^0

1. Identify the malocclusion?

    (A) Angle's class I malocclusion
    (B) Angle's class II division I subdivision malocclusion
    (C) Angle's class II division 2 malocclusion
    (D) Angle's class II division 1 malocclusion

2. What is true regarding chevron sticks?

    (A) Used during clinical examination for measuring lip protrusion
    (B) Introduced in orthodontics by Dr Ricketts
    (C) Used for measuring dental compensation needed in orthodontic camouflage
    (D) Both b & c are correct

3. The indications of first premolar extraction in upper arch only includes all **except**?

    (A) Lower arch with minimal crowding
    (B) As an alternative to orthognathic surgery for non growing class II patients
    (C) In class II cases where headgear and functional appliance therapy has failed to achieve class I canine relation
    (D) Absence of mandibular deficiency

4. All of the following measures can be employed to minimise friction during retraction of canine by sliding mechanics except?

    (A) Using stainless steel brackets
    (B) Using stainless steel wire during retraction phase
    (C) Providing at least 2 mil clearance between archwire and bracket
    (D) Using 017×025 TMA wire

5. What is false regarding class II elastics?

    (A) Engaged from maxillary canine to mandibular molar
    (B) Also known as Baker's elastics
    (C) Engaged from mandibular canine to maxillary molar
    (D) Cause lingual tipping of maxillary anteriors

Answers:

1. D

    Angle's class II molar relationship, large overjet of 10mm and deepbite, convex facial profile are classic features of Angle's class II division 1 malocclusion. [1]

2. C

    In the Steiner analysis the ideal relationship of the incisors is expected when the ANB angle is 2 degree. If the ANB angle is different from 2 degrees the different positioning of the incisors given by the inclination and protrusion figures will produce a dental compromise that leads to correct occlusion despite the jaw discrepancy. Chevron sticks or Steiner's sticks are graphical representation of inclination of incisors at different ANB angle.[2]

3. D

    The indications of first premolar extraction in upper arch only is relative mandibular deficiency.[3]

4. D

    TMA wire shows the greatest friction.[4]

5. C

    Class II elastics are engaged from maxillary canine to mandibular molars while class III elastics runs from mandibular canine to maxillary molars. [5]

References:

1. Kharbanda OP. Management of class II malocclusion with fixed appliance. In: Orthodontics: Diagnosis and Management of Malocclusion and Dentofacial Deformities. 2nd Ed. Elsevier, 2013: 534

2. Proffit WR, Fields F W, Sarver D M. Orthodontic diagnosis: the problem oriented approach. Contemporary orthodontics. 5th Ed. Elsevier, 2013: 210

3. Kharbanda OP. Management of class II malocclusion with fixed appliance. In: Orthodontics: Diagnosis and Management of Malocclusion and Dentofacial Deformities. 2nd Ed. Mosby Elsevier, 2013: 532

4. Proffit WR, Fields F W, Sarver D M. Mechanical principles in orthodontic force control. Contemporary orthodontics. 5th Ed. Mosby Elsevier, 2013: 328

5. Kharbanda OP. Management of class II malocclusion with fixed appliance. In: Orthodontics: Diagnosis and Management of Malocclusion and Dentofacial Deformities. 2nd Ed. Mosby Elsevier, 2013: 536

Class II Division 2 Malocclusion

Dr Gyan P Singh, Associate Professor; Dr Pradeep
Tandon, Professor & Head and Dr. Gulshan K. Singh, Professor,
Department of Orthodontics and Dentofacial Orthopaedics

A 10 year old female patient reported to the OPD with history of early loss of milk teeth due to caries. She had a pleasing profile with competent lips and bilateral end on molar relationship. There was excessive deep bite with retroclination of maxillary central incisors.

1. What is the most likely diagnosis of the malocclusion?

    (A) Angle's Class I
    (B) Angle's Class II Div.1
    (C) Angle's Class II Div.2
    (D) Angle's Class III

2. The Angle's class II Div.2 malocclusion has mostly?

    (A) Skeletal Class I with Horizontal growth pattern
    (B) Skeletal Class I with Vertical growth pattern
    (C) Angle's Class II with Horizontal growth pattern
    (D) Skeletal class II with Vertical growth pattern

3. The most appropriate treatment plan for the above mentioned patient is?

    (A) Camouflage by extraction of teeth
    (B) Orthognathic surgery
    (C) Distalization of molars
    (D) Reproximation of selective teeth

4. These are various distalization appliances **except**?

    (A) Distal jet
    (B) Pendulum
    (C) Headgear with face bow
    (D) Face mask

5. If the patient has backward shift during closure of mouth from centric relation to the centric occlusion, then it is?

    (A) Unfavorable with bad prognosis
    (B) Favorable with good prognosis
    (C) Unfavorable with good prognosis
    (D) Favorable with bad prognosis

Answers:

1. C

   The Angle's Class II div.2 malocclusion has distinguishing feature of lingual inclination of maxillary central incisors with labial inclination of lateral incisors.[1]

2. A

   The mandibular growth vector is horizontally oriented, with a flat mandibular plane, giving the appearance of a hypodivergent facial pattern.[2]

3. C

   Alignment of the buccal segments is achieved with distalization of the maxillary buccal dentition for correction of class II malocclusion.[3]

4. D

   Face mask is used for protraction of maxilla in correction of Class III malocclusion. [4]

5. B

   The logical sequencing of early treatment is to resolve functional problems and the maxillary arch length development. With correction of incisor inclination, mandible becomes free to come forward and helps in establishing the molar in class I relationship. [5]

References:

1. Graber T M, Classification of malocclusion. Orthodontics- Principles and Practice; 3rd edition,W.B. Saunders company;1992: 241

2. Kharbanda OP. Class II division 2 malocclusion. In: Kharbanda OP: Orthodontics: Diagnosis and Management of Malocclusion and Dentofacial Deformities; 2nd edition, Mosby Elsevier; 2013: 539

3. Kharbanda OP. Class II division 2 malocclusion. In:: Orthodontics: Diagnosis and Management of Malocclusion and Dentofacial Deformities; 2nd edition, Mosby Elsevier; 2013: 542

4. Darendeliler MA, Kharbanda OP. Class III malocclusion in growing patients. In: Kharbanda OP: Orthodontics: Diagnosis and Management of Malocclusion and Dentofacial Deformities;2nd edition, Mosby Elsevier; 2013: 550

5. Kharbanda OP. Class II division 2 malocclusion. In: Kharbanda OP: Orthodontics: Diagnosis and Management of Malocclusion and Dentofacial Deformities; 2nd edition, Mosby Elsevier; 2013: 541

Ectopic Canine

Dr. Noshi, Junior Resident; Dr Pradeep Tandon, Professor &
Head and Dr Gyan P. Singh, Associate Professor, Department
of Orthodontics and Dentofacial Orthopaedics

A 12 years old female patient presents with buccally erupted maxillary left canine. Extraoral examination shows mildly convex facial profile, euryprosopic facial form and dental midline shifted to patient's left. Intraorally both the molars are in end on position, mild crowding in lower arch and deepbite. Study models analysis revealed 5mm discrepancy in maxilla. Cephalometric analysis shows ANB= 4^0, $\underline{1}$ to NA=1mm/21^0, $\overline{1}$ to NB= 1mm/12^0. FMA = 16^0. PtV to first molar= 16mm.

1. Which of the following is not an indication of molar distalization?

    (A) Less than 4-5 mm of required space per side
    (B) Lip and maxillary dental protrusion should be minimal
    (C) Vertical face dimension should be normal or with a short face tendency
    (D) Openbite

2. What is true regarding timing of molar distalization?

    (A) Recommended time for maxillary molar distalization is during early
    (B) Anchorage loss is same whether distalization is performed prior to or after 2nd molar eruption
    (C) Molar distalization is impossible after eruption of 2nd molar
    (D) The most appropriate time for maxillary molar distalization is before eruption of 2nd molars

3. Pendex appliance is used for?

    (A) Maxillary expansion
    (B) Maxillary molar distalisaton
    (C) Both A & B
    (D) Space regaining appliance

4. Which of the following is not a molar distalization appliance?

    (A) Jone's jig
    (B) T-rex appliance
    (C) C-rex appliance
    (D) Distal jet

Answers:

1. D

   The overbite should be somewhat greater than normal due to bite opening mechanics. [1]

2. D

   The most appropriate time for molar distalization is during mixed or late mixed dentition before the eruption of 2nd molars. Problems of anchorage loss is more when molars are distalized after 2nd molar eruption.[2]

3. C

   Pendex is a modification of pendulum appliance that is used for maxillary expansion and molar distalisation.[3]

4. C

   Jones jig and distal jet and T-rex (a modification of pendulum appliance) are all molar distalizing appliance [4]

References:

1. Proffit WR, Fields FW, Sarver DM. Complex nonskeletal problems in preadolescent children: preventive and interceptive treatment. Contemporary orthodontics: 5th edition, Mosby Elsevier: 2013: 462

2. Kharbanda OP. Nonextraction treatment. In: Kharbanda OP: Orthodontics: Diagnosis and Management of Malocclusion and Dentofacial Deformities: 2nd Edition, Mosby Elsevier: 2013: 452

3. Kharbanda OP. Nonextraction treatment. In: Kharbanda OP: Orthodontics: Diagnosis and Management of Malocclusion and Dentofacial Deformities: 2nd Edition, Mosby Elsevier: 2013: 452

4. Kharbanda OP. Nonextraction treatment: Chapter 3In: Kharbanda OP: Orthodontics: Diagnosis and Management of Malocclusion and Dentofacial Deformities: 2nd Edition, Mosby Elsevier: 2013: 452

Ugly Duckling

Dr. Sunil Singh, Senior Resident; Dr Pradeep Tandon,
Professor & Head and Dr. Amit Nagar, Professor, Department
of Orthodontics and Dentofacial Orthopaedics

A female patient aged 9 years came to the department with the chief complaint of spacing between upper front teeth. Medical and dental history was irrelevant. On examination patient had apparently bilateral symmetrical face (mesoprosopic type) and mesocephalic head type with normal growth status with age. Intraoral examination showed patient was in mixed dentition with only permanent incisors and permanent first molars. Maxillary central incisors was disto-angular rotated with 2mm of midline diastema. Maxillary frenum and oral hygiene normal. Radiographic findings on orthopantomogram shows erupting canines and premolars with restored deciduous second molars.

1. The "Ugly Duckling" stage of the transitional dentition is characterized by all of the following **except?**

   (A) Flared and spaced anteriors
   (B) Distoangular axial inclination of the maxillary incisors.
   (C) Maxillary lateral incisors erupting lingual to the mandibular incisors.
   (D) Midline diastema

2. The ugly duckling stage is seen at the age of?

   (A) 4-6 years
   (B) 6-7 years
   (C) 9-10 years
   (D) 12-14 years

3. Term 'Ugly duckling stage' was given by?

   (A) Broadbent
   (B) Nance
   (C) Lawrence F Andrews
   (D) Calvin Case

4. The best line of treatment for the above mentioned case will be?

   (A) Fixed appliance
   (B) Removable appliance
   (C) Inclined plane
   (D) No treatment, observation of patient

5. Dolichocephalic, mesocephalic and brachycephalic classification of head type was given by?

 (A) Sheldon
 (B) Martin and Saller
 (C) Le Fouloun
 (D) Kjelgren

Answers:

1. C

 Maxillary lateral incisor erupting lingual to mandibular incisor is the case of anterior cross bite. All other features are the clinical features of Ugly duckling stage.[1]

2. C

 Dental appearance at age 9-10 shows flared incisors with spacing, which is due to pressure exerted on the roots of lateral incisors by the canine. This can be seen on OPG of patient.[2]

3. A

 "Ugly duckling stage" seen in mixed dentition, a term given by Broadbent. It also known as "Broadbent phenomenon"[3]

4. D

 The spaces tend to close as the permanent canines erupt. The greater the amount of spacing, the less the likelihood that a maxillary central diastema will totally close on its own. As a general guideline, a maxillary central diastema of 2 mm or less will probably close spontaneously, while total closure of a diastema initially greater than 2 mm is unlikely.[4]

5. B

 The ratio (in percentage) of the maximum breadth to the maximum length of the skull or head is known as cephalic index. Long and narrow head below 75% (dolicocephalic), average from 75% to 79.9% (mesocephalic) and broad more than 80% (brachycephalic).[5]

References:

1. Proffit WR, Fields FW, Sarver DM. Early Stages Of Development. Contemporary Orthodontics; 4th Edition, St. Louis, Missouri: Mosby Elsevier; 2007: 100

2. Proffit WR, Fields FW, Sarver DM. Early Stages Of Development: Contemporary Orthodontics; 4th Edition, St. Louis, Missouri: Mosby Elsevier; 2007: 101

3. Graber TM. Interceptive orthodontics. Orthodontics Principles and Practice; 3rd Edition, W.B.Saunders Company; 1992: 675

4. Proffit WR, Fields F W, Sarver D M. Early Stages Of Development: Contemporary Orthodontics; 4th Edition. St. Louis, Missouri: Mosby Elsevier; 2007: 100

5. Rakosi T, Jonas I, Graber TM. Diagnostic Procedures. Rateitschak KH, Wolf HF. Color Atlas Of Dental Medicine Orthodontic-Diagnosis. New York: Thieme Medical Publishers; 1999: 108.

Developing Class III Malocclusion

Dr. Gyan P. Singh, Associate Professor; Dr. Pradeep Tandon, Professor
& Head and Dr. Alka Singh, Associate Professor, Department
of Orthodontics and Dentofacial Orthopaedics

An 8 years old boy presented with chief complaint of reverse bite of anterior teeth. Clinical examination revealed a concave profile with a maxillary deficiency. The deciduous second molar relationship was in mesial step, negative overjet of 2 mm and the overbite was 4 mm. The intra -oral frontal photograph shown below:

1. The above malocclusion is called as?

    (A) Apertognathia

    (B) Open-bite

    (C) Telescopic bite

    (D) Anterior cross-bite

2. The preferred treatment plan for the above condition is?

    (A) Observation

    (B) Orthognathic surgery

    (C) Growth modification with correction of cross-bite

    (D) Distalization

3. Based on the clinical findings following appliances can be used except?

    (A) Delaire face-mask

    (B) Chin- cup therapy

    (C) Reverse Twin Bock

    (D) Head gear with face-bow

4. Developing cross- bite can lead to which kind of malocclusion in due course of time?

    (A) Angle's Class II Div.2

    (B) Angle's Class II Div.1

    (C) Angle's Class III

    (D) Angle's Class I open-bite

5. Early correction of the anterior cross-bite can help the patient except?

    (A) Can avoid the orthognathic surgery

    (B) Promotes the normal growth of the jaws

    (C) No improvement in the mastication

    (D) Economical and less traumatic

Answers:

1. **D**

   In this condition the lower incisors are overlapping the upper incisors in centric occlusion and hinder the normal growth and development of the maxilla.[1]

2. **C**

   Upon elimination of these interferences, which are mainly due to incisors retroclination, the maxilla and mandible return to a normal class I relationship.[2]

3. **D**

   Head gear with face-bow is used to control the growth of maxilla, anchorage augmentation and distalization of the molars.[3]

4. **C**

   The anterior cross-bite may be the result of a pre-maxillry dentoalveolar deficiency or a functional problem where occlusal interferences create an anterior shift. If it is left unattended, a functional class III malocclusion is likely to develop into a skeletal malocclusion.[4]

5. **C**

   Early correction of anterior cross bite restores the normal growth of maxilla in harmony with mandible.[5]

References:

1. Kharbanda OP. Class III malocclusion in growing patients. In: Kharbanda OP: Orthodontics: Diagnosis and Management of Malocclusion and Dentofacial Deformities;2nd edition, Mosby Elsevier; 2013:548

2. Kharbanda OP. Class III malocclusion in growing patients. In:Kharbanda OP: Orthodontics: Diagnosis and Management of Malocclusion and Dentofacial Deformities; 2nd edition, Mosby Elsevier; 2013:548

3. Kharbanda OP. Dentofacial orthopaedics for class II malocclusion with vertical maxillary excess. In:Kharbanda OP: Orthodontics: Diagnosis and Management of Malocclusion and Dentofacial Deformities; 2nd edition, Mosby Elsevier; 2013:527

4. Kharbanda OP. Class III malocclusion in growing patients. In:Kharbanda OP: Orthodontics: Diagnosis and Management of Malocclusion and Dentofacial Deformities;2nd edition, Mosby Elsevier; 2013: 548

5. Kharbanda OP. Class III malocclusion in growing patients. In:Kharbanda OP: Orthodontics: Diagnosis and Management of Malocclusion and Dentofacial Deformities; 2nd edition, Mosby Elsevier; 2013: 555

Pseudo-Class III Malocclusion

Dr Alka Singh, Associate Professor, Dr. Pradeep Tandon, Professor & Head and Dr. Gyan P. Singh, Associate Professor, Department of Orthodontics and Dentofacial Orthopaedics

An 11 year old female patient came to the department with the chief complaint of coming out of her lower front teeth. On taking history no one in her family had a similar malocclusion. On extra oral examination, she had concave profile with maxillary retrusion. On intraoral examination she had anterior crossbite, mild midline assymetry and class III molar relationship. The functional examination in postural rest and at first contact showed that the mandible was closing in a normal class I relation. Her cephalometric readings were: SNA-78°, SNB-80°, ANB- -2°

1. Patient may be diagnosed as?

    (A) Angle's class III type 1 malocclusion
    (B) Angle's class III type 2 malocclusion
    (C) Angle's class III type 3 malocclusion
    (D) Pseudo class III malocclusion

2. The most likely cause of the malocclusion is?

    (A) Excessive growth of mandible
    (B) Occlusal interferences leading to forward posture of mandible
    (C) Deficient growth of maxilla and excessive growth of mandible
    (D) Deficient growth of maxilla and normal mandible

3. What should be the ideal treatment for this patient?

    (A) Chin cap
    (B) Protraction face mask therapy
    (C) Rapid Maxillary Expansion
    (D) Rapid Maxillary Expansion followed by protraction face mask therapy

4. Force used for maxillary protraction should be in the range of?

    (A) 200gram on each side for 10-12 hours everyday with direction of force 300 below the occlusion plane
    (B) 200gram on each side for 24 hours everyday with direction of force 300 below the occlusion plane
    (C) 200gram on each side for 24hours everyday direction of force 300 above the occlusion plane
    (D) 200 gram on each side for 10-12 hours everyday with direction of force 300 above the occlusion plane

5. The appliance of choice for functional retention after protraction is?

   (A) Schwartz plate
   (B) Hawley's appliance with potential bite plate
   (C) Frankel regulator 3
   (D) Swed appliance

Answers:

1. D

   Presentation of pseudo-class III is similar to true class III but the functional examination in postural rest and at first contact shows that the mandible is closing in a normal class I relation.[1]

2. B

   The main cause of pseudoclass III is occlusal interferences which leads to forward posture of mandible.[2]

3. D

   Patient has deficient maxilla, so Rapid Maxillary Expansion should be done for loosening of cranio-maxillary sutures before protraction of maxilla[3]

4. A

   Recommended force is 200-250gm on each side for 10-12 hrs everyday initially which can be increased till 400-500gms on each side gradually. The line of force should pass 15 mm above and directed 30^0 below the occlusion plane.[4]

5. C

   After active treatment is finished with protraction appliance, it is absolutely vital to maintain the outcome either with a Class III bionator or a Frankel FR 3.[5]

References:

1. Kharbanda OP. Classification and method of recording malocclusion. In: Kharbanda OP: Orthodontics: Diagnosis and Management of Malocclusion and Dentofacial Deformities; 2nd Edition, Mosby Elsevier: 2013: 47

2. Kharbanda OP: Classification and method of recording malocclusion. In: Kharbanda OP: Orthodontics: Diagnosis and management of Malocclusion and Dentofacial Deformities, 2nd edition, Mosby Elsevier: 2013:46

3. Kharbanda OP. Class IIImalocclusion in growing patient. In: Kharbanda OP: Orthodontics Diagnosis and Management of Malocclusion and Dentofacial Deformities; 2nd Edition, Mosby Elsevier: 2013: 407

4. Kharbanda OP, ClassIII malocclusion in growing patients. In:Kharbanda OP: Orthodontics: Diagnosis and Management of Malocclusion and Dentofacial Deformities; 2nd Edition, Mosby Elsevier: 2013: 551

5. Kharbanda OP, Class IIImalocclusion in growing patient. Kharbanda OP: Orthodontics: Diagnosis and Management of Malocclusion and Dentofacial Deformities; 2nd Edition, Mosby Elsevier: 2013: 405

Skeletal Class III Malocclusion

Dr. Noshi, Junior Resident, Dr. Pradeep Tandon, Professor & Head and
Dr. Alka Singh, Associate Professor, Department of
Orthodontics and Dentofacial Orthopaedics

An 11 year old male patient presented with anterior and bilateral posterior crossbite, with no functional shift. The facial profile shows concavity. Cephalometric readings are SNA = 75^0, SNB= 80^0 and FMA is 30^0.

1. When should the treatment for crossbite be started in this patient?

    (A) After completion of permanent dentition

    (B) As soon as possible

    (C) After eruption of first premolars

    (D) All of the above

2. Which kind of maxillary expansion would you prefer in this patient?

    (A) Banded Rapid Maxillary Expansion

    (B) Bonded Rapid MaxillaryExpansion

    (C) Removable maxillary expansion plate with midline expansion screw

    (D) Coffin spring

3. Which of the following is not a treatment option for growing class III patients?

    (A) Functional appliance

    (B) Facemask therapy

    (C) Class III elastics to skeletal anchors

    (D) Maxillary advancement surgery

4. The overall result of rapid verses slow expansion is?

    (A) In rapid expansion, 80% skeletal and 20% dental effects are achieved finally

    (B) In slow expansion 40% skeletal and 60% dental effects are there

    (C) Both rapid and slow expansion, overall result is 50% skeletal and 50% dental effects are there

    (D) In rapid palatal expansion, there is always more skeletal effects than slow expansion

Answers:

1. C

Palatal expansion should be started as soon as possible, before the end of adolescent growth spurt. In the late mixed dentition, root resorption of primary molars may have reached the point that these teeth offer little resistance and it may be wise to wait for eruption of the first premolars before beginning expansion.[1]

2. B

In the late mixed dentition, sutural expansion requires placing a relatively heavy force directed across the suture to move the halves of the maxilla apart. A fixed jackscrew appliance (either banded or bonded) is required. A bonded appliance that covers the occlusal surface of the posterior teeth may be a better choice for a child with a long face tendency by producing less mandibular rotation than a banded appliance.[2]

3. D

Option of surgery is considered after completion of growth.[3]

4. C

Initially, after 2 weeks of Rapid Maxillary Expansion, there is 80% skeletal and 20 % dental effects. But after 2 weeks there is skeletal relapse, finally there is 50% skeletal and 50% dental relapse. In slow expansion, skeletal and dental effects are equal from the beginning.[4]

References:

1. Proffit WR, Fields F W, Sarver D M. Treatment of skeletal problems in children. In: John Dolan (ed), Contemporary orthodontics. 4th Ed. Mosby Elsevier, 2007: 499

2. Proffit WR, Fields F W, Sarver D M. Treatment of skeletal problems in children. In: John Dolan (ed), Contemporary orthodontics. 4th Ed. Mosby Elsevier, 2007:499

3. Proffit WR, Fields F W, Sarver D M. Treatment of skeletal problems in children. In: John Dolan (ed), Contemporary orthodontics. 4th Ed. Mosby Elsevier, 2007: 498

4. Proffit WR, Fields F W, Sarver D M. Orthodontic treatment planning: From problem list to specific plan. Contemporary orthodontics. 5th Ed. Mosby Elsevier, 2013: 228

Mid Face Deficiency

Dr. Jyoti S. Pandhare, Junior Resident; Dr Pradeep Tandon, Professor & Head and
Dr. Gulshan K. Singh, Professor, Department of
Orthodontics and Dentofacial Orthopaedics

The parents of a 9 years old boy came to the department with chief complaint of abnormal placement of front teeth. On clinical examination he had concave profile with average lower facial height. Intraoral examination showed class III molar relationship with reverse overjet of 4mm. Cephalometric analysis revealed SNA= 77⁰, SNB= 80⁰, ANB= -3⁰, Wits= -5mm and FMA= 21⁰. No centric relation-centric occlusion discrepancy. There was no family history.

1. Best treatment option in this case is?

    (A) Class III elastics
    (B) Twin block
    (C) RME and protraction facemask
    (D) Camouflage

2. Elastic traction from intraoral hook to protraction facemask should be given at?
    (A) 1-50 from the occlusal plane
    (B) 15-300 from the occlusal plane
    (C) 60-700 from the occlusal plane
    (D) 50-600 from the occlusal plane

3. Modified protraction headgear is given in order to?

    (A) Decrease proclination of maxillary incisors
    (B) To prevent retroclination of lower incisors
    (C) To counteract counterclockwise rotation of maxilla
    (D) To counteract clockwise rotation of maxilla

4. Greatest amount of maxillary changes was observed in?

    (A) 7-9 years of age group
    (B) 9- 11 years of age group
    (C) 11-13 years of age group
    (D) 4-7 years of age group

5. According to Hata and Lee the centre of resistance of maxilla is located?

    (A) 5mm above the palatal plane and 15 mm above occlusal plane
    (B) Between roots of maxillary premolars
    (C) 5 to 10 mm below orbitale on zygomatic bone
    (D) Posteriosuperior aspect of zygomaticomaxillary sutures

Answers:

1. C

   This is a growing patient with skeletal class III mainly because of retrognathic maxilla. To achieve maximum skeletal effects, RME with protraction facemask is a optimum treatment plan.[1]

2. B

   As protraction force is applied below center of resistance of maxilla, counterclockwise rotation of maxilla occurs to prevent this elastic pull, at 15-30° to occlusal plane.[2]

3. C

   In modified protraction headgear, line of action of force is through the center of resistance of maxilla, to prevent counterclockwise rotation of maxilla.[3]

4. A

   7-9 age group shows maximum changes in maxillary protraction.[4]

5. A

   Hata and Lee did the study in which they found that centre of resistance of maxilla is located 5mm above the palatal plane and 15 mm above occlusal plane.[5]

References:

1. Kharbanda OP. Class III malocclusion in growing patient. In: Kharbanda OP: Orthodontics: Diagnosis and Management of Malocclusion and Dentofacial Deformities; 2nd Edition, Mosby Elsevier; 2013: 549

2. Kharbanda OP. Class III malocclusion in growing patient. In: Kharbanda OP: Orthodontics: Diagnosis and Management of Malocclusion and Dentofacial Deformities; 2nd Edition, Mosby Elsevier; 2013: 551

3. Kharbanda OP. Class III malocclusion in growing patient. In: Kharbanda OP: Orthodontics: Diagnosis and Management of Malocclusion and Dentofacial Deformities; 2nd Edition, Mosby Elsevier; 2013: 551

4. Kharbanda OP. Class III malocclusion in growing patient. In: Kharbanda OP: Orthodontics: Diagnosis and Management of Malocclusion and Dentofacial Deformities; 2nd Edition, Mosby Elsevier; 2013:554

5. Kharbanda OP, Class IIImalocclusion in growing patient: Chapter 4In:Kharbanda OP: Orthodontics: Diagnosis and Management of Malocclusion and Dentofacial Deformities; 2nd Edition, Elsevier: 405, Mosby Elsevier: 551

Serial Extraction

Dr. Amit Nagar, Professor, Dr. Pradeep Tandon, Professor &
Head and Dr. Gyan P Singh, Associate Professor, Department
of Orthodontics and Dentofacial Orthopaedics

A child between 8-9 years of age in mixed dentition stage presented with mild crowding. His OPG and model analysis predicted that there will not be enough space in the jaws to accommodate all permanent teeth in their proper alignment. It is also established that at this age there are lesser chances of increase in distance from mesial aspect of molar of one side to molar of other side. However there are still chances of losing space in the form of "Leeway space" for correction of 'flush terminal plane'.

1. Which of the following is not an indication for serial extraction?

    (A) Tooth size –arch length discrepancy.
    (B) Ankylosis of deciduous teeth.
    (C) Ectopic eruption of permanent teeth.
    (D) Spacing among the deciduous dentition

2. Serial extraction is contraindicated in?

    (A) Altered eruption sequence in primary teeth
    (B) Lingual eruption of upper lateral incisors
    (C) In cleft lip and palate cases
    (D) Premature exfoliation of deciduous canine especially in lower arches

3. In Dewel's method of serial extraction the sequence is?

    (A) CD4
    (B) DC4
    (C) C4D
    (D) D4C

4. In Nance Method of serial extraction which tooth is extracted first?

    (A) C
    (B) D
    (C) 4
    (D) None of the above

5. Which of the following is not a method of gaining space?

    (A) Proximal stripping
    (B) Proclination
    (C) Retraction
    (D) Distalization

Answers:

1. D

   For serial extraction the dental arches must not have any spaces and should be slightly crowded. Other indications include altered eruption sequence, arch length tooth size discrepancy, abnormal root resorption pattern, abnormal exfoliation pattern, ectopic eruption of permanent teeth, and ankylosis of primary teeth.[1]

2. C

   In patients of cleft lip and palate, the eruption sequence is disturbed due to abnormal jaw growth pattern and presence of cleft. Many teeth are impacted and submerged also. In such cases the serial extractions should not be attempted. [2]

3. A

   In Dewel's method objective for the extraction of primary canine first is to facilitate alignment of incisors, after that deciduos first premolars are extracted to facilitate eruption of first permanent premolars before the eruption of canines and in the last step first permanent premolars are extracted to facilitate eruption of canine [3]

4. B

   In Nance method deciduos first molars are extracted first in order to facilitate eruption of first premolar before the eruption of canine, in second step first premolars are extracted to facilitate the eruption of canines and in the last deciduos canines are extracted to create the space for permanent canines [4]

5. C

   The methods of gaining space in an arch are mainly Extraction, Expansion,3. Molar distalization, 4.Reproximation Proclination Derotaion of posterior teeth.[5]

References:

1. Phulari B S. Interceptive Orthodontics. Orthodontics Principles and practice; 1st edition, Jaypee; 2011:252

2. Phulari B S. Interceptive Orthodontics. Orthodontics Principles and practice; 1st edition, Jaypee; 2011:252

3. Phulari B S. Interceptive Orthodontics. Orthodontics Principles and practice; 1st edition, Jaypee; 2011:254

4. Phulari B S. Interceptive Orthodontics. Orthodontics Principles and practice; 1st edition, Jaypee; 2011: 254

5. Phulari B S.Methods of gaining space. Orthodontics Principles and practice;1st edition, Jaypee;2011:303

Non Extraction Treatment

Dr. Noshi, Junior Resident, Dr. Pradeep Tandon, Professor and Head and Dr. Alka Singh, Associate Professor, Orthodontics & Dentofacial Orthopaedics

A 13 year old male patient reported with 5mm crowding in maxillary arch. Facial profile was straight with obtuse nasolabial angle. Intraoral examination showed narrow maxillary arch, unilateral posterior crossbite, no functional shift of mandible and Class I molar relationship. Cephalometric analysis shows FMA = 26.

1. Best treatment plan for this patient?
    (A) Extraction of maxillary first premolars
    (B) Extraction of maxillary 2nd premolars
    (C) Maxillary expansion
    (D) Molar distalization

2. Which of the following is not used for maxillary expansion?
    (A) Quad helix
    (B) Coffin spring
    (C) W- arch
    (D) Z spring

3. With expansion gain in arch length for every 1mm increase in posterior arch width?
    (A) 0.8mm
    (B) 0.7mm
    (C) 0.6mm
    (D) 1mm

4. Which of the following is not a method of space regaining?
    (A) Reproximation
    (B) Derotation of posterior teeth
    (C) Molar distalisation
    (D) Derotation of anterior teeth

Answers:

1. C

The case is presenting moderate crowding where extraction and nonextraction both treatment options are possible. Unilateral crossbite reveals transverse maxillary deficiency which should be treated by maxillary expansion.[1]

2. D

Quad helix, coffin spring and W arch all are used for maxillary expansion while Z spring are used for labial movement of teeth. [2]

3. B

According to Adkins, for every 1mm gain in posterior arch width there is 0.7mm increase in arch length. [3]

4. D

Derotation of anterior teeth require space while derotation of posterior teeth gives space [4]

References:

1. Proffit WR, Fields F W, Sarver D M. Orthodontic Treatment planning: From Problem List to Specific Plan Contemporary orthodontics. Contemporary orthodontics.5th edition. Mosby, Elsevier, 2013: 226

2. Fields F W, Proffit WR.Treatment of skeletal problems in children and preadolescents. In: Proffit WR, Fields F W, Sarver D M.Contemporary Orthodontics 5th edition. Mosby Elsevier, 2013: 476

3. Fields F W, Proffit WR. Moderate Nonskeletal Problems in Preadolescent Children. In: Proffit WR, Fields F W, Sarver D M.Contemporary Orthodontics.5th edition. Mosby Elsevier, 2013: 403

4. Kharbanda OP. Nonextraction treatment. Orthodontics: Diagnosis and Management of Malocclusion and Dentofacial Deformities. 2nd Edition, Mosby Elsevier, 2013: 444

Molar Distalization

Dr. Sunil Singh, Senior Resident; Dr. Pradeep Tandon, Professor & Head and
Dr Gulshan K. Singh, Professor, Orthodontics & Dentofacial Orthopaedics

A 12 year old male patient came to the department with the chief complaint of extra
teeth erupted in the upper jaw. Patient was having straight and pleasing profile. On
examination patient had retained both deciduous canines in maxillary arch, labially
impacted maxillary permanent right canine as well as labially erupted permanent
maxillary left canine. Molars are in End-On relation on both sides. Cephalometric
readings are in normal range.

1. What is the best time for maxillary 1st molar distalization?

   (A) Before eruption of maxillary canine
   (B) Before eruption of maxillary 2nd molar
   (C) Before eruption of mandibular 1st molar
   (D) Before eruption of mandibular 2nd molar

2. Which is the primary objective of molar distalization?

   (A) To distalize the mesially migrated maxillary molars due to their premature
       mesial drift
   (B) To correct class II dental relationship of no more than half cusp severity and
       mild dentoalveolar protrusion
   (C) In class I occlusion patients it may be indicated to gain space to resolve minor
       crowding in the anterior segments
   (D) All of the above

3. The best method of evaluating canine impaction is?

   (A) CBCT
   (B) Lateral cephalogram
   (C) Orthopantomogram
   (D) IOPA X-ray

4. Which of the following is not a molar distalization appliance?

   (A) Distal jet
   (B) Pendulum appliance
   (C) First class appliance
   (D) Facemask

5. Force generated when activation of pendulum appliance is done for molar distalization?

    (A) 75 gms
    (B) 125 gms
    (C) 200 gms
    (D) 150 gms

Answers:

1. B

    Recommended time for maxillary molar distalization is either during mixed or late mixed dentition and sometimes in permanent dentition. The most appropriate time for maxillary molar distalization is before eruption of maxillary second molars.[1]

2. D

    The primary objective of molar distalization is to treat mild crowding, Class II molar relationship and misally migrated molar due to premature exfoliation of deciduous molars. Molar distalization is generally done in cases having mandibular arch well aligned or requires minimal orthodontic treatment.[2]

3. A

    IOPA X-ray, lateral cephalogram, OPG are all used in diagnosis of canine impaction but the main drawback is two dimensional view of canine with all these diagnostic aids. CBCT is modern diagnostic aid which provides three dimensional view of canine and gives exact position of canine in bone which helps in surgery and treatment planning.[3]

4. D

    Facemask is used in cases having maxillary retrusion. In Class III cases forward traction to maxilla is applied with Facemask to correct the skeletal maxillary retrusion. Distal jet, pendulum appliance and first class appliance are all intraoral maxillary molar distalization appliance.[4]

5. C

    In patients treated to a super-Class I molar relationship with the pendulum appliance, it is activated to produce 200 to 250 grams force.[5]

References:

1. Kharbanda OP. Nonextraction treatment. Orthodontics: Diagnosis and Management of Malocclusion and Dentofacial Deformities. 2nd Edition, Mosby Elsevier, 2013: 454.

2. Kharbanda OP. Nonextraction treatment. Orthodontics: Diagnosis and Management of Malocclusion and Dentofacial Deformities. 2nd Edition, Mosby Elsevier, 2013: 449.

3. Proffit WR, Sarver DM, Ackerman JL. Orthodontic Diagnosis. The Problem-Oriented Approach. In: Proffit WR, Fields HW, Sarver DM. Contemporary Orthodontics, 5th Edition. St. Louis, Missouri: Mosby Elsevier; 2013: 199

4. Kharbanda OP. Nonextraction treatment. Orthodontics: Diagnosis and Management of Malocclusion and Dentofacial Deformities. 2nd Edition, Mosby Elsevier, 2013: 454.

5. Proffit WR, Fields F W, Sarver D M. The Second Stage Of Comprehensive Treatment: Correction Of Molar Relationship And Space Closure. Contemporary Orthodontics; 4th Edition, St. Louis, Missouri: Mosby Elsevier; 2007: 580.

Functional Appliance

Dr. Dipti Shastri, Senior Resident; Dr. Pradeep Tandon, Professor & Head and
Dr. Gyan P. Singh, Associate Professor, Orthodontics & Dentofacial Orthopaedics

A 12 year old male presented with chief complaint of forward placement of his teeth. Extraoral examination of the patient revealed convex profile with retrognathic mandible. Intraoral examination showed Angle's Class II molar relation on both side, 9mm overjet, deep overbite and spacing maxillary arch. Cephalometric values of the patient shows skeletal Class II relationship as SNA of the patient is 82 and SNB is 7Cervical Vertebrae Maturity Indicator of the patient shows stage III. Twin Block appliance was given to the patient for the treatment.

1. Twin block appliance given to the patient is a?

   (A) Fixed appliance
   (B) Separator
   (C) Myofunctional appliance
   (D) Retainer

2. Twin block uses forces of occlusion through the?

   (A) Bite blocks with70 degree inclination
   (B) Bite block with 90 degree inclination
   (C) Bite block with 120 degree inclination
   (D) Bite block with 150 degree inclination

3. Twin block are designed to be worn?

   (A) 1 hour per day
   (B) 10 hours per day
   (C) 15 hours per day
   (D) 24 hours per day

4. While doing bite registration for the twin block, sagittal advancement should not exceed?

   (A) 50% of maximum protrusive limit of mandible
   (B) 70% of maximum protrusive limit of mandible
   (C) 80% of maximum protrusive limit of mandible
   (D) 90% of maximum protrusive limit of mandible

5. The first twin block appliance were fitted on?

   (A) 7th Sep, 1977
   (B) 7th Sep, 1980
   (C) 7th Sep, 1982
   (D) 7th Sep, 1987

Answers:

1. C

   Twin Block is a myofunctional appliance and among the myofunctional appliance twin block is the best because it is two piece appliance that does not interfere with the normal function of oral cavity.[1]

2. A

   Twin block uses force of occlusion through the 70^0 inclined plane as the functional mechanism for the correction of malocclusion.[2]

3. D

   Twin blocks are designed to be worn 24 hours per day to take full advantage of all functional forces applied to the dentition.[3]

4. B

   During bite registration, sagittal advancement should not exceed 70% of maximum protrusive limit of mandible.[4]

5. A

   First twin block appliance was fitted on 7 th Sep. 1977.[5]

References:

1. Clark W J. Introduction to Twin Block, Twin Block Functional Therapy; Application in Dentofacial Orthopaedics. 2nd ed. Mosby.2002: 8

2. Clark W J. Introduction to Twin Block. Twin Block Functional Therapy. Application in Dentofacial Orthopaedics. 2nd ed. Mosby.2002: 5

3. Clark W J. Introduction to Twin Block. Twin Block Functional Therapy; Application in Dentofacial Orthopaedics. 2nd ed. Mosby.2002: 6

4. Clark W J. Introduction to Twin Block. Twin Block Functional Therapy; Application in Dentofacial Orthopaedics. 2nd ed. Mosby.2002: 6

5. Clark W J. Introduction to Twin Block. Twin Block Functional Therapy; Application in Dentofacial Orthopaedics. 2nd ed. Mosby.2002: 8

Bonding

Dr. Dipti Shastri, Senior Resident; Dr. Pradeep Tandon, Professor & Head and
Dr. Alka Singh, Associate Professor, Orthodontics & Dentofacial Orthopaedics

Initially orthodontic brackets on tooth surface were welded on a steel gauge mesh much larger than bracket base. In 1954 Buonocore first time suggested that etching enamel with 85% phosphoric acid solution resulted in adhesion of acrylic resin. In 1960s banding was replaced by bonding and marked the beginning of a new era in the history of orthodontics. Now a days available bonding agents offer bond strength of 12-20 MPa which exceeds the minimum shear bond strength requirements of orthodontic attachments.

1. Who replaced orthodontic banding with bonding?

    (A) Buonocore
    (B) Newman
    (C) Maijer
    (D) Smith

2. Acid etching removes approximately?

    (A) 10 micrometer of enamel
    (B) 15 micrometer of enamel
    (C) 20 micrometer of enamel
    (D) 25micrometer of enamel

3. What is the minimum bond strength of ideal bonding system?

    (A) 5-12 Mpa
    (B) 12-20 Mpa
    (C) 7-15 Mpa
    (D) 20-25 MPa

4. All are alternative method of acid etching except?

    (A) Crystal growth technique
    (B) Moisture insensitive primer
    (C) Bonding with self etching primer
    (D) All of the above

5. During etching surface energy of the enamel?

    (A) Doubled
    (B) Four times
    (C) Six times
    (D) Eight times

Answers:

1. B

    Buonocore first time suggested etching enamel with 85% phosphoric acid solution resulted in adhesion of acrylic resin. Newman replaced banding with bonding. Maijer and Smith introduced crystal growth technique.[1]

2. A

    Acid etching removes approximately 10 micrometer of enamel surface and creates a morphologically porous layer of 5-50 micrometer deep on the enamel.[2]

3. C

    Ideal bonding agent should generate minimum bond strength of 7-15 MPa. Currently available bonding agents offer bond strength of 12-20 MPa which exceeds the minimum shear bond strength requirements of orthodontic attachments.[3]

4. D

    Crystal growth technique and bonding with self etching primer are alternative methods of acid etching. Moisture insensitive primer has been developed for bonding in difficult situations where achieving total moisture controls is not possible.[4]

5. A

    With etching surface energy is doubled, and as a result the fluid resin contacts the surface and is attracted to the interior of these microporosities created by conditioning through capillary attraction.[5]

References:

1. Gupta A, Kharbanda OP. Orthodontic adhesives and bonding technique. In:Kharbanda OP, Orthodontics: Diagnosis and Management of Malocclusion and Dentofacial Deformities. 2nd Ed. Mosby Elsevier, 2013: 346

2. Gupta A, Kharbanda OP. Orthodontic adhesives and bonding technique. In:Kharbanda OP, Orthodontics: Diagnosis and Management of Malocclusion and Dentofacial Deformities. 2nd Ed. Mosby Elsevier, 2013: 347

3. Gupta A, Kharbanda OP. Orthodontic adhesives and bonding technique. In:Kharbanda OP, Orthodontics: Diagnosis and Management of Malocclusion and Dentofacial Deformities. 2nd Ed. Mosby Elsevier, 2013: 346

4. Gupta A, Kharbanda OP. Orthodontic adhesives and bonding technique. In:Kharbanda OP, Orthodontics: Diagnosis and Management of Malocclusion and Dentofacial Deformities. 2nd Ed. Mosby Elsevier, 2013: 346

5. Gupta A, Kharbanda OP. Orthodontic adhesives and bonding technique. In:Kharbanda OP, Orthodontics: Diagnosis and Management of Malocclusion and Dentofacial Deformities. 2nd Ed. Mosby Elsevier, 2013: 347

Debonding and Retention

Dr. Jitesh Haryani, Junior Resident; Dr. Pradeep Tandon, Professor & Head and Dr. Gyan P. Singh, Associate Professor, Orthodontics & Dentofacial Orthopaedics

A 15 year old boy has been given an appointment for debonding of his upper and lower fixed braces. He was treated for a Class II division 1 malocclusion by orthodontic camouflage with extraction of upper 1st premolars. The upper anteriors were retracted 5.5 mm and lower incisors were proclined 2.2 mm for correction of overjet. The final occlusion achieved is acceptable and esthetics is pleasing. Debonding by mechanical method is planned with fixed retainers.

1. What is the final canine relation in this case?

    (A) Class I
    (B) Class II
    (C) Class III
    (D) None

2. Retention period required for lower incisors in this case is?

    (A) 6 months
    (B) 1 year
    (C) Permanent retention
    (D) Any of the above

3. A CPP-ACP (Casein Phosphoprotein-Amorphous Calcium Phosphate) containing dental cream is prescribed to the patient for 3 months. The use of this cream is?

    (A) To treat gingival enlargement
    (B) To remineralize the white spot lesions
    (C) For enhancing healing of ulcerated mucosa
    (D) Tooth desensitization

4. Which chemical agent has been suggested to facilitate mechanical debonding?

    (A) Peppermint oil
    (B) Sodium lauryl sulphate
    (C) Stannous fluoride
    (D) None

Answers:

1. A

   Camouflage treatment of full cusp Class II division 1 malocclusion with only upper premolar extraction is aimed at finishing the molars in full cusp Class II and canines in Class I.[1]

2. C

   As a general guideline, if more than 2 mm of forward repositioning of the lower incisors occurred during treatment, permanent retention will be required.[2]

3. B

   Use of dental cream containing casein phosphoprotein – amorphous calcium phosphate (CPP-ACP) for 3 months shows significant reduction of White Spot Lesions after debonding. [3]

4. A

   Post debonding agent (GAC) and P-de-A (Oradent) are both derivatives of peppermint oil applied around the bracket base before debonding.[4]

References:

1. Kharbanda OP. Management of class II malocclusion with fixed appliance. In: Kharbanda OP, Orthodontics: Diagnosis and Management of Malocclusion and Dentofacial Deformities; 2nd ed. Mosby Elsevier, 2013: 532

2. Proffit WR. Retention. In: Proffit WR, Fields F W, Sarver D M.Contemporary orthodontics.5th ed. Mosby Elsevier, 2013: 609

3. Kharbanda OP. Post orthodontic care and management of white spot lesions. In:Kharbanda OP, Orthodontics: Diagnosis and Management of Malocclusion and Dentofacial Deformities; 2nd ed. Mosby Elsevier, 2013: 738

4. Kharbanda OP. Debanddebracketing and delivery of retention appliance. In: Kharbanda OP, Orthodontics: Diagnosis and Management of Malocclusion and Dentofacial Deformities; 2nd ed. Mosby Elsevier, 2013: 734

Fixed Functional Appliance

Dr. Jyoti S. Pandhare, Junior Resident; Dr Pradeep Tandon, Professor
& Head and Dr Alka Singh, Associate Professor, Department
of Orthodontics and Dentofacial Orthopaedics

A 15 year old male reported with chief complaint of forward placement of upper front teeth. On clinical examination patient had convex profile, positive visual treatment objective, competent lips and average lower facial height. Intraoral examination revealed overjet of 8mm with 90% overbite, well aligned arches, full cusp class II molar relationship. Cephalometric analysis revealed SNA- 81, FMA- 24, lower 1 to A Pog- 1mm. Cervical vertebrae showed concavities at the lower border of C2, C3 and C4. Patient was having mainly external motivation for treatment and expected to have poor compliance.

1. Diagnosis for this patient will be?

    (A) Class I with bimaxillary protrusion
    (B) Class II Div 1
    (C) Class II Div 2
    (D) Class III

2. Most efficient treatment option will be?

    (A) Fixed Functional appliance
    (B) Class II elastics
    (C) First premolar extraction
    (D) Headgear

3. Which of the following is rigid fixed functional appliance?

    (A) Jasper jumper
    (B) Twin force bite corrector
    (C) Herbst appliance
    (D) FORSUS

4. According to growth relativity theory of Voudouris which of the following factors induce growth modification?

    (A) Displacement, Lateral pterygoid hyperactivity, transduction
    (B) Displacement, Viscoelasticity, Transduction
    (C) Displacement, Masseter hyperactivity, Transduction
    (D) Displacement, relaxation of diagastric, Transduction

5. What is the main disadvantage of Herbst appliance?

    (A) Relies on patient's cooperation
    (B) Lateral movement is restricted
    (C) Deep bite
    (D) Generation of intrusive forces on molars and incisors

Answers:

1. B

    Convex profile, class II molar relationship, increased overjet are the clinical findings associated with class II div 1 malocclusion [1]

2. A

    Patient is 15 years old with cervical vertebrae stage 4 which coincides with deceleration phase of maturity index. To achieve maximum skeletal changes fixed functional appliance is a best option to utilize remaining little growth to maximum advantage.[2]

3. C

    As Herbst appliance provides limited jaw movements, it falls under rigid fixed functional category.[3]

4. B

    Vodourious proposed growth relativity theory in which for condyle -glenoid fossa remodelling, displacement of condyle from glenoid fossa occurs, which leads to stretch of viscoelastic tissues and bone formation at distant location i.e. transduction.[4]

5. **B**

    Herbst appliance is rigid fixed functional appliance and its main disadvantage is limited jaw movement [5]

References:

1. Kharbanda OP.Class II division 1 malocclusion:features and early intervention of growing maxillary excess. In:Kharbanda OP, Orthodontics: Diagnosis and Management of Malocclusion and Dentofacial Deformities.2nd Edition, Mosby Elsevier,2013: 459

2. Kharbanda OP. Interception and treatment of mandibular retrusion with non-compliant fixed functional appliance. In: Kharbanda OP,Orthodontics: Diagnosis and Management of Malocclusion and Dentofacial Deformities. 2nd Edition. Mosby Elsevier, 2013: 500

3. Kharbanda OP. Interception and treatment of mandibular retrusion with non-compliant fixed functional appliance. In: Kharbanda OP,Orthodontics: Diagnosis and Management of Malocclusion and Dentofacial Deformities. 2nd Edition. Mosby Elsevier, 2013: 500

4. Kharbanda OP. Mode of action of functional appliance. In: Kharbanda OP, Orthodontics: Diagnosis and Management of Malocclusion and Dentofacial Deformities. 2nd Edition, Mosby Elsevier,2013: 513

5. Singh G. Functional Appliances. Textbook of orthodontics. 3rd edition. Jaypee, 2015: 543

Cleft Lip & Palate

Dr. Alka Singh, Associate Professor; Dr. Pradeep Tandon,
Professor & Head and Dr. Gyan P. Singh, Associate Professor,
Department of Orthodontics and Dentofacial Orthopaedics

A 13 year old female patient came to the department with chief complaint of wrong placement of anterior teeth. She had history of two previous surgeries, one for the lips and one for the palate for closure of cleft lip & palate. On examination her right lateral incisor was missing, right canine and left lateral incisor were palatally placed with crossbite of anterior teeth. Her maxillary arch was also constricted.

1. Cleft of the lip occurs because of failure of fusion between?

   (A) Medial nasal process, lateral nasal process & the maxillary process
   (B) Medial nasal process & lateral nasal process
   (C) Lateral nasal process & maxillary process
   (D) Medial nasal process & maxillary process

2. Cleft of lip/palate occurs in?

   (A) Third developmental stage
   (B) Fifth developmental stage
   (C) Fourth developmental stage
   (D) Second developmental stage

3. Closure of secondary palate occurs by elevation of palatal shelves during?

   (A) 6to 8 weeks
   (B) 8 to 12 weeks
   (C) 12to 15 weeks
   (D) 17to 20 weeks

4. In some patient, clefts of lip and alveolus may have bands of soft tissue bridging across the two sides called?

   (A) Molar bands
   (B) Intermediate plexus
   (C) Simonarts bands
   (D) epithelial tissue bands

5. What is the correct sequence of treatment in these type of cases?

   (A) Expansion $\Rightarrow$ secondary alveolar bone grafting $\Rightarrow$ eruption of canine
   (B) Secondary alveolar bone grafting $\Rightarrow$ eruption of canine $\Rightarrow$ expansion
   (C) Expansion $\Rightarrow$ eruption of canine $\Rightarrow$ secondary alveolar bone grafting
   (D) Eruption of canine $\Rightarrow$ expansion $\Rightarrow$ secondary alveolar bone grafting

Answers:

1. D

   Upper lip is formed by the fusion of medial nasal processand the maxillary process. [1]

2. C

   Fusion of Processes occurs during fourth developmental stage.[2]

3. B

   Closure of the lip & alveolus occurs during 6th wk of intrauterine life followed by closure of secondary palate which starts at the 8th wk (when elevation of palatal shelves occures & tongue falls down) and continued till 12th wk. The direction of closure is from anterior to posterior.[3]

4. C

   Simonarts 's band[4]

5. A

   Orthodontic expansion should be done before secondary alveolar bone grafting so that the canine will erupt through the graft.[5]

References:

1. Wadhawan N, Nanda RS, Kharbanda OP. Prenatal development of the Foetus with reference tocraniofacial region. In:Kharbanda OP, Orthodontics: Diagnosis and Management of Malocclusion and Dentofacial Deformities; 2nd Edition, Mosby Elsevier 2013: 715

2. Proffit WR, Fields F W. Early stages of Development. Contemporary Orthodontics. 3th edition, Mosby, St Louis, 2000: 66

3. Proffit WR, Fields F W. Early stages of Development. Contemporary Orthodontics. 3th edition. Mosby, St Louis, 2000: 67

4. Kharbanda OP. Historic treatment approach in the interdisciplinary management of cleft lip and palate. Orthodontics, Diagnosis and management of Malocclusion and Dentofacial Deformities. 1st edition. Mosby, Elsevier, 2009: 492

5. Kharbanda OP. Historic treatment approach in the interdisciplinary management of cleft lip and palate. Orthodontics, Diagnosis and management of Malocclusion and Dentofacial Deformities. 1st edition, Mosby, Elsevier, 2009: 509

Obstructive Sleep Apnoea

Dr. Jitesh Haryani, Junior Resident; Dr. Pradeep Tandon,
Professor & Head and Dr. Alka Singh, Associate
Professor, Department of Orthodontics and Dentofacial Orthopaedics

A 44 year old obese male has a chief complaint of excessive day time sleepiness and loud snoring. His lateral cephalogram shows decreased posterior airway space, a retrognathic mandible and increased distance of hyoid to mandibular plane. His Apnea/hypopnea index is 44.5 and Epsworth sleepiness scale value of 24.

1. Patient is suffering from?

    (A) Sleep bruxism
    (B) Obstructive sleep apnea
    (C) Upper respiratory tract infection
    (D) Asthma

2. What kind of oral appliances are used for management of this disease?

    (A) Mandibular advancement devices
    (B) Tongue retaining devices
    (C) Palatal lift appliances
    (D) All of the above

3. What is the gold standard investigation for the diagnosis of this problem?

    (A) MRI
    (B) CT scan
    (C) Polysomnography
    (D) EMG

4. One of the most widely used fixed mandibular advancement device in the management of this disease is?

    (A) Karwetzky activator
    (B) Van beek activator
    (C) Aveo device
    (D) Twin block

Answers:

1. B

   Obstructive sleep apnea refers to occurrence of atleast 5 apnea hypopnea per sleep hour.[1]

2. D

   Oral appliances include: Mandibular advancement devices like Karwetzky activator, bionator, removable Herbst etc and Tongue retaining devices[2]

3. C

   Polysomnography is considered as the gold standard test for diagnosis of OSA.[3]

4. A

   Karwetzky activator is one of the most widely used fixed mandibular advancement device in management of OSA.[4]

References:

1. Jayan B, Kharbanda OP. Orthodontist's role in upper airway sleep disorders. In:Kharbanda OP, Orthodontics: Diagnosis and Management of Malocclusion and Dentofacial Deformities; 2nd Edition, Mosby Elsevier 2013: 709

2. Jayan B, Kharbanda OP. Orthodontist's role in upper airway sleep disorders. In:Kharbanda OP, Orthodontics: Diagnosis and Management of Malocclusion and Dentofacial Deformities; 2nd Edition, Mosby Elsevier 2013: 715

3. Jayan B, Kharbanda OP. Orthodontist's role in upper airway sleep disorders. In:Kharbanda OP, Orthodontics: Diagnosis and Management of Malocclusion and Dentofacial Deformities; 2nd Edition, Mosby Elsevier 2013: 713

4. .Jayan B, Kharbanda OP. Orthodontist's role in upper airway sleep disorders. In:Kharbanda OP, Orthodontics: Diagnosis and Management of Malocclusion and Dentofacial Deformities; 2nd Edition, Mosby Elsevier 2013: 715

Orthognathic Surgery

Dr. Gulshan K. Singh, Professor; Dr. Alka Singh, Associate Professor and Dr. Dipti Shastri, Senior Resident, Orthodontics & Dentofacial Orthopaedics

A 25 year old female patient reported with large lower jaw was having following features: concave profile, retruded maxilla, retruded upper lip, increased anterior facial height, prominent chin, reverse overjet approximately 8mm, retroclined mandibular anterior teeth, mesiobuccal cusps of maxillary 1st molars falls in between embrasure of 1st and 2nd permanent mandibular molars. Her Cephalometric readings were ANB -8^0, SNA 79^0, SNB 87^0, Wit's appraisal was 7mm. During speech she is not able to pronounce sounds like S,F,V and B. Her parents were having similar type of facial pattern.

1. What is your probable diagnosis?

   (A) Super class I M.O.
   (B) Skeletal class III M.O.
   (C) Pseudo class III M.O.
   (D) Skeletal class III Type I M.O.

2. Orthognathic surgery should be performed?

   (A) As early as possible
   (B) After the completion of Growth of Individual
   (C) After the completion of Pubertal Growth spurt
   (D) May be performed at any time

3. Which surgical procedure will be more suitable for above case?

   (A) Mandibular Distraction Osteogenesis.
   (B) Genioplasty
   (C) Bilateral sagittal split osteotomy -BSSO for reduction of Mandibular Length
   (D) Surgical expansion of Maxila.

4. Orthodontist can perform Post-surgical Orthodontics after?

   (A) 6-8 weeks of Surgery
   (B) 1-2 weeks of Surgery
   (C) 6-8 Days of Surgery
   (D) 3-4 Months of Surgery

5. The single most frequent and significant complication of Bilateral sagittal split osteotomy is?

(A) Avascular necrosis

(B) Acute/postoperative condylar resorption

(C) Velopharyngeal Insufficiency

(D) Injury to Inferior alveolar nerve

Answers:

1. B

ANB angle is used to assess the sagittal relationship between the maxillary and mandibular base. If ANB angle is smaller than 2^0, then it is referred as small ANB angle. It indicates class III skeletal tendency. Concave facial profile- possible type of malocclusion- class III malocclusion. [1]

2. B

Orthognathic surgery should be delayed till adulthood so that the skeletal growth is completed and deformity is fully expressed.[2]

3. C

BSSO of the mandible is a good option for reduction in mandible. [3]

4. A

Post surgical orthodontics phase typically begins 6-8 weeks after surgery when patient is seen in the orthodontic clinic (office).At this stage the patient would have recovered from most of his facial oedema. [4]

5. D

Injury to inferior alveolar nerve is the single most frequent and significant complication of Bilateral sagittal split osteotomy.[5]

References:

1. Phulari BS. Cephalometrics in Orthodontics. Orthodontics : Principles and practice. First edition. Jaypee, 2011 :195.

2. Kharbanda OP, Darendeliler MA. Ortho-surgical management of skeletal malocclusion. In: Kharbanda OP,Orthodontics: Diagnosis and Management of Malocclusion and Dentofacial Deformities. 2nd Edition, Mosby Elsevier, 2013: 650

3. Kharbanda OP, Darendeliler MA. Ortho-surgical management of skeletal malocclusion. In: Kharbanda OP,Orthodontics: Diagnosis and Management of Malocclusion and Dentofacial Deformities. 2nd Edition, Mosby Elsevier, 2013: 655

4. Kharbanda OP, Darendeliler MA. Ortho-surgical management of skeletal malocclusion. In: Kharbanda OP,Orthodontics: Diagnosis and Management of Malocclusion and Dentofacial Deformities. 2nd Edition, Mosby Elsevier, 2013: 656

5. Kharbanda OP, Darendeliler MA. Ortho-surgical management of skeletal malocclusion. In: Kharbanda OP, Orthodontics: Diagnosis and Management of Malocclusion and Dentofacial Deformities. 2nd Edition. Mosby Elsevier, 2013: 664

Distraction Osteogenesis

Dr. Gulshan K. Singh, Professor; Dr. Alka Singh, Associate Professor and Dr. Dipti Shastri, Senior Resident, Department of Orthodontics and Dentofacial Orthopaedics

A 20 year female patient reported with forward placement of upper front teeth. On clinical examination she had convex facial profile, severely retruded chin, incompetent lips, lip trap, proclined maxillary anterior teeth, increased overjet (more than 14 mm), deep overbite and narrow arches. No other family members have similar facial pattern and malocclusion. Cephalometric evaluation of patient revealed: SNA= 83^0, SNB= 73^0, ANB =10^0 along with increased anterior facial height.

1. What is the exact diagnosis of this case?

    (A) Class I type 2 malocclusion

    (B) Class II div 1 malocclusion

    (Ç) Class II subdivision malocclusion

    (D) Class II div 2 malocclusion

2. Which cephalometric analysis was specially developed for Orthognathic surgery?

    (A) Downs analysis

    (B) Steiner analysis

    (C) Wit's analysis

    (D) COGS analysis

3. Which surgical procedure will be more suitable for above case?

    (A) Le fort I surgery

    (B) Le fort II surgery

    (C) Mandibular Distraction Osteogenesis.

    (D) Advancement Genioplasty

4. Before Orthognathic surgery following procedures are required?

    (A) Presurgical Orthodontics

    (B) Mock surgery

    (C) Premedication

    (D) All of above.

5. What is Template?

    (A) A Surgical splint

    (B) A Cephalometric tracing

    (C) A mock surgery

    (D) A surgical procedure.

Answers:

1. B

   ANB angle is used to assess the sagittal relationship between the maxillary and mandibular base. If ANB angle is greater than normal it is known as large ANB angle. It indicates class II skeletal tendency. [1]

2. D

   COGS Cephalometric analysis was specially develop for Orthognathic surgery by Burstone and colleagues in 1978.[3]

3. C)

   Conventional osteotomy techniques have several limitations. Distraction osteogenesis is developed to overcome these limitations.[4]

4. D

   Alignment and levelling of arches within respective jaws is a prerequisite to most of Orthognathic surgeries. A mock model surgery can be attempted to view the final outcome of the occlusion and extend of surgical movement required.[5]

5. B

   Cephalometric template can be used to predict the type and extent of the surgical movement required.[6]

References:

1. Phulari BS. Cephalometrics in Orthodontics. Orthodontics : Principals and Practice .First Edition. Jaypee, 2011 : 159

2. Kharbanda OP Darendeliler MA. Ortho-surgical management of skeletal malocclusion. In: Kharbanda OP,Orthodontics: Diagnosis and Management of Malocclusion and Dentofacial Deformities. First Edition, Mosby Elsevier, 2013: 445

3. Tsahannerr, Zakaullah S,Phulari BS. Surgical Orthodontics .In :Phulari BS Orthodontics : Principals and Practice. First Edition. Jaypee 2011:588.

4. Kharbanda OP, Darendeliler MA. Ortho-surgical management of skeletal malocclusion. In: Kharbanda OP, Orthodontics: Diagnosis and Management of

Malocclusion and Dentofacial Deformities. Ist Edition, Mosby Elsevier, 2009: 452-453

5. Kharbanda OP, Darendeliler MA. Ortho-surgical management of skeletal malocclusion. In: Kharbanda OP, Orthodontics: Diagnosis and Management of Malocclusion and Dentofacial Deformities. Ist Edition, Mosby Elsevier, 2009: 453.

Chapter - 4

Oral Medicine and Radiology

Ankyloglossia

Dr. Ranjit kumar Patil, Prof & Head, Department of Oral Medicine

Patient was 19 year old male with unclear speech since childhood. Notching of tip of tongue noticed with 2mm tongue protrusion. Lingual frenum with high attachment noticed. Speech of the patient was affected.

Investigations: No specific test

Brief treatment history: Frenectomy of lingual frenum was done under local anasthesia

Diagnosis: Ankyloglossia

1. Ankyloglossia is associated with which syndrome
   - (A) Facial hemiatrophy
   - (B) Cheilitis glandularis
   - (C) Van der woude syndrome
   - (D) Cleft lip & palate

2. A 20 year old male comes to the OPD with a short lingual frenum resulting in limitation of tongue movement. A diagnosis of tongue tie is made. What other feature is associated with this anomaly
   - (A) Anterior open bite
   - (B) Posterior open bite
   - (C) Anterior cross bite
   - (D) Posterior cross bite

Answers:

1. C.

   Van Der Woude syndrome is a genetic disorder characterized by the combination of lower lip pits, cleft lip with or without cleft palate, and cleft palate alone (CP). Ankyloglossia can sometimes be component of the syndrome. (1)

2. A.

   Tongue tie leads to orthodontic problems including anterior open bite. (1)

Reference:

1. Shafer, Hine, Levy. Textbook of Oral Pathology Elsevier publication 7th edition

Verrucous Carcinoma

Dr. Ranjit kumar Patil, Prof & Head, Department of Oral Medicine

55 year old male presented with a growth on right cheek since 6 years. History revealed a slow and persistent growth without pain. On examination a single proliferative lesion 3 x 2 cm^2 was present on right buccal mucosa. The lesion was white in colour and Bleeding was noted from the lesion. The patient gave history of tobacco chewing habit for past 30 years.

Investigations: Routine Blood investigations were in normal range. There were no radiographic changes noted in the OPG and IOPAR of 45,46

Brief treatment history: Wide Surgical Excision of lesion

Diagnosis: Verrucous Carcinoma

1. Which of the following has least potential to metastasize

    (A) Malignant melanoma
    (B) Squamous cell carcinoma
    (C) Verrucous carcinoma
    (D) Sarcoma

2. Keratins plugs are seen in

    (A) Verrucous carcinoma
    (B) Squamous cell carcinoma
    (C) Verruca vulgaris
    (D) Condyloma accuminatum

3. What would be the line of treatment for Verrucous Carcinoma

    (A) No treatment
    (B) Chemotherapy only
    (C) Excision of lesion
    (D) Wide excision of lesion

Answers:

1. (C)

    Verrucous carcinoma has least tendency to metastasize. (1)

2. (A)

    Abundance of keratin is seen in Verrucous carcinoma on surface and it dips down with invaginating epithelium and produces keratins plugs.(1)

3. (D)

    Wide surgical excision has been recommended treatment for many years. Close & continued post surgical surveillance is obligatory. (1)

Reference:

1. Wood & Goaz. Differential diagnosis of Oral & Maxillofacial region. Mosby publication 5th ed. Year 1997 page 113-115

TMJ Ankylosis

Dr. Ranjit kumar Patil, Prof & Head, Departmene of Oral Medicine

A seventeen year old girl presented with decreased mouth opening since 07 years of age. Patient gives a history of fall at 06 years of age. Deviation of mandible was towards left side. Bilateral antegonial notching evident. Interincisal mouth opening of 08 mm noticed.

Investigations: Panoramic radiograph and Cone Beam Computed Tomography

Brief treatment history: Condylectomy followed by reconstruction

Diagnosis: TMJ Ankylosis left side

1. Most common cause of TMJ ankylosis is

   (A) Bacterial Infection
   (B) Rheumatoid Arthritis
   (C) Trauma
   (D) Psoriasis

2. Most common type of dislocation of the mandibular condyles is

   (A) Anterior
   (B) Posterior
   (C) Cranial
   (D) Basal

3. Which of the following is not seen in TMJ ankylosis

   (A) Reduced mandibular movement
   (B) Deviation of mandible to affected side on mouth opening
   (C) Facial asymmetry
   (D) Deviation of mandible to unaffected side on mouth opening

Answers:

1. C.

   Trauma to the jaw during developmental years is common cause of ankylosis of joint (1)

2. A.

   Self explanatory (1)

3. D

   The most common cause of TMJ ankylosis is trauma in younger age group with anterior dislocation Clinical feature includes deep antegonial notch on affected side with restricted mouth opening and deviation of mandible towards affected side.(2)

References:

1. Shafer, Hine, Levy. Textbook of Oral Pathology Elsevier publication 7th edition page 741-742

2. Greenberg MS, Glick M Burkett's Oral Medicine: Diagnosis and Treatment. (11stedn), BC Decker, Hamilton, Canada. Pg 254

Stafne's Cyst

Dr. Ranjit kumar Patil, Prof. & Head, Department of Oral Medicine

A 56 year old male patient reported with pain left lower back teeth since 04 days. Multiple root stumps and missing teeth were noticed. Tender root stump of left mandibular second molar noticed. Patient was adviced for orthpantomogram.

Investigations: orthopantomogram: besides other findings, revealed single radiolucency below the inferior alveolar canal of right mandible of 05 x 04 cm in size.

No treatment was required for the right mandibular radiolucency. Left mandibular 2nd and 3rd molars were extracted.

Diagnosis: Stafne's Cyst

1. Stafne's Cyst is usually located

   (A) Between angle of mandible and 1st Molar above the level of inferior alveolar nerve

   (B) Between angle of mandible and 1st Molar below the level of inferior alveolar nerve

   (C) Between angle of mandible and 2nd Molar above the level of inferior alveolar nerve

   (D) Between angle of mandible and 2nd Molar below the level of inferior alveolar nerve

2. A 25 year old male reported with radiolucent lesion near angle of mandible. A biopsy confirms the presence of normal salivary gland tissue. What would be the probable diagnosis?

   (A) Traumatic bone cyst

   (B) Static bone cyst

   (C) Sialadenosis

   (D) Pleomorphic adenoma

3. Most common etiology for Stafne's cyst

   (A) Developmental

   (B) Pressure of Submandibular Gland

   (C) Trauma

   (D) Infection

Answers:

1. (B)

   It is a depression in the mandible caused by sub-mandibular salivary gland. Stafne's cyst is accidental finding usually located below the inferior alveolar canal. (1-3)

2. (B)

   Stafne's cyst and static bone cyst are synonym. (1-3)

3. (B)

   Stafne's cyst is also known as static bone cyst and it has aberrant salivary gland tissue inside it. (1-3)

References:

1. Greenberg MS, Glick M (2003) Burkett's Oral Medicine: Diagnosis and Treatment. (11stedn), BC Decker, Hamilton, Canada page 200

2. Neville BW, Damm DD, Allen CM, Bouquot JE (2002) Oral and Maxillofacial Pathology. (2stedn), WB Saunders, Philadelphia, London, Toronto. Page 24

3. Tsui SH, Chan FF. Lingual mandibular bone defect: case report and review of the literature Aust Dent J 1994;39:368–71

Carcinoma Buccal Mucosa

Dr. Ranjit kumar Patil, Prof & Head, Department of Oral Medicine

Patient presented with a ulcerative growth at the right angle of lip. Patient noticed a very small proliferation in the region about two years back which slowly grew to present stage.

No history of pain in the region. History of infrequent bleeding from the lesion was reported. No history of paraesthesia in the region.

Investigations: Incisional biopsy, Routine blood investigations, Orthopatomograph.

Brief treatment history: Incisional biopsy followed by excisional biopsy of the lesion was performed.

Diagnosis: Squamous cell carcinoma of buccal mucosa

1. Oral Squamous cell carcinoma of buccal mucosa is more in patients
   (A) Using tobacco quid
   (B) In smokers
   (C) In alcoholic patients
   (D) Same in all above

2. In western countries least common site for intra oral carcinoma is
   (A) Posterior surface of tongue
   (B) Soft palate
   (C) Gingiva
   (D) Buccal mucosa

3. Which amongst the following lesions has the highest malignant transformation potential
   (A) Nicotina palatinus in reverse smokers
   (B) Erthyroplakia
   (C) OSMF
   (D) Erthyro-leukoplakia

Answers:

1. A

    Tobacco quid habit is prevalent in many geographical locations leading to rise of buccal mucosal cancers (1)

2. D

    This could be due to difference of habits (2)

3. A

    In reverse smoking, the burning end is kept in the oral cavity (3)

References:

1. Chen PC, Kuo C, Pan CC, Chou MY. Risk of oral cancer associated with human papillomavirus infection, betel quid chewing, and cigarette smoking in Taiwan— an integrated molecular and epidemiological study of 58 cases. J Oral Pathol Med 2002;31:317 – 322

2. Neville BW, Damm DD, Allen CM, Bouquot JE (2002) Oral and Maxillofacial Pathology. (2nd Edn), WB Saunders, Philadelphia, London, Toronto. Page 415

3. Neville BW, Damm DD, Allen CM, Bouquot JE (2002) Oral and Maxillofacial Pathology. (2stedn), WB Saunders, Philadelphia, London, Toronto. Page 410

Pyogenic Granuloma

Dr. Ranjit Kumar Patil, Prof & Head, Department of Oral Medicine

A 63 year old male presented with painless growth of lower jaw since 15 years. Patient noticed a small nodular growth 15 year back which slowly grew to the present stage. The growth is painless. On examination the growth was non tender, mobile, pedunculated.

Investigations: Orthopantomography was done with no significant relevant finding.

Brief treatment history: Antibiotic therapy followed by surgical excision of the lesion

Diagnosis: Pygenic granuloma with secondary infection

1. Pyogenic Granuloma are
    (A) Pus containing lesion
    (B) Benign tumor
    (C) Inflammatory hyperplasia lesion
    (D) Granulomatous lesion

2. New histological terminology for pyogenic granuloma
    (A) Lobular Capillary malformation
    (B) Lobular capillary hemangioma
    (C) Lobular capillary granuloma
    (D) Lobular Arteriovenous malformation

3. Cause of pyogenic Granuloma is
    (A) Infection
    (B) Chronic irritation
    (C) Genetic
    (D) Developmental

Answers:

1. C.

    Pyogenic granuloma is an inflammatory hyperplasia lesion that becomes ulcerated. Necrotic part resembles pus prompted the clinicians to refer it as pyogenic granuloma (1)

2. B

    This new term because of the significant vascular component. (2)

3. B

    This lesion is always associated with local factors like calculus and plaque, causing chronic irritation. (2)

References:

1. Wood & Goaz. Differential diagnosis of Oral & Maxillofacial region. Mosby publication 8th ed. Year 1997 page 138

2. Neville BW, Damm DD, Allen CM, Bouquot JE (2002) Oral and Maxillofacial Pathology. (2nd edn), WB Saunders, Philadelphia, London, Toronto.

Carcinoma floor of mouth

Dr. Vikram Khanna, Assistant Professor, Department of Oral Medicine

Patient presented with ulceration of floor of mouth since 05 months. The patient noticed a small growth of floor of mouth 06 month back which ulcerated 05 month back. History of 3-4 bleeding episodes from the lesion. On examination a single ulcero-proliferative growth of midline of floor of mouth, round in shape, of about 4 cm diameter, non tender with granular floor of ulcer and raised borders. Two palpable sub-mental lymph nodes which were firm and non tender.

Investigations: Incisional biopsy, Routine blood investigations, Orthopatomograph.

Brief treatment history: Incisional biopsy followed by excisional biopsy of the lesion was performed.

Diagnosis: Squamous cell carcinoma of floor of the mouth

1. Most common site affected by Squamous cell carcinoma in oral mucosa

    (A) Buccal mucosa
    (B) Gingival
    (C) Labial mucosa
    (D) Floor of the mouth

2. Major reason for floor of mucosa to be affected by Squamous cell carcinoma is

    (A) Thick mucosal epithelium
    (B) Thin mucosal epithelium
    (C) Tobacco quid is placed under tongue
    (D) Most deposition of calculus in lingual aspect of lower anterior which can cause chronic irritation

3. Which of the following location of oral carcinoma has more chance to metastasize to regional lymph node

    (A) Lip
    (B) Hard palate
    (C) Floor of mouth
    (D) Maxillary gingival

Answers:

1. D

    The ventral surface of the tongue and the floor of the mouth are the sites most commonly affected by SCC because they are lined by thin non-keratinised epithelium. (1)

2. B

    The ventral surface of the tongue and the floor of the mouth are the sites most commonly affected by SCC be-cause they are lined by thin non-keratinised epithelium. (1)

3. C

    Floor of mouth is obscured location with close proximity to vascularity and lymphatics. (2)

References:

1. B. W. Neville and T. A. Day, "Oral Cancer and Precan-cerous Lesions," *CA: A Cancer Journal for Clinicians*, Vol. 52, No. 4, 2002, pp. 195-215.

2. J. P. Shah and Z. Gil, "Current Concepts in Management of Oral Cancer-Surgery," *Oral Oncology*, Vol. 45, No. 4, 2009, pp. 394-401.

Peripheral Giant Cell Granuloma

Dr. Vikram Khanna, Assistant Professor, Department of Oral Medicine

The patient reported with swelling of left upper jaw since 18 months. The swelling was non tender with slow persistent enlargement. No history of parasthesia of region. History of mobility and extraction of left upper teeth about 01 year back.

Investigations: Routine blood test, Free and bound serum calcium, OPG x-ray, Serum alkaline phosphatase.

Brief treatment history: Excision of the lesion was done under local anesthesia. No history of recurrence since 05 months.

Diagnosis: Peripheral giant cell granuloma

1. Radiologically peripheral giant cell granuloma is presented as
   (A) Multilocular radiolucency
   (B) Peripheral cupping
   (C) Unilocular radiolucency
   (D) No findings

2. Peripheral giant cell granuloma is often associated with
   (A) Hyperthyroidism
   (B) Hypothyroidism
   (C) Hyperparathyroidism
   (D) Hypoparathyroidism

3. Peripheral giant cell lesion is
   (A) Inflammatory lesion
   (B) Reactive lesion
   (C) Infection
   (D) Developmental lesion

Answers:

1. B

   Peripheral giant cell granuloma causes lateral pressure on the bone. (1)

2. B

   Peripheral giant-cell granuloma is an <u>oral pathologic</u> condition that appears in the <u>mouth</u> as an <u>overgrowth</u> of <u>tissue</u> due to <u>irritation</u> or <u>trauma</u>. (1)

3. B

   Peripheral giant cell granuloma or the so-called "giant cell epulis" is the most common oral giant cell lesion. It normally presents as a soft tissue purplish-red nodule consisting of multinucleated giant cells in a background of mononuclear stromal cells and extravasated red blood cells. (2,3)

References:

1. Dayan D, Buchner A, Spirer S. Bone formation in peripheral giant cell granuloma. J Periodontol. 1990;61:444–6

2. Smith BR, Fowler CB, Svane TJ. Primary hyperparathyroidism presenting as a "peripheral" giant cell granuloma. J Oral Maxillofac Surg. 1988;46:65–9

3. Carvalho YR, Loyola AM, Gomez RS, Araujo VC. Peripheral giant cell granuloma. An immuno-histochemical and ultrastructural study. Oral Dis. 1995;1:20–5.

Nasopharyngeal Carcinoma

Dr. Vikram Khanna, Assistant Professor, Department of Oral Medicine

A 63 year old male complained of bleeding from oral cavity since three weeks. History of palatal perforation since two months. Patient also gives history of nasal bleeding two weeks ago which stopped with nasal packing.

Investigations: Maxillary occlusal view, CT scan axial

Brief treatment history: Incisional biopsy

Diagnosis: Nasopharyngeal carcinoma

1. Nasopharyngeal carcinoma may be associated with
   (A) HSV
   (B) HPV
   (C) HZV
   (D) EBV

2. Radiotherapy of which of the following may cause radiation exposure of all of the salivary gland with severe xerostomia
   (A) Nasopharyngeal carcinoma
   (B) Squamous cell carcinoma of tongue
   (C) Carcinoma of thyroid gland
   (D) None of the above

Answers:

1. D

    Nasopharyngeal carcinoma is caused by a combination of factors: viral, environmental influences, and heredity. The viral influence is associated with infection with Epstein-Barr virus. (1)

2. A

    Radiotherapy in Nasopharyngeal carcinoma patient, may expose all the major salivary glands due to anatomical position.(2,3)

References:

1. Greenberg MS, Glick M Burkett's Oral Medicine: Diagnosis and Treatment. (11stedn), BC Decker, Hamilton, Canada.

2. Neville BW, Damm DD, Allen CM, Bouquot JE (2002) Oral and Maxillofacial Pathology. (2nd edn), WB Saunders, Philadelphia, London, Toronto. pg 428-429

3. Neville BW, Damm DD, Allen CM, Bouquot JE (2002) Oral and Maxillofacial Pathology. (2nd edn), WB Saunders, Philadelphia, London, Toronto. pg 428-429

Irritational Fibroma

Dr. Vikram Khanna, Assistant Professor, Department of Oral Medicine

The patient presented with a nodular growth right lateral border of tongue since 6 month. It slowly grew in size to present stage. It was painless. Non tender, firm, mobile on palpation, pedunculated.

Investigations: Excisional biopsy

Brief treatment history: Excisional biopsy

Diagnosis: Irritational fibroma

1. Which one of the following is incorrect about irritational fibroma
   (A) It is the common benign tumor of oral cavity
   (B) It is usually solitary lesion
   (C) It has high malignant rate
   (D) It is associated with any trauma/friction

2. Which one of the following would not be included in differential diagnosis of the irritational fibroma on buccal mucosa
   (A) Squamous Papilloma
   (B) Peripheral giant cell granuloma
   (C) Pyogenic granuloma
   (D) Hairy leukoplakia

3. The radiographic appearance of irritational fibroma is:
   (A) Well differentiated radiopaque lesion
   (B) Poorly differentiated radiopaque lesion
   (C) Well differentiated radiolucent lesion
   (D) No significant radiographic changes

Answers:

1. C

    Irritational fibroma is benign growth caused by repeated trauma (1)

2. D

    Hairy leukoplakia occurs on lateral border of tongue in immune-compromised individual (1)

3. D

    It is a soft tissue lesion (1)

Reference:

1. Neville BW, Damm DD, Allen CM, Bouquot JE (2002) Oral and Maxillofacial Pathology. (2nd edn), WB Saunders, Philadelphia, London, Toronto. Pg 507-509

Herpes-Zoster

Dr. Vikram Khanna, Assistant Professor, Department of Oral Medicine

56 year old male reported of right face vesicular eruptions and swelling of right eye since 03 days. Patient also reported of intra oral vesicles of right palate. Patient gives history of fever for one day before the occurrence of the lesion.

Investigations: Tzanck smear

Brief treatment history: Topical and systemic antiviral medication

Diagnosis:Herpes-zoster

1. After primary infection of VZV, it becomes latent in the
   (A) Dorsal root ganglia of spinal nerves or extra medullary ganglion of cranial nerves
   (B) In the marginal gingiva
   (C) In the saliva & other body fluid
   (D) None of the above

2. The most commonly involved nerve in herpes zoster infection is
   (A) Facial nerve
   (B) Trigeminal 1st branch
   (C) Trigeminal 2nd branch
   (D) Trigeminal 3rd branch

3. What is zoster sine herpete
   (A) Zoster without rash
   (B) Zoster vesicles on face
   (C) Shiny vesicles in oral cavity
   (D) Shiny vesicles on whole body

Answers:

1. A

   The virus travels along the nerve to get lodged in ganglion (1)

2. B

   Herpes zoster infection commonly involves ophthalmic division of trigeminal nerve (1)

3. A

   Some patients may have prodromal symptoms without developing the characteristic rash. This situation is known as zoster sine herpete. (1)

References:

1. Neville BW, Damm DD, Allen CM, Bouquot JE (2002) Oral and Maxillofacial Pathology. (2nd edn), WB Saunders, Philadelphia, London, Toronto. pg 252-253

Gingival Hyperplasia

Dr. Vikram Khanna, Assistant Professor, Department of Oral Medicine

Presenting features: A 27 year old female complained of burning sensation of mouth since 08 months. Patient visited several consultants with no relief. No history of skin lesions.

1. Which one of the following type of lichen planus is more common?

   (A) Erosive lichen planus
   (B) Reticular lichen planus
   (C) Papular lichen planus
   (D) Bullous lichen planus

2. Which one of the following type of oral lichen planus has more malignant potential?

   (A) Lichenoid reaction
   (B) Erosive Lichen planus
   (C) Reticular lichen planus
   (D) Fordyces granules

3. A 35 year old female presented with atrophic, erythematous areas with central ulcerations and periphery of the atrophic region bordered by fine, white radiating striae on left buccal mucosa and tongue. The most probable diagnosis would be

   (A) Reticular lichen planus
   (B) Erosive lichen planus
   (C) Lichenoid reaction
   (D) Aphthous ulcer major

4. Which one of the following is immune mediated:

   (A) Fordyces granules
   (B) Erosive lichen planus
   (C) Chemical burn
   (D) Atrophic candidiasis

Answers:

1. B

   reticular lichen planus is the commonest variety of lichen planus (1)

2. B

   erosive lichen planus has highest malignant potential due to thinning of mucosa, thereby increased absorption of carcinogens (1)

3. B

   the mentioned features are of erosive lichen planus (1)

4. B

   only lichen planus is immune mediated disorder (1)

Reference:

1. Neville BW, Damm DD, Allen CM, Bouquot JE (2002) Oral and Maxillofacial Pathology. (2nd edn), WB Saunders, Philadelphia, London, Toronto. Pg 782-788

Condylar Hyperplasia

Dr. Vandana Singh, Lecturer, Department of Oral Medicine

23 year old male complained of deviation of lower jaw to the right side since two years. Patient noticed slow and progressive deviation to the right side. No history of pain on mouth opening.

Investigations: OPG showed enlargement of left condyle.

1. Incorrect about unilateral condylar hyperplasia
    (A) The chin is deviated to the unaffected side
    (B) The chin is deviated to the affected side
    (C) Chin is not deviated
    (D) None of the above

2. Condylar neoplasm can be differentiated from condylar hyperplasia as
    (A) Radigraphically there is normal cortical thickness & trabecular pattern in condylar hyperplasia.
    (B) Condylar hyperplasia is more painful
    (C) Hyperplastic condyle shows hereditary predilection.
    (D) Hyperplastic condyle is more irregular in shape

3. Which of the following manifestation is not seen in condylar hyperplasia
    (A) Facial asymmetry
    (B) Prognathism
    (C) Open bite
    (D) Impacted tooth

4. Which of the following may be included in the differential diagnosis of condylar hyperplasia
    (A) Osteochondroma of condyle
    (B) Myofacial pain dysfunction syndrome
    (C) Condyloma Accuminatum
    (D) TMJ arthritis

Answers:

1. A

    The chin deviates toward unaffected side due to increase in the vertical dimension of ramus. There is normal anatomical & functional development of opposite side condyle in unilateral condylar hyperplasia. (1)

2. A

    condylar neoplasm will break cortical margins and demonstrate haphazard trabeculation (1)

3. D

    impacted tooth is unrelated to condylar hyperplasia (1)

4. A

    Ostechondroma is a benign tumor of condyle where there is irregular and uncontrolled growth of condyle occurs. Other entities do not show condylar over growth. (1)

Reference:

1. White and pharaoh oral radiology principles and interpretation 6th ed 2008 pg 481-483

Carcinoma Antrum

Dr. Vandana Singh, Lecturer, Department of Oral Medicine

A 40 year female reported with swelling on l side of face since 2 months. H/o frequent Sinusitis and bleeding from nose 10 days ago. H/o change in the voice present. O/E swelling noticed on left side maxillary sinus region. I/o mobility noticed in 25, 26, 27.

Investigations: Complete blood examination. Radiographic Investigations: water's view and CT scan of the Head & Neck region. Incisional Biopsy

Brief treatment history: Hemimaxillectomy and radiotherapy with chemotherapy.

Diagnosis: Carcinoma Left maxillary Antrum

1. The cause of consequent delay in the diagnosis of Carcinoma antrum is because of
   (A) Antrum is closed and concealed site, neoplasm within it can reach a considerable size
   (B) Lack of diagnostic methods
   (C) Carcinoma antrum does not cause any sign and symptom at all
   (D) None of the above

2. A patient with carcinoma antrum will have worst prognosis if the path of spread is:
   (A) Along the orbital wall
   (B) Posterior spread
   (C) Inferior spraed
   (D) Medial spread

3. The radiographic finding of carcinoma antrum is
   (A) "Cloudy" antrum, a diffuse opacity or an irregular soft tissue outline with bony erosions
   (B) No significant radigraphic changes
   (C) A smooth radiopaque well circumscribed lesion
   (D) Tear drop appearance

4. Which of the following imaging technique is not indicated for CA antrum
   (A) Water's view
   (B) USG antrum
   (C) CT head
   (D) OPG

Answers:

1. A

    Anotomically maxillary antrum is a pyramidal shaped closed air cavity, neoplasm within it spread rapidly and reaches upto considerable size before any sign and symptom. (1)

2. B

    Posterior spread will involve base of the skull quickly. (1)

3. A

    The antrum has cloudy apperance as the antrum is filled with soft tissue proliferative mass and inflammatory. There may be bony involvement (erosion). (1)

4. B

    USG antrum is not useful in CA antrum as this cannot give the picture of bony involvement and spread of the carcinoma. The other radiographic methods and CT antrum are indicated for CA antrum. (1)

Reference:

1. Neville BW, Damm DD, Allen CM, Bouquot JE (2002) Oral and Maxillofacial Pathology. (2nd edn), WB Saunders, Philadelphia, London, Toronto. pg 782-788

Hemangioma Tongue

Dr. Vandana Singh, Lecturer, Department of Oral Medicine

A 29 year old male patient reported with swelling in tongue since childhood. Swelling increased to present size gradually with no history of pain. O/E intraorally on palpation the swelling was reducible and compressible. Pulsation can also be felt on palpation. Diascopy test was positive.

Investigations: Ultrasonography with Doppler examination. MRI of Tongue

Brief treatment history: Sclerotherapy followed by surgery

Diagnosis: Haemangioma of tongue

1. Which one of the following is incorrect about hemangioma
   (A) They are usually present at birth but commonly manifest in childhood or adolescence.
   (B) The most common sites in oral cavity are anterior two third of the tongue, palate, and gingiva and buccal mucosa
   (C) These are the lesions with direct communications between an artery and a vein
   (D) They are more common to AV malformation

2. Which one is true about hemangiomas
   (A) Hemangiomas are low flow lesions
   (B) They are not present at birth
   (C) hemangiomas always occur extraosseous
   (D) hemangioma has no significant radiographic changes

3. The radiographic appearance of intrabony hemangiomas
   (A) Well defined, corticated multilocular radiolucent lesion
   (B) Diffuse radipaque lesion
   (C) Diffuse cyst like radiolucent lesion
   (D) No significant radiographic changes.

Answers:

1. C

   This feature is related to AV Malformations (1)

2. A

   Hemangiomas are vascular lesions. They are classified as low flow (1)

3. A

   A tortuous and enlarged vessel in bone gives such appearance.(1)

Reference:

1. White and pharaoh, oral radiology principles and interpretation 6th ed 2008 pg 592-593

Anug

Dr. Vandana Singh, Lecturer, Department of Oral Medicine

A 30 year old male patient reported with pain in gums since 3 weeks. H/o of frequent sensitivity in teeth with bleeding was present. H/o of bidi smoking and poor oral hygiene. O/E punched out lesions of attached gingival was noticed in lower anterior with recession in gingival. Papillary swelling was present

Investigations: Direct microsopy emanination

Brief treatment history: H_2O_2 debridement of the lesion followed by curettage of lesion. Regular follow up

Diagnosis: Acute Necrotic Ulcerative Gingivitis

1. A patient presents with the pseudomembrane on gingival which cannot be peeled off; smear shows spirochaetal infestation and it responds to antibiotic. It can be:
    (A) ANUG
    (B) Diptheritic lesion
    (C) Desqamative gingivitis
    (D) Secondary stage of syphilis

2. Hiv associated gingivitis is best described by the term:
    (A) Juvenile gingivitis
    (B) Acute necrotizing ulcerative gingivitis
    (C) Ulcerative gingivitis
    (D) Linear gingival erythema

3. A patient 17 y.o. complains on pain in the oral cavity, intense bleeding of gums, and putrid smell from a mouth, and general weakness during 72 hours. Objective examination: the patient is pale, regional lymphatic nodes are enlarged, painful during palpation, the mucous membrane of gums on both jaws is swollen, hyperemic, covered by a grey pseudomembrane, painful and bleeding. What is the most probable diagnosis?
    (A) Acute necrotizing Ulcerative gingivitis
    (B) Catarrhal gingivitis
    (C) Generalised periodontitis
    (D) Herpetic gingivostomatitis

Answers:

1. A

   ANUG is caused by fuso-spirochaetal organism [1]

2. D

   This is characteristic lesion of HIV along with necrotizing ulcerative gingivitis and necrotizing ulcerative periodontitis [1]

3. A

   Features of ANUG are mentioned [1]

Reference:

1. Neville BW, Damm DD, Allen CM, Bouquot JE (2002) Oral and Maxillofacial Pathology. (2nd edn), WB Saunders, Philadelphia, London, Toronto. pg157-159

Pigmented Lichen Planus

Dr. Anurag Tripathi, Assistant Professor, Department of Oral Medicine

A 50 year old female reported with blackish discoloration of the buccal mucosa since 4 months. H/o white non-scrapable lesions in bilateral buccal mucosa associated with burning sensation. H/o of treatment of the same. O/e black pigmentation is noticed in bilateral buccal mucosa with no atrophic areas.

Brief treatment history: patient is kept under observation and follow up after every 3 months

Diagnosis: Pigmented Oral Lichen Planus

1. Koebners phenomenon is seen in:
    (A) Lichen planus
    (B) Psoriasis
    (C) Icthyosis
    (D) Phemphigus

2. Which of the following is pruritic:

    (A) Lichen planus
    (B) Psoriasis
    (C) Icthyosis
    (D) Secondary syphilis

3. Pterygium of nail is characteristically seen in:
    (A) Lichen planus
    (B) Psoriasis
    (C) Tinea unguium
    (D) Alopecia areata

Answers:

1. A

    The **Koebner phenomenon**, also called the isomorphic response, refers to the appearance of lesions along a site of injury. This **phenomenon** is seen in a variety of conditions; for example, lichen planus, warts, molluscum contagiosum, psoriasis, lichen nitidus, and the systemic form of juvenile rheumatoid arthritis. Koebners phenomenon is seen on the skin lesions of lichen [1]

2. A

    skin lesions of lichen planus are pruritic in nature, consists of multiple polygonal papule with shiny scale [1]

3. A

    Lichen Planus can involve the proximal nail folds with bluish-red discoloration. Nail-plate changes include thinning, onychorrhexis, brittleness, crumbling or fragmentation, and accentuation of surface longitudinal ridging. All these features are secondary to disease affecting the matrix, which can also produce transient or permanent longitudinal melanonychia or leukonychia as a post inflammatory phenomenon [1]

Reference:

1. Neville BW, Damm DD, Allen CM, Bouquot JE (2002) Oral and Maxillofacial Pathology. (2nd edn), WB Saunders, Philadelphia, London, Toronto. pg 782-788

Smokers Palate

Dr. Anurag Tripathi, Assistant Professor, Department of Oral Medicine

Patient came with complaint of unsighted appearance of teeth since 05 years. History of smoking 04 bundles of beedi per day since past 26 years. On examination stains of teeth observed. Grayish discoloration of flat noticed with reddish pin point openings of minor salivary gland ducts of the palate and angular cheilitis observed. Leukoplakic patches of right and left buccal mucosa noticed.

Brief treatment history: patient was motivated to stop the habit

Diagnosis: Nicotina Stomatitis

1. In a patient white keratotic patches are seen on hard palate with reddish spots. The patient can be
    (A) Pipe smoker
    (B) Tobacco chewer
    (C) Snuff chewer
    (D) Cigar smoker

2. Which of the following is true about smokers palate
    (A) It is irreversible
    (B) It is precancerous lesion
    (C) It is caused by heat from smoke
    (D) It shows dysplastic changes

Answers:

1. A

    Thermal insult of smoke leads to grayish appearance of palatal mucosa with inflammation of ductal opening of palatal minor salivary gland ducts [1]

2. C

    above explanation holds true [1]

Reference:

1. Neville BW, Damm DD, Allen CM, Bouquot JE (2002) Oral and Maxillofacial Pathology. (2nd edn), WB Saunders, Philadelphia, London, Toronto. pg 403-404

Traumatic Ulcer

Dr. Anurag Tripathi, Assistant Professor, Department of Oral Medicine

62 year old male presented with ulceration of right maxillary buccal vestibule in the maxillary tuborosity region since 03 days. History of partial denture wearing since 04 months.

Brief treatment history: topical anaesthetic agent, multivitamin, patient advised to stop denture usage for two weeks for healing of lesion.

1. Commonest ulcer of oral cavity is
    (A) malignant ulcer
    (B) marjoli's ulcer
    (C) traumatic ulcer
    (D) tuberculous ulcer

2. Sign of healing ulcer is
    (A) lack of bleeding
    (B) slough on the floor
    (C) granulation tissue
    (D) desmoplasia of base

3. Margin of traumatic ulcer is
    (A) regular
    (B) irregular
    (C) raised
    (D) everted

Answers:

1. C

   traumatic ulcer is commonest ulcer of oral cavity due to mechanical, chemical and thermal injuries [1]

2. C

   pink granulation tissue on the floor of ulcer shows healing ulcer [1]

3. B

   Traumatic ulcers have irregular margin [1]

Reference:

1. Neville BW, Damm DD, Allen CM, Bouquot JE (2002) Oral and Maxillofacial Pathology. (2nd edn), WB Saunders, Philadelphia, London, Toronto. pg 287-289

Minor Salivary Gland Tumor

Dr. Anurag Tripathi, Assistant Professor, Department of Oral Medicine

A 48 years old female patient reported with swelling in palate since 6 months, Swelling started as small one and progressed to present size in 6 months. No H/o pain or fever. O/e Swelling was present on the right side hard palate region with well defined margins and firm in consistency. The surface over the swelling in smooth with no discoloration.

Investigations: FNAC followed by CT Scan, Incisional Biopsy

Brief treatment history: Surgical management but never turned up for surgery

Diagnosis: Minor Salivary gland Tumor (Pleomorphic adenoma)

1. Most common salivary gland tumor is

    (A) Basal cell adenoma
    (B) Mixed cell carcinoma
    (C) Pleomorphic carcinoma
    (D) Pleomorphic adenoma

2. Most common salivary gland malignancy in palatal region is

    (A) Adenoid cystic carcinoma
    (B) Warthin's tumor
    (C) Pleomorphic adenoma
    (D) Mucoepidermoid carcinoma

3. Which salivary gland tumor spreads along nerve sheath
    (A) Mucoepidermoid carcinoma
    (B) Pleomorphic carcinoma
    (C) Acinic cell carcinoma
    (D) Adenoid cystic carcinoma

Answers:

1. D

    Pleomorphic adenoma is a common benign salivary gland neoplasm characterised by neoplastic proliferation of parenchymatous glandular cells along with myoepithelial components, having a malignant potentiality. It is the most common type of salivary gland tumor and the most common tumor of the parotid gland. [1]

2. C

    The incidence of salivary gland neoplasms peaks in the fifth decade of life. The most common benign tumor is the benign mixed tumor, or **pleomorphic adenoma**. [1]

3. D

    It is the third most common malignant salivary gland tumor overall (after mucoepidermoid carcinoma and polymorphous low grade adenocarcinoma). It represents 28% of malignant submandibular gland tumors, making it the single most common malignant salivary gland tumor in this region. It demonstrates perineural spread [1]

Reference:

1. Neville BW, Damm DD, Allen CM, Bouquot JE (2002) Oral and Maxillofacial Pathology. (2nd edn), WB Saunders, Philadelphia, London, Toronto. Pg 471-499

Fibrous Dysplasia

Dr. Anurag Tripathi, Assistant Professor, Department of Oral Medicine

A male patient of 34 years old presented with swelling on left side of face since 1 and half year. Swelling is not associated with pain. Swelling started as small which progressed to present size in 1 and half years time. O/E swelling was hard in consistency with diffuse margins and non tender. No ulcerative lesion or sinus opening was noticed over the skin. Intraorally expansion of the palate on left side was noticed

Investigations: CT scan followed by incisional biopsy

Brief treatment history: Surgical shaving of the lesion with regular follow up

Diagnosis: Fibrous dysplasia of the left maxilla

1. Syndrome related to fibrous dysplasia is
   (A) Hunters syndrome
   (B) Albright syndrome
   (C) Moellers syndrome
   (D) Gorlin's syndrome

2. Peut de orange appearance of radiograph is seen in
   (A) Hand schuller christian's disease
   (B) Pagets disease
   (C) Fibrous dysplasia
   (D) Marble bone disease

3. Café au lait pigmentation is seen in
   (A) Peutz jhegers syndrome
   (B) Albright syndrome
   (C) Gardeners syndrome
   (D) Malignant melanoma

Answers:

1. B

    McCune–Albright syndrome is suspected when two of the three following features are present: Autonomous <u>endocrine</u> hormone excess, such as in <u>precocious puberty</u>, <u>Polyostotic fibrous dysplasia</u>, Unilateral <u>café au lait spots</u> [1]

2. C

    Peau d'orange (<u>French</u> for "orange peel skin" or, more literally, "skin of an orange") describes imaging with the appearance and dimpled texture of an <u>orange</u> peel. [1]

3. B

    Café au lait spots or café au lait macules are flat, pigmented <u>birthmarks</u>. The name <u>café au lait</u> is French for "coffee with milk" and refers to their light-brown color. They are also called "giraffe spots" or "coast of Maine spots". They are caused by a collection of pigmented-producing melanocytes in the epidermis of the skin. [1]

Reference:

1. Neville BW, Damm DD, Allen CM, Bouquot JE (2002) Oral and Maxillofacial Pathology. (2nd edn), WB Saunders, Philadelphia, London, Toronto. pg 635-640

Von Der Woude Syndrome

Dr. Anurag Tripathi, Assistant Professor, Department of Oral Medicine

A 12-year-old male patient reported to the Department with drainage of fluid from depression on the lower lip since birth. The watery discharge was continuous and was aggravated during eating.

Past surgical history revealed that the patient had undergone surgical correction of upper cleft lip and cleft palate at the age of 10 month. The family history did not reveal consanguineous marriage of his parents.

On examination the left feet showed complete syndactyly of second and third toe while partial syndactyly of second and third toe was evident in right feet. No popliteal webbing was noted and the scrotum and testes were absent. Dental examination revealed missing maxillary lateral incisors (hypodontia) and malpositioned teeth (13 and 24).

1. Van der woude syndrome consists of

    (A) Micrognathia +high arched palate +enlarged tongue
    (B) Congenital Lip pits+ cleft lip/palate
    (C) Facial paralysis+scrotal tongue + chelitis granulomatosa
    (D) None of the above

2. Double lip is seen in

    (A) Ascher's syndrome
    (B) Van der woude syndrome
    (C) Baelz's disease
    (D) Peutz jeghers syndrome

Answers:

1. B

   Van Der Woude syndrome is a genetic disorder characterized by the combination of lower lip pits, cleft lip with or without cleft palate, and cleft palate alone, hypodontia, syndactyly of the hands, polythelia, ankyloglossia, and adhesions between the upper and lower gum pads. [1]

2. B

   Ascher's syndrome, or Laffer-Ascher Syndrome, is a rare disorder first described in 1920. It is characterized by repeated episodes of lip and eyelid edema and occasionally euthyroid goiter. Double Upper lip has Swelling which causes duplication between the inner and outer parts of the upper lip. Occasionally the lower lip is involved [1]

Reference:

1. Neville BW, Damm DD, Allen CM, Bouquot JE (2002) Oral and Maxillofacial Pathology. (2nd edn), WB Saunders, Philadelphia, London, Toronto. pg 526

Calcifying Epithelial Odontogenic Tumor

Dr. Akhilanand Chaurasia, Assistant Professor, Department of Oral Medicine

A 45 yrs complaint of swelling in right side of jaw progressively increasing in size and causing facial asymmetry.

Radiological findings-

1. Panoramic radiograph showing a multilocular mixed lesion extending from distal surface of mandibular second molar anteriorly to full length of ramus causing complete replacement and obliteration of coronoid process and coronoid notch sparing the head of condyle and angle of mandible. There are multilocular spaces with multiple small density highly suggestive of Pindborg's tumor.

2. PA skull shows showing complete obliteration of inferior border of mandible and condyle extending mesially to floor of right maxillary sinus.

3. CT shows anill defined expansile osteolytic lesion with soft tissue component and multiple calcified densities seen in body, alveolar process, coronoid, condyloid, ramus of mandible. The soft tissue component is seen extending into left infra-temporal fossa causing infiltration of right temporalis and lateral pterygoid muscles. The lesion is causing marked thinning of posterior wall of maxillary sinus and its remodeling. The lesion is infiltrating right retromolar trigone, right upper gingivo-buccal sulcus and lateral pterygoid muscle.

1. What is another name for calcifying epithelial odontogenic tumour?
    (A) ameloblastoma
    (B) gorlin cyst
    (C) pindborg tumour
    (D) odontoma

2. Which of the following is true about pindborg's tumour?
    (A) middle age tumour
    (B) mandible: maxilla::2:1
    (C) found most commonly in molar ramus area of jaw
    (D) all the above

Answers:

1. C [1]

1. D

    The calcifying epithelial odontogenic tumor, also known as a Pindborg tumor or CEOT, is an odontogenic tumor first recognized by the Danish pathologist Jens Jørgen Pindborg in 195[2]

2. B

    It is a typically benign and slow growing, but invasive neoplasm. Intraosseous tumors (tumors within the bone) are more likely (94%) versus extraosseus tumors (6%). It is more common in the posterior mandible of adults, typically in the 4th to 5th decades. [2]

References:

1. Greenberg MS, Glick M Burkett's Oral Medicine: Diagnosis and Treatment. (11stedn), BC Decker, Hamilton, Canada. pg 150

2. Shafer, Hine, Levy. Textbook of Oral Pathology Elsevier publication 7th edition pg 283- 285

3. Shafer, Hine, Levy. Textbook of Oral Pathology Elsevier publication 7th edition pg 284

4. Shafer, Hine, Levy. Textbook of Oral Pathology Elsevier publication 7th edition pg 285

5. Shafer, Hine, Levy. Textbook of Oral Pathology Elsevier publication 7th edition pg 285

Complex Odontome

Dr. Akhilanand Chaurasia, Assistant Professor, Department of Oral Medicine

A 10 year old boy complaint of non-eruption of teeth in left posterior region of mandible as well swelling causing mild facial asymmetry in left side of face since 4 month.

Radiological findings-

1. The intraoral periapical radiograph shows a irregular radio-opaque mass of 1x1 cm overlying over crown of mandibular left 1st premolar region having well defined and regular borders. There is retained deciduous left canine. The whole radio-opacity is surrounded by well defined capsule.

2. Panoramic radiograph showing a well defined radio-opacity overlying over crown of mandibular left 1st premolar region having well defined and regular borders. The radio-opacity has tooth like density and surrounded by well defined capsule causing noneruption of mandibular 1st premolar and impaction of mandibular left canine. Due to impaction there is retention of deciduous left canine and spacing between teeth noted.

1. Which of the following is true about compound composite odontome?
   (A) it is mixed tumour (odontogenic epithelium with odontogenic ectomesenchyme)
   (B) it shows predilection for anterior maxilla
   (C) histologically characterised by production of enamel dentin cementum pulp
   (D) all the above

2. All are types of odontome except?
   (A) complex composite odontome
   (B) compound composite odontome
   (C) dilated odontome
   (D) hyperplastic odontome

3. Composite complex odontome
   (A) are found most frequently in posterior mandible
   (B) appears on radiographs as radiopaque mass
   (C) treatment requires surgical excision
   (D) all the above

Answers:

1. D

    A compound odontoma still has the three separate dental tissues (enamel, dentin and cementum), but may present a lobulated appearance where there is no definitive demarcation of separate tissues between the individual "toothlets" (or denticles). It usually appears in the anterior maxilla. [1]

2. D

    In addition to the above forms, the dilated odontoma is an infrequent developmental alteration that appears in any area of the dental arches and can affect deciduous, permanent and supernumerary teeth. The most extreme form of dens invaginatus is known as dilated odontoma. [3]

3. D

    the complex odontome type is unrecognizable as dental tissues, usually presenting as a radioopaque area with varying densities. It usually appears in the posterior maxilla or in the mandible and requires surgical correction [4]

References:

1. White and pharaoh, oral radiology principles and interpretation, 6th edition pg 378

2. White and pharaoh, oral radiology principles and interpretation, 6th edition pg 378

3. Greenberg MS, Glick M Burkett's Oral Medicine: Diagnosis and Treatment. (11stedn), BC Decker, Hamilton, Canada. pg 151

4. Greenberg MS, Glick M Burkett's Oral Medicine: Diagnosis and Treatment. (11stedn), BC Decker, Hamilton, Canada. pg 151

5. Shafer, Hine, Levy. Textbook of Oral Pathology Elsevier publication 7th edition pg 293

Dens Invaginatus

Dr. Akhilanand Chaurasia, Assistant Professor, Department of Oral Medicine

A 26 year old male patient complaint of pain and swelling in right upper anterior palatal region since 2 month.

Radiographic findings

The intraoral periapical radiograph of right maxillary lateral incisor with oehlers' Type IIIA dens invaginatus. The pulp canal with an adjacent invagination is opening into periodontal ligament space causing a periapical radiolucency.

Maxillary Anterior Occlusal Radiograph showing right maxillary lateral incisor with oehlers' Type IIIA dens invaginatus causing a periapical radiolucency.

Panoramic Radigraph showing right maxillary lateral incisor with oehlers' Type IIIA dens invaginatus causing a periapical radiolucency superimposing on roots of right maxillary central incisor and right maxillary canine.

1. Which of the following is not the synonym of dens invaginatus?

    (A) dens in dente
    (B) dilated composite odontome
    (C) both a and b
    (D) evaginated odontome

2. Which of the teeth is most commonly affected by dens invaginatus?

    (A) maxillary premolar
    (B) maxillary lateral incisor
    (C) mandibular third molar
    (D) mandibular premolar

3. What is the most important clinical importance of dens invaginatus?

    (A) risk of pulpal infection
    (B) external resorption
    (C) crown fracture
    (D) none of the above

Answers:

1. D

   Dens invaginatus, also known as dens in dente ("tooth within a tooth") is a condition found in <u>teeth</u> where the outer surface folds inward. There are <u>coronal</u> and <u>radicular</u> forms, with the coronal form being more common. [1]

2. B

   Teeth most affected are <u>maxillary</u> lateral <u>incisors</u> and bilateral occurrence is not uncommon. [2]

3. A

   dens invaginatus may act like a pathway for pulpal infection [3]

References:

1. Shafer, Hine, Levy. Textbook of Oral Pathology Elsevier publication 7th edition pg 42

2. Shafer, Hine, Levy. Textbook of Oral Pathology Elsevier publication 7th edition pg 43

3. White and pharaoh, oral radiology principles and interpretation, 6th edition pg 305

4. White and pharaoh, oral radiology principles and interpretation, 6th edition pg 305

5. Shafer, Hine, Levy. Textbook of Oral Pathology Elsevier publication 7th edition pg 43

Intra Osseous Carcinoma

Dr. Akhilanand Chaurasia, Assistant Professor, Department of Oral Medicine

1. A 66 year old male patient complaint of a swelling associated with pain and paresthesia in left side of face since 3 months.

2. Panoramic radiograph showing unilocular radiolucency with poorly defined margin and ragged border with moth eaten appearance and infiltrative osteolysis in the left mandibular 2nd premolar extending till 1st molar of the mandible. The lamina dura of 2nd premolar adjacent to the lesion was lost.

3. Lateral oblique view(Modified) showing unilocular radiolucency with poorly defined margin and ragged border with moth eaten appearance and infiltrative osteolysis in mandibular 2nd premolar region eroding the inferior border of mandible.

4. Contrast Enhanced Computed tomography showing perforation of labial and buccal cortical plate of the mandible and a soft tissue mass with contrast enhancement extending through the labial and buccal cortical plate of the mandible into adjacent soft tissue. Breaching in inferior border is also noted.

1. Primary intraosseous carcinoma of jaw is also referred as
   (A) central squamous cell carcinoma
   (B) primary epithelial tumour of jaw
   (C) both of above
   (D) none of above

2. All are true about intraosseous carcinoma of jaw except
   (A) always associated with peripheral soft tissue component
   (B) shows resorption of bone cortex canal sinus boundaries
   (C) osteomyelitis is included in differential diagnosis
   (D) most commonly found in mandible as compared to maxilla

3. Intraosseous carcinoma of jaw arises from
   (A) intraosseous remnants of odontogenic epithelium
   (B) odontogenic cyst
   (C) distant metastasis
   (D) none of above

Answers:

1. A

   It has been referred to by a variety of names such as primary carcinoma of the mandible, primary epithelial tumor of the jaw, intraalveolar carcinoma of the jaw, primary intraalveolar epidermoid carcinoma, primary intraosseous carcinoma, primary intraalveolar squamous cell carcinoma (SCC) of the mandible, malignant primary intraosseous carcinoma and central SCC of the mandible. [1]

2. A

   It is not associated with peripheral component. [3]

3. A

   It arises denovo from remnants of trapped epithelium within bone [4]

References:

1. White and pharaoh, oral radiology principles and interpretation, 6th edition pg 409

2. White and pharaoh, oral radiology principles and interpretation, 6th edition pg 409

3. Wood & Goaz. Differential diagnosis of Oral & Maxillofacial region. Mosby publication 5th ed. Year 1997 page 360-361

4. White and pharaoh, oral radiology principles and interpretation, 6th edition pg 409

5. White and pharaoh, oral radiology principles and interpretation, 6th edition pg 409

Osteochondroma

Dr. Akhilanand Chaurasia, Assistant Professor, Department of Oral Medicine

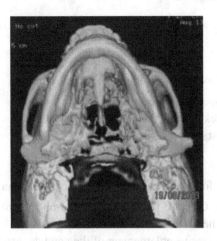

A 27 year old female patient complaint of a swelling in left parotid region since 2 years. it was slowly increasing in size. There was clicking sound and pain in left TMJ region since 4 month. There was mild facial asymmetry. On jaw movements mandible was deviated towards right side.

Radiological Findings-

1. In panoramic view on left side, an irregular radiolucent mass of 1.5cm x 1.5cm surrounded by well defined radio-opaque margin was present superimposing on anterior end of neck of condyle.

2. The CT (coronal sections) showed an abnormal, well defined pedunculated rounded bony outgrowth arising from the neck of left mandibular condyle extending anteriorly, laterally and medially into infratemporal fossa having dimension of 1.5x1x1cm. The cortex and medulla of the lesion were continuous with same structures of the mandibular condyle, a feature that is considered diagnostic of osteochondromas.

3. CT with 3D reconstruction showed rounded bony mass projects out from the lateral cortex of upper end of the neck of left mandibular condyle.

1. Which of the following are symptoms of osteochondroma of TMJ?
    (A) pain and decrease range of motion
    (B) malocclusion
    (C) deviation of mandible movements
    (D) all the above

2. Which of the following are considered in differential diagnosis of osteochondroma of jaw?

   (A) condylar hyperplasia
   (B) osteoma
   (C) both of above
   (D) none of above

3. Which of the following is true about ostechondroma?

   (A) it is benign neoplasm of cartilage
   (B) it shows no sex predilection and is slow growing
   (C) its radio-resistant
   (D) all the above

4. Which one of the following is true about Osteochondroma of jaw?

   (A) The condylar OCs are frequently situated on the antero-medial surface of the condylar head
   (B) causes a progressive enlargement of the condyle, usually resulting in facial asymmetry, prognathic deviation of chin, TMJ dysfunction
   (C) CT scans can easily demonstrate the continuity of cortex and medulla of the bone tumor and is considered the best tool to demonstrate calcified cartilage
   (D) all the above

Answers:

1. D

   Progressive enlargement of the condyle, usually resulting in facial asymmetry, temporo mandibular joint dysfunction, limited mouth opening and malocclusion. [1]

2. C

   Osteochondroma should be differentiated from unilateral condylar hyperplasia, osteoma, chondroma, chondroblastoma, benign osteoblastoma, giant cell tumor, myxoma, fibro-osteoma, fibrous dysplasia, fibrosarcoma, and chondrosarcoma. [2]

3. D

   Osteochondroma of temporo mandibular joint is a rare, slow growing, benign tumor that causes a progressive enlargement of the condyle being slow growing hard tissue tumor, it is radio-resistant. [3]

4. D

Osteochondroma of temporo mandibular joint is a rare, slow growing, benign tumor that causes a progressive enlargement of the condyle, usually resulting in facial asymmetry, temporo mandibular joint dysfunction, limited mouth opening and malocclusion. [5]

References:

1. White and pharaoh, oral radiology principles and interpretation, 6th edition pg 500

2. White and pharaoh, oral radiology principles and interpretation, 6th edition pg 501

3. Shafer, Hine, Levy. Textbook of Oral Pathology Elsevier publication 7th edition pg 153

4. Shafer, Hine, Levy. Textbook of Oral Pathology Elsevier publication 7th edition pg 153

5. More CB, Gupta S. Osteochondroma of mandibular condyle: A clinic-radiographic correlation. Journal of Natural Science, Biology, and Medicine. 2013;4(2):465-46doi:10.4103/0976-9668.116969.

Osteoma

Dr. Akhilanand Chaurasia, Assistant Professor, Department of Oral Medicine

A 22-year-old male patient complained of a swelling on the left inner side of the mandible for the past 6 months, slowly increasing in size and causing difficulty in chewing food. The swelling was approximately 1.5x1 cm, located below the first molar and firm to hard in consistency with a smooth surface.

Radiological findings-

1. Intra-oral periapical radiograph showing a radio-opaque mass superimposing proximal on the mesial and distal root of the left first mandibular molar tooth.

2. Mandibular True Occlusal radiograph showing a circumscribed oval radio-opaque mass of 1x1 cm on the left attached to the lingual cortex of the body of the mandible in the first molar region extending posteriorly to the mesio-lingual surface of the second molar.

1. Which of the following bones is most commonly involved with osteoma in head and neck?
   (A) maxilla
   (B) mandible
   (C) nasal bone
   (D) sphenoid bone

2. Which of the following conditon is associated with multiple osteomas?
   (A) melkerson rosenthal syndrome
   (B) cleidocranial dysostosis
   (C) gardners syndrome
   (D) Down syndrome

3. Which of the following is not related to osteoma?
   (A) it is benign tumour characterised by proliferation of compact or cancellous bone
   (B) it is slow growing and usually asymptomatic
   (C) it is associated with nonvital teeth
   (D) it is one of the features of gardners syndrome

Answers:

1. B

    Peripheral osteoma is an uncommon lesion, mostly occurring in young adults, which affects equally men and women. It mainly affects the frontal bone, mandible, and paranasal sinuses. Mandibular cases occur in the angle or condyle, followed by the molar area of the mandibular body and ascending ramus. (1)

2. C

    Gardner syndrome, also known as familial colorectal polyposis, is an autosomal dominant form of polyposis characterized by the presence of multiple polyps in the colontogether with tumors outside the colon. The extracolonic tumors may include osteomas of the skull, thyroid cancer, epidermoid cysts and fibromas (2)

3. C

    osteoma is unrelated to non-vital teeth (3)

References:

1. White and pharaoh, oral radiology principles and interpretation, 6th edition pg 393

2. White and pharaoh, oral radiology principles and interpretation, 6th edition pg 393

3. White and pharaoh, oral radiology principles and interpretation, 6th edition pg 394

4. Shafer, Hine, Levy. Textbook of Oral Pathology Elsevier publication 7th edition pg 155

5. Shafer, Hine, Levy. Textbook of Oral Pathology Elsevier publication 7th edition pg 155

Chapter - 5

Oral Pathology & Microbiology

Verrucous Carcinoma

Prof. Shaleen Chandra, Dept. of Oral Pathology & Microbiology

A 42 year old female patient reported with a chief complains of pain in the left side of mouth since 7 days. Patient noticed a small, painless growth over the left buccal mucosa 1 year back, which gradually grew to the present size. Patient had a history of chewing quid since 15 years. On examination solitary proliferative verrucous growth with well-defined but irregular margins Surface was with finger like projections in pinkish white color

1. What is the most probable diagnosis of above patient?

   (A) Tobacco pouch keratosis
   (B) Verrucous carcinoma
   (C) Leukoplakia
   (D) All of the above

2. Ackerman's tumor is also known as

   (A) Keratoacanthoma
   (B) Verrucous carcinoma
   (C) Malocclusion
   (D) None of the above

3. Verrucous carcinoma is characterized histologically by

   (A) Para keratin plugging
   (B) Spinous plugging
   (C) Basal cell plugging
   (D) Keratin pearl formation

4. Treatment of verrucous carcinoma

   (A) Conservative
   (B) Chemotherapy only
   (C) Surgical excision with wide margins
   (D) Surgical excision with neck dissection

5. Fate of verrucous carcinoma if not treated for long time.

   (A) Turn into squamous cell carcinoma
   (B) Regress spontaneously
   (C) Turn into verrucous hyperplasia
   (D) None of the above

Answers:

1. B

   cauliflower like hyperkeratotic lesion is most common diagnostic sign of verrucous carcinoma.

2. B

   another name of verrucous carcinoma.

3. A

   broad and bulbous rete pegs minimal dysplasia along with parakeratin plugging is the striking features of verrucous carcinoma.

4. C

   most accepted treatment method of verrucous carcinoma is surgical excision with wide margins.

5. A

   it will progress like verrucous carcinoma or can be develop into squamous cell carcinoma.

Reference:

1. Neville BW, Damn DD, Allen CM, Bouquot JE.Oral & Maxillofacial Pathology, 2nd Ed.New Delhi:Elsevier:2005.

Neurofibroma

Prof. Shaleen Chandra, Dept. of Oral Pathology & Microbiology

A 24 year old female patient reported with a pedunculated growth in her buccal mucosa since last one year. She does not have any pain and discomfort with this progressive growth. After surgical excision with wide base tissue was sent for histopathology. And patient was asymptomatic after one year of surgery.

1. Which of the following lesions are seen in von Recklinghausen's disease of skin:

    (A) hemangioma
    (B) ameloblastoma
    (C) neurofibroma
    (D) giant cell fibroma

2. An inflamed capillary hemangioma of the oral cavity looks similar to a:

    (A) nevus
    (B) neurofibroma
    (C) pyogenic granuloma
    (D) angiosarcoma

3. Which of the following conditions is characterized by café-au-spots, non-encapsulation and potential for malignant transformation:

    (A) neurilemmoma
    (B) neurofibroma
    (C) Traumatic neuroma
    (D) Solitary plasmacytoma

4. Stori form pattern of fibrous tissue is seen in:

    (A) Fibrosarcoma
    (B) Malignant fibrous histiocytoma
    (C) Neurofibroma
    (D) Ameloblastic fibroma

5. Which of the following is most malignant:

    (A) Neurilemmoma
    (B) Neurofibroma
    (C) Neurogenic fibroma
    (D) Traumatic neuroma

Answers:

1. C

   von Recklinghausen's disease is associated with neurofibromatosis on skin of face and extremities.

2. C

   pyogenic granuloma is associated with marked vascularity.

3. B

   neurofibroma is characterized by café-au-spots, non-encapsulation and potential for malignant transformation

4. B

   malignant fibrous histiocytoma is a malignant tumor of fibrous tissue and histiocytes.

5. B

   neurofibroma is characterized by café-au-spots, non-encapsulation and potential for malignant transformation

Reference:

1. Rajendran R., Sivapathasundharam B.: Shafer's Text Book of Oral Pathology.6th Ed.New Delhi: Elsevier; 2009-2010.

Eruption Cyst

Prof. Shaleen Chandra, Dept. of Oral Pathology & Microbiology

An 8 year old boy reported with 1.5 × 2.0 cm gingival lesions appeared as bluish-black, circumscribed, fluctuant swellings on the gingiva over the buccal side of un-erupted regional tooth. History revealed that it was appearing 2 weeks back as translucent swellings over normal mucosa and it slowly increased to its present size. The color of the lesions also slowly changed from its normal red mucosa to the present bluish black color 1 week back. No fluid discharge or any other associated symptoms were associated. The overlying mucosa was smooth and no ulceration was present. X-rays of the lesions confirmed no signs of bone involvement or any radiolucency surrounding this tooth.

1. What is the most probable diagnosis of the case?

    (A) Hamartoma
    (B) Lymphangioma
    (C) Eruption cyst
    (D) hemangioma

2. What treatment you suggest in the above case

    (A) Wait and watch
    (B) Incision and drainage
    (C) Antibiotic therapy
    (D) Surgical enucleation

3. Lesion that does not necessarily need treatment

    (A) mamelons
    (B) eruption hematoma
    (C) perikymata
    (D) All of the above

4. What type of cyst is eruption hematoma according to (shear 1992,) occurring in soft tissue

    (A) OKC
    (B) Radicular cyst
    (C) Dentigerous cyst
    (D) Lateral periodontal cyst

5. Eruption cyst is clinically visible as
   (A) Non mobile mass on the alveolar bone
   (B) Bluish mass on the alveolar bone
   (C) Soft mass on the alveolar bone
   (D) Soft fluctuant mass on the alveolar bone

Answer:

1. C

   lymphangioma and hemangioma are hamartoma of lymphatic and vascular origin respectively.

2. A

   eruption cyst regress after the eruption of involved teeth.

3. D

   mameleons are nodular protuberances over the incisal edges of newly erupted incisors

4. C

   eruption hamartoma is histologically resemble to dentigerous cyst

5. D

   A soft fluctuant mass over alveolar ridge, which histologically resemble to dentigerous cyst is nothing buteruption hamartoma.

Reference:

1. Rajendran R., Sivapathasundharam B.: Shafer's Text Book of Oral Pathology.6th Ed.New Delhi:Elsevier; 2009-2010.

Epistein Pearls:

Prof. Shaleen Chandra, Dept. of Oral Pathology & Microbiology

Benign nodules, which range from one to three millimeters in size (less than a tenth of an inch) and appear on the roof of a baby's mouth just behind her gums, are perfectly harmless. Similar-looking cysts can appear in other areas of the child mouth, in which case they are known as Bohn's nodules. These cysts contain epithelial cells as well as mucous membranes. The same combination is seen in the layers of moist tissue that line the baby's urogenital, digestive, and respiratory tracts.

1. Epstein pearls are

    (A) Benigntumor
    (B) Malignant tumor
    (C) Developmental anomaly
    (D) Foreign body

2. Epstein pearls are typically present as

    (A) Multiple masses
    (B) Doubles masses
    (C) Single mass
    (D) Scattered masses

3. The degenerated keratin in cystic lumen of palatal cyst are arranged in form of

    (A) Onion rings
    (B) Concentric ring
    (C) Lamellations
    (D) Both a&b

4. Palatal cyst remains intact deeply in the submucosal stroma for how many months before rupture

    (A) 6 to 8 months
    (B) 3 to 4 months
    (C) 1 to 2 months
    (D) 1 year

5. Following is true in the case of palatal cyst

    (A) No treatment is required
    (B) Surgical treatment is required
    (C) Conservative treatment is required
    (D) Radiotherapy is required

Answers:

1. C

   Developmental cysts of mid palatal region.

2. A

   Developmental cysts of mid palatal region.

3. D

   Cystic lumen filled with lamellations of keratin

4. A

   Cystic lumen filled with lamellations of keratin which will be expelled after 6-8 months.

5. A

   No treatment required for Epstein pearls as self-correcting anomaly.

Reference:

1. Rajendran R., Sivapathasundharam B.: Shafer's Text Book of Oral Pathology.6th Ed.New Delhi: Elsevier; 2009-2010.

Mucocele

Prof. Shaleen Chandra, Dept. of Oral Pathology & Microbiology

A13 years old female child was panicy about a soft, fluctuant and palpable, painless swelling in the lower lip since 2 days; progressive in nature on lower lip in the 34, 35 region. Her parents noticed that she had a habit of lip biting. The treatment planning consisted of Oral prophylaxis followed by surgical removal. The lesion was excised by placing an incision vertically, therefore splitting the overlying mucosa and then aspirating the fluid which was mucous, separating the lesion from the mucosa by placing a suture and resecting from the base so that chances of reoccurrence were less.

1. What will be your first diagnosis for a whitish blue swelling over the lower lip?

    (A) Mucocele
    (B) Hemangioma
    (C) Lymphangioma
    (D) All of the above

2. Mucous retention cyst is

    (A) True cyst
    (B) Pseudo cyst
    (C) Not a cyst at al
    (D) All of the above depends upon etiology

2. Most accepted etiology of mucocele is

    (A) Pooling of mucous
    (B) Traumatic origin
    (C) Inflammation of salivary acini
    (D) Myoepithelial cell origin

3. Most common site for mucocele is

    (A) Lower lip
    (B) Upper lip
    (C) Buccal mucosa around second molar
    (D) Buccal mucosa around first molar

4. Mucous extravasation is most commonly associated with

    (A) Parotid gland
    (B) Submandibular salivary glands
    (C) Sub lingual glands
    (D) Minor salivary glands

5. What treatment you suggest in the mucocele cases to prevent recurrence
   (A) Incisional biopsy
   (B) Surgical Excisional
   (C) Incision and drainage
   (D) Excision of salivary acini along with cyst

Answers:

1. A

   Mucocele is the most common diagnosis for a blue or pink swelling over the lower lip.

2. B

   Mucocele does not have any epithelial lining so it is not true cyst.

3. B

   Mucocele is the most common diagnosis for a blue or pink swelling over the lower lip.

4. D

   Minor salivary glands are usually involved.

5. D

   Local excision of cystic growth along with regional minor salivary glands is treatment of choice for mucocele.

Reference:

1. Rajendran R., Sivapathasundharam B.: Shafer's Text Book of Oral Pathology.6th Ed.New Delhi:Elsevier; 2009-2010.

Retention Cyst

Prof. Shaleen Chandra, Dept. of Oral Pathology & Microbiology

One biopsy specimen was sent to us which was taken from the floor of mouth of a 25 year lady. She was having a bluish colored dome shaped lump which increases and decrease in size before and after mastication respectively. It was non painful and no history of surface ulceration. Histopathology reveals a fluid filled cavity lined by single layer of flat to cuboidal epithelial cells, also visualized salivary gland acini.

1. Most common etiologic factor for mucous retention cyst

    (A) Calculi deposition in the ducts
    (B) Trauma to ductal system
    (C) Trauma to nearby connective tissue of acinars and their ductal system
    (D) Idiopathic etiology

2. Retention cyst is

    (A) True cyst
    (B) Pseudo-cyst
    (C) Depends on location of the cyst
    (D) All of the above

3. Histologic features of mucous retention cyst

    (A) Mucous spillage in the soft tissue
    (B) Mucous filled spaces in the epithelial tissue
    (C) Mucous pooled in salivary gland duct
    (D) Mucous pooled in salivary gland acini

4. Radiological appearance of mucous retention cyst

    (A) Well defined radiolucent area
    (B) Well defined radiopaque area
    (C) Superficial erosion of bone
    (D) No radiographic findings

5. Treatment of mucous retention cyst

    (A) Puncture of the lesion
    (B) Excision of the cyst
    (C) No treatment is necessary as it regresses after short period
    (D) Anti-inflammatory medication

Answers:

1. A

    traumatic rupture of salivary duct for extravasation and any blockage for retention are considered as etiology for mucocele.

2. A

    mucous extravasations does not have any epithelial lining so it is not true cyst.

3. C

    retention cyst is due to pooling of mucous in the salivary gland duct.

4. D

    sialography is the radiologic investigation of choice for salivary gland pathology.

5. B

    local excision of cystic growth along with regional minor salivary glands is treatment of choice.

Reference:

1. Rajendran R., Sivapathasundharam B.: Shafer's Text Book of Oral Pathology.6th Ed.New Delhi:Elsevier; 2009-2010.

Extravassation Cyst

Prof. Shaleen Chandra, Dept. of Oral Pathology & Microbiology

One biopsy was taken from the lower lip of a 12 year boy from internal aspect in relation to 31 and 4He was having a bluish colorederuption which was non painful and no history of surface ulceration. He reported that sometimes it regresses after expelling some fluid but it reappears again after some time. Histopathology reveals an area of mucous spillage and some mucinophages, overlying mucosa was non dysplastic and non -ulcerated. Also visualized few salivary gland acini.

1. Most common etiologic factor for mucous extravasation cyst

    (A) Calculi deposition in the ducts
    (B) Trauma to ductal system
    (C) Trauma to nearby connective tissue of acinars and their ductal system
    (D) Idiopathic etiology

2. Mucous extravasation cyst is

    (A) True cyst
    (B) Pseudo-cyst
    (C) Depends on location of the cyst
    (D) All of the above

3. Histologically extravasation cyst is lined by

    (A) Compressed fibrous wall
    (B) Single cell layer of epithelium
    (C) Dilation of ruptured duct
    (D) Arrangement of acini around cystic cavity

4. Radiological appearance of mucous retention cyst

    (A) Well defined radiolucent area
    (B) Well defined radiopaque area
    (C) Superficial erosion of bone
    (D) No radiographic findings

5. Treatment of mucous retention cyst

    (A) Puncture of the lesion
    (B) Excision of the cyst
    (C) No treatment is necessary as it regresses after short period
    (D) Anti-inflammatory medication

Answers:

1. B

   a traumatic rupture of salivary duct for extravasation and any blockage for retention are considered as etiology for mucocele.

2. B

   a mucous extravasations does not have any epithelial lining so it is not true cyst

3. A

   mucous pooled in the connective tissue lined by compressed fibrous tissue is the histological presentation of extravasations cyst.

4. D

   It is a soft tissue phenomenon producing no radiological changes

5. B

   local excision of cystic growth along with regional minor salivary glands is treatment of choice for mucocele.

Reference:

1. Rajendran R., Sivapathasundharam B.: Shafer's Text Book of Oral Pathology.6th Ed.New Delhi: Elsevier; 2009-2010.

Ranula

Prof. Shaleen Chandra, Dept. of Oral Pathology & Microbiology

A 22 year old male patient reported to the outpatient department with a chief complaint of painless swelling below the tongue on the right side, for the past one month. History revealed that the swelling has gradually increased in size to the present size. No history of any pain was reported. His past history revealed that he had undergone endodontic treatment in 46.

1. Special form of mucous retention cyst located at the floor of mouth is called as

    (A) Mucocele
    (B) Morula
    (C) Ranula
    (D) Blastula

2. Ranula is

    (A) True cyst
    (B) Pseudo-cyst
    (C) Depends on location of the cyst
    (D) All of the above

3. Histologically ranula is lined by

    (A) Compressed fibrous wall
    (B) Single cell layer of epithelium
    (C) Dilation of ruptured duct
    (D) Arrangement of acini around cystic cavity

4. Treatment of ranula is

    (A) Puncture of the lesion
    (B) Excision of the cyst along with affected gland
    (C) No treatment is necessary as it regresses after short period
    (D) Anti-inflammatory medication

Answers:

1. C

    ranula is the retention cyst under the tongue.

2. A

    mucous extravasations does not have any epithelial lining so it is not true cyst

3. B

    ranula is lined by ductal epithelium of salivary gland

4. B

    local excision of cystic growth along with regional minor salivary glands is treatment of choice for ranula.

Reference:

1. Rajendran R., Sivapathasundharam B.: Shafer's Text Book of Oral Pathology.6th Ed.New Delhi:Elsevier; 2009-2010.

Pleomorphic Adenoma

Prof. Shaleen Chandra, Dept. of Oral Pathology & Microbiology

A 45 year old male complaining of slow growing painless incidence of parotid tumor is about 2.4 in defined mass, with a firm and non-tender mass on the right side elevating ear lobe and was not attached to the skin. There was no symptom suggestive of facial gland and is seldom encountered in the nerve involvement. Tumor on histological evaluation shows areas of chondroid, myxoid and osseous changes. No complications were observed after surgical removal of pleomorphic adenoma and four months of follow up.

1. Pleomorphic adenoma also known as

    (A) Mixed tumor
    (B) Adenolymphoma
    (C) Acinic cell carcinoma
    (D) Oxyphilic adenoma

2. Cells involved in pleomorphic adenoma is

    (A) Epithelial cells
    (B) Mesenchymal
    (C) Both
    (D) None of the above

3. Pleomorphic adenoma most commonly occur in

    (A) Males
    (B) Females
    (C) Both
    (D) None of the above

4. Borders of pleomorphic adenoma are

    (A) Well defined
    (B) Corrugated
    (C) Diffused
    (D) None of the above

5. In TNM staging Nx denotes

    (A) Regional nodes cannot be assessed
    (B) No regional node metastasis
    (C) Both
    (D) No distant metastasis

Answers:

1. A

   pleomorphic adenoma is a mixed benign tumor of salivary gland origin.

2. C

   pleomorphic adenoma is a mixed benign tumor of salivary gland origin.

3. B

   all salivary gland tumors have female predilection for their occurrence.

4. A

   pleomorphic adenoma is pseudo-encapsulated tumor.

5. A

   Nx denotes for uncertainty about lymph nodes or cannot be assessed.

Reference:

1. Rajendran R., Sivapathasundharam B.: Shafer's Text Book of Oral Pathology.6th Ed.New Delhi:Elsevier; 2009-2010.

Warthin Tumour

Prof. Shaleen Chandra, Dept. of Oral Pathology & Microbiology

A 69-year-old male patient visited the dental clinic, complaining of swelling on his left cheek. He had been aware of this swelling for 2 years but had not sought medical help since it had not caused any pain or discomfort. Recently, however, he found that the swelling was worsening and consequently visited the clinic. Clinician planned to excise the lump and send it for histopathologic examination. There is lots of epithelium lined spaces filled with eosinophiliccoagulum and their wall contain lymphoid follicles.

1. Warthin's tumor is also known as

    (A) Adenolymphoma
    (B) Papillary cyst adenoma
    (C) Both
    (D) None of the above

2. Warthin's tumor first recognized by

    (A) ALBRECHT in 1910
    (B) Warthin's in 1929
    (C) Foote in 1954
    (D) None

3. Warthin's tumor is a disease of

    (A) Man
    (B) Women
    (C) Children
    (D) All of the above

4. Tumor made up of histological component of

    (A) Epithelial cell
    (B) Lymphoid cell
    (C) Both
    (D) None of the above

5. Warthin's tumor contains of

    (A) Strawcolour fluid
    (B) Clear fluid
    (C) Cloudy fluid
    (D) None of the above

Answers:

1. C

    histologic nomination of Warthin'stumor is papillary cyst adenoma lymphomatosum.

2. A

    named after Warthin for his significant contribution.

3. A

    this is the only salivary gland tumor having male predilection and exclusively found in major salivary glands.

4. C

    histologic nomination of Warthin'stumor is papillary cyst adenoma lymphomatosum

5. B

    cystic space is filled with eosinophilic coagulum.

Reference:

1. Rajendran R., Sivapathasundharam B.: Shafer's Text Book of Oral Pathology.6ᵗʰ Ed.New Delhi:Elsevier; 2009-2010.

Adenoid Cystic Carcinoma

Prof. Shaleen Chandra, Dept. of Oral Pathology & Microbiology

A 35 year female presented with a chief complaint of a swelling in the upper back jaw region for the past six months. She had difficulty in mastication and deglutition. On extra oral examination a diffuse ill-defined swelling was noticed in the left side of the face causing facial asymmetry. The nasolabial fold was obliterated. The skin over the swelling was stretched and smooth. No lymph nodes were palpable.

1. Adenoid cystic carcinoma arises from

   (A) Epithelium
   (B) Plasma cells
   (C) Both
   (D) Salivary gland epithelium

2. Commonest intraoral site for ACC

   (A) Lip
   (B) Buccal mucosa
   (C) Both
   (D) Gingiva

3. Growth pattern of ACC

   (A) Solid
   (B) Papillary cystic pattern
   (C) Follicular pattern
   (D) All of the above

4. Adenoid cystic carcinoma is also known as

   (A) Epithelioma
   (B) Adenoepithelioma
   (C) Cylindroma
   (D) Rhomboidoma

5. Histologically adenoid cystic carcinoma looking like

   (A) Dysplastic cells making Concentric ring pattern
   (B) Dysplastic cells making Swiss cheese pattern
   (C) Dysplastic cells making cylindrical pattern
   (D) Non-dysplastic cells making cylindrical pattern

Answers:

1. D

   malignant salivary gland tumor arising from epithelial cells.

2. C

   origin from minor salivary glands of oral cavity is common.

3. D

   histologic variants includes Solid, Papillary cystic pattern, and Follicular pattern

4. C

   due to its growth also called as cylindroma

5. B

   Histologically adenoid cystic carcinoma looking like dysplastic cells making Swiss cheese pattern

Reference:

1. Rajendran R., Sivapathasundharam B.: Shafer's Text Book of Oral Pathology.6th Ed.New Delhi:Elsevier; 2009-2010.

Central Giant Cell Granuloma

Prof. Shaleen Chandra, Dept. of Oral Pathology & Microbiology

A 25 year old female reported with a progressive 4X4 cm swelling and intermittent pain in the lower jaw across the midline since 1 year. There was no history of trauma, neurological deficit, fever, loss of appetite, loss of weight. On extra oral examination a single, diffuse swelling was seen on the right side of the face in the region of anterior maxilla. On intra oral examination swelling was firm in consistency, showed no secondary changes and was slightly tender on palpation. An incisional biopsy done and sample was sent for histopathological examination which reveals multinucleated giant cells.

1. What are the most common lesions crossing the midline

   (A) Ossifying fibroma
   (B) Radicular cyst
   (C) Central giant cell granuloma
   (D) All of the above

2. Type of giant cells present in central giant cell granuloma

   (A) Foreign body type
   (B) Langhans type
   (C) Tuton giant cells
   (D) All of the above

3. Most common radiological presentation of central giant cell granuloma

   (A) Unilocular/Multilocular radiolucency
   (B) Unilocular/Multilocular radiopacity
   (C) Both of the above depending upon stages
   (D) None of the above it depends upon stages

4. Point to differentiate central giant cell granuloma and giant cell tumor

   (A) On the basis of giant cells
   (B) On the basis of inflammatory changes
   (C) Both of the above
   (D) None of the above

5. What is the treatment you suggest in the above case

   (A) Antibiotic therapy
   (B) Curettage
   (C) Enucleation
   (D) Wait and watch

Answers:

1. C

central giant cell granuloma is giant cell lesion inside the bone

2. A

central giant cell granuloma is giant cell lesion containing foreign body giant cells inside the bone

3. A

Usual presentation is unilocular radiolucency inside the bone.

4. C

Giant cell tumor is the tumor of giant cell origin while granuloma is a reactive lesion containing giant cells

5. C

Local excision is the treatment of choice.

Reference:

1. Neville BW, Damn DD, Allen CM, Bouquot JE.Oral & Maxillofacial Pathology, 2nd Ed.New Delhi:Elsevier:2005.

2. Ghom AG.text book of oral pathology, 2nd Ed.New Delhi:Jaypee:2013.

Hemangioma

Prof. Shaleen Chandra, Dept. of Oral Pathology & Microbiology

A 17-year old female presented with a swelling on anterior 2/3rd of the tongue since one and half years which gradually increased to the present size1.5 x 2 cm. swelling was soft to firm in consistency, non-mobile, non-tender and bluish purple in color, surface appeared to be smooth and granular with well- defined borders. There were no associated features of pain & fever.

1. What is the most probable diagnosis of the lesion?

   (A) Pyogenic granuloma

   (B) Hemangioma

   (C) Lymphangioma

   (D) All of the above

2. Hemangioma is

   (A) Tumor of blood vessels

   (B) Tumor of capillaries

   (C) Tumor of arterioles

   (D) Hamartomatous growth only

3. Treatment of hemangioma is

   (A) Sclerosing agent application

   (B) wide surgical excision

   (C) steroid therapy

   (D) all of the above

4. Hemangioma appears

   (A) At birth

   (B) In first year of life

   (C) After any trauma in adolescent age

   (D) After many year of trauma in adulthood

5. To see the origin of vascular lesion most accurate diagnostic aid is

   (A) Digital palpation for feeding vessel

   (B) CT scan

   (C) Angiography

   (D) Orthopentomographic examination

Answers:

1. B

   Pyogenic granuloma is a pedunculated growth arising from gingival.

2. D

   Hamartomas are malformation of native cells of that site.

3. D

   Steroids, sclerosing agents and surgery all can be done in hemangiomas depending upon stage of lesion.

4. B

   Appears within one year after birth.

5. C

   Angiography is the investigation of choice to see the feeding vessel.

Reference:

1. Neville BW, Damn DD, Allen CM, Bouquot JE.Oral & Maxillofacial Pathology, 2nd Ed.New Delhi:Elsevier:2005.

Mandibular Tori

Prof. Shaleen Chandra, Dept. of Oral Pathology & Microbiology

A 54-year-old male patient complaining of bony growth on his lower jaw below the tongue. He had noticed this growth 2 years ago gradually increasing to attain the present size. On examination bilateral sublingual bony growth covered with normal oral mucosa in the premolar & 1st molar region was found. The growths were non tender and were no lymphadenopathy.

1. Most common location of mandibular tori

    (A) Incisal region
    (B) canine region
    (C) premolar region
    (D) Molar region

2. What should be the complain of patient having mandibular tori

    (A) occasional Pain
    (B) Difficulty in chewing
    (C) Difficulty in swallowing
    (D) All of the above

3. Treatment of mandibular tori

    (A) wait and watch
    (B) wide surgical excision
    (C) surgical recon touring
    (D) mandibulectomy

4. Histologically mandibular tori presents similar to

    (A) Ossifying fibroma
    (B) Juvenile Ossifying fibroma
    (C) Cemento-ossifying dysplasia
    (D) Normal bone

5. To see the lingual extension of mandibular tori best radiograph will be

    (A) Bite wing radiograph
    (B) Standard occlusal radiograph
    (C) Intra oral periapical radiograph
    (D) Ortho pentomograph

Answers:

1. C

   Lingual side on premolar region of mandible is the most common location of tori.

2. D

   Pain difficulty in mastication, and speaking problems are most commonly encountered with tori

3. C

   Surgical recon touring is usually done.

4. D

   These appears as normal osseous tissue in H&E sections.

5. B

   Standard occlusal view of mandible is the radiograph of choice in these cases.

Reference:

1. Neville BW, Damn DD, Allen CM, Bouquot JE.Oral & Maxillofacial Pathology, 2nd Ed.New Delhi:Elsevier:2005.

Schwanoma

Prof. Shaleen Chandra, Dept. of Oral Pathology & Microbiology

25-year-old presented a lump in the right lateral border of tongue, which was increasing in size for the last six months. The tumor was radically removed, and the sections were stained with Hematoxylin-Eosin. The tumor was encapsulated and showed two different pattern of growth. Antoni A areas displayed spindle cells closely packed together with palisading of nuclei. Verocay bodies, which were presented in Antoni A areas, are whorled formations of palisading tumor cells.

1. What is the most probable diagnosis for the lesion presented above?

    (A) Pleomorphic Antony carcinoma
    (B) Bimorphic antony carcinoma
    (C) Schwanoma
    (D) Neurofibroma

2. Verocay bodies are found in

    (A) Pleomorphic Antony carcinoma
    (B) Bimorphic antony carcinoma
    (C) Neurilemmoma
    (D) Neurofibroma

3. Most common site of neurilemmoma

    (A) Buccal mucosa
    (B) Tongue
    (C) Floor of mouth
    (D) lip

4. Most probable treatment option for schwanoma

    (A) Wait and watch
    (B) Surgical excision
    (C) Modified radical neck dissection
    (D) Topical steroid application

5. What is the difference between Antony A and Antony B

    (A) Antony a shows irregular arrangement of spindle cells
    (B) Antony b shows irregular arrangement of spindle cells
    (C) Antony a shows irregular arrangement of round cells
    (D) Antony b shows irregular arrangement of round cells

Answers:

1. C

    two types of patterns in one lesion is most commonly indicate neurilemmoma.

2. C

    these are larger eosinophilic areas found in neurilemmoma.

3. B

    tongue is the most common site.

4. B

    it is benign tumor of neural tissue origin so can be excised surgically.

5. B

    Antony b shows irregular arrangement of spindle cells while antony A shows palisading arrangement.

Refernce:

1. Neville BW, Damn DD, Allen CM, Bouquot JE.Oral & Maxillofacial Pathology, 2nd Ed.New Delhi:Elsevier:2005.

Idiopathic Gingival Enlargement

Dr. Shalini Gupta, Associate Prof, Dept of Oral Pathology

A 23-year-old man reported with complaining pain and swelling in the gums and continuously increased spacing, tooth mobility with migration of upper front teeth. Intraoral examination revealed moderate-to-severe gingival overgrowth of a firm, dense and fibrotic consistency that involved both the maxillary and mandibular arches. He had, especially of the upper anterior teeth.

1. Most probable diagnosis of the condition is

    (A) Gingival enlargement
    (B) Gingival inflammation
    (C) Bony exotoxins
    (D) Elephantiasis

2. Etiology of the gingival enlargement

    (A) Idiopathic
    (B) Drug consumption
    (C) Hormonal imbalance
    (D) All of the above

3. Drug does not causing gingival enlargement

    (A) Nifidipine
    (B) Phenytoin
    (C) cyclosporin
    (D) cephaperazone

4. Treatment of gingival enlargement is

    (A) Surgical excision
    (B) Gingivectomy
    (C) Removal of causing agent
    (D) All of the above

5. What do you mean by Dilantin Hyperplasia?

    (A) Hyperplasia caused by dilute alcohol
    (B) Hyperplasia caused by anti-epileptic drugs
    (C) Hyperplasia caused by nicotine consumption
    (D) None of the above

Answers:

1. A

   Gingival enlargement clinically present with disturbed scalloping of gingival contour.

2. D

   Gingival enlargement can be without any etiology, can be Phenytoin induced or can be due to pregnancy.

3. D

   Since only Cephaparazone is Third generation Cephalosporin group antibiotic.

4. D

   Gingival enlargement can be treated according to its aetiology.

5. B

   Antiepileptic drugs induce gingival enlargement due to increased amount of extracellular matrix.

Reference:

1.   Rajendran R., Sivapathasundharam B.: Shafer's Text Book of Oral Pathology.6th Ed.New Delhi:Elsevier; 2009-2010.

Hypercementosis

Dr. Shalini Gupta, Associate Prof, Dept of Oral Pathology

A 45 year old patient reported with pain in left lower back region of jaw after extraction. On clinical examination of extracted tooth, the root appear larger in diameter than normal with presence of rounded apices. On Radiographic examination of the tooth thickening and blunting of root was found.

1. Hypercementosis is..
    (A) Increase in thickness of cementum on root surfaces
    (B) Decrease in thickness of cementum on root surfaces
    (C) Excessive cementogenesis on root surfaces
    (D) a) and c)

2. Hypercementosis is not caused by
    (A) Periapical inflammation
    (B) Mechanical stimulation
    (C) paget's disease of bone
    (D) functionless or unerupted tooth

3. Hypercementosis is more common in
    (A) teeth subjected to wear and tear
    (B) Patients with Paget's disease
    (C) teeth associated with chronic inflammation
    (D) All the above

4. Hypercementosis is also called
    (A) Dentin hyperplasia
    (B) Cementum hyperplasia
    (C) Pulp hyperplasia
    (D) Enamel hyperplasia

Answers:

1. A

   formation is not defective, there is only increased width of cementum.

2. D

   Excessive deposition of secondary cementum on the root of a tooth, which may be caused by localized trauma or inflammation, excessive tooth eruption, or osteitis deformans, or may occur idiopathically but not in unerupted tooth.

3. D

   Hypercementosis can occur as a reactionary process or in diseased condition.

4. B

   Cementum Hyperplasia is abnormal increase in volume of the tissue caused by the formation and growth of new normal cells.

Reference:

1. Rajendran R., Sivapathasundharam B.: Shafer's Text Book of Oral Pathology.6th Ed.New Delhi:Elsevier; 2009-2010.

Internal Resorption

Dr. Shalini Gupta, Associate Prof, Dept of Oral Pathology

A 25 year old patient reported with pain in upper on upper front region of tooth since 1 month. On clinical examination pink hued area was found on the crown of the tooth. On radiographic examination a round radiolucent area was seen in the central region of the tooth associated with pulp but not with external surface of the tooth.

1. 'PINK SPOT' is referred as
   (A) External resorption
   (B) Internal resorption
   (C) ankyloses
   (D) Hypercementosis

2. Internal resorption is caused by
   (A) Resorption of enamel
   (B) Resorption of dentin
   (C) Resorption of cementum
   (D) all of the above

3. 'Pink tooth of mummery' is characteristic feature of
   (A) Internal resorption
   (B) External resorption
   (C) Erosion
   (D) Hypercementosis

4. Internal resorption is treated by
   (A) Extraction of the tooth
   (B) Surgery
   (C) Extirpation of pulp tissue & conventional endodontic therapy
   (D) A) and c)

Answers:

1. B

   The first evidence of the lesion may be the appearance of a pink-hued area on the crown of the tooth; the hyperplastic, vascular pulp tissue filling in the resorbed areas

2. B

   Internal resorption is an unusual condition where the dentin and pulpal walls begin to resorb centrally within the root canal.

3. C

   If the condition is discovered before perforation of the crown or root has occurred, endodontic therapy (root canal therapy) may be carried out with the expectation of a fairly high success rate.

Reference:

1. Rajendran R., Sivapathasundharam B.: Shafer's Text Book of Oral Pathology.6th Ed.New Delhi:Elsevier; 2009-2010.

Erosion

Dr. Shalini Gupta, Associate Prof, Dept of Oral Pathology

A 28 year old patient reported with sensitivity and loss of tooth structure. Patient also gives history of overconsumption of soft drinks and fruit juices. On clinical examination incisal grooving with dentin exposure, increased incisal translucency, wear on non-occluding surfaces was found.

1. Erosion is caused by..

   (A) Tooth to tooth wear
   (B) Progressive dissolution of tooth structure by exposure to acids
   (C) Overvigorous tooth brushing & use of dentifrices
   (D) Smoking

2. Saucer shaped defects on enamel is associated with

   (A) Attrition
   (B) Erosion
   (C) Abrasion
   (D) Internal resorption

3. A man working in a chemical industry is more likely to have

   (A) Erosion
   (B) Attrition
   (C) Abrasion
   (D) Internal resorption

4. Chronic regurgitation of gastric secretions can cause

   (A) Erosion
   (B) Abrasion
   (C) Attrition
   (D) Chronic pulpitis

Answers:

1. B

progressive dissolution of tooth structure by exposure to acids present in foods and drinks with a pH below 5.0–5.7 have been known to trigger dental erosion effects.

2. B

Due to erosion of enamel layer.

3. A

Due to consistent exposure to chemicals and chemical fumes.

4. A

regurgitation of gastric acids chelates enamel layer.

Reference:

1. Rajendran R., Sivapathasundharam B.: Shafer's Text Book of Oral Pathology.6th Ed.New Delhi:Elsevier; 2009-2010.

Abrasion

Dr. Shalini Gupta, Associate Prof, Dept of Oral Pathology

A 45 years old patient reported to department of conservative and endodontics with loss of tooth structure from the neck of the tooth and sensitivity sometimes. On clinical examination abrading surface was present on the cervical region of the teeth leaving deep grooves with exposed dentin which is shiny and smooth.

1. Abrasion is.

    (A) Physiological wearing of tooth structure
    (B) Chemical wearing of tooth structure
    (C) Mechanical wearing of tooth structure
    (D) External resorption

2. Abrasion is seen mostly on...

    (A) Cervical area
    (B) Incisal surface
    (C) Cervical and incisal surface
    (D) Lingual surface

3. Abrasion is caused by..

    (A) Vigorous brushing and use of dentifrices
    (B) Overconsumption of soft drinks and fruit juices
    (C) Bruxism
    (D) Flossing

4. Shiny and polished surface is seen in

    (A) Erosion
    (B) Dental Caries
    (C) Abrasion
    (D) Hypercementosis

Answers:

1. C

   Abrasion is the loss of tooth structure by mechanical forces from a foreign element.

2. A

   force begins at the cementoenamel junction, then progression of tooth loss can be rapid since enamel is very thin in this region of the tooth

3. A

   Possible sources of this wearing of tooth are toothbrushes, toothpicks, floss, and any dental appliance frequently set in and removed from the mouth.

4. C

   Erosion causes planning and smoothening of tooth surface.

Reference:

1. Rajendran R., Sivapathasundharam B.: Shafer's Text Book of Oral Pathology.6th Ed.New Delhi: Elsevier; 2009-2010.

Attrition

Dr. Shalini Gupta, Associate Prof, Dept of Oral Pathology

A 30 year old patient reported to the department of oral medicine & radiology with complain of loss of tooth structure and sensitivity in lower anteriors. On clinical examination wear facets were seen along with mobile teeth and tenderness in muscles of mastication.

1. Attrition is due to..

    (A) tooth to tooth wear
    (B) trauma from occlusion
    (C) Exposure to acids
    (D) vigorous brushing

2. Bruxism is associated with..

    (A) Erosion
    (B) Attrition
    (C) Abrasion
    (D) Internal resorption

3. A patient with bruxism shows all of these except..

    (A) Noise during grinding
    (B) Wear facets
    (C) Tenderness of masticatory muscles on palpation
    (D) Discoloration of tooth

4. Pain dysfunction syndrome is often linked with

    (A) Bruxism
    (B) Erosion
    (C) Abrasion
    (D) Hypercementosis

Answers:

1. B

    Dental attrition is a type of tooth wear caused by tooth-to-tooth contact, i.e. Trauma due to occlusion;resulting in loss of tooth tissue, usually starting at the incisal or occlusal surfaces.

2. B

    The pathological wear of the tooth surface can be caused by bruxism, which is clenching and grinding of the teeth

3. D

    Bruxism is a completely devoid of any muscular involvement.

4. A

    Bruxism is the para-functional movement of the mandible, occurring during the day or night causing pain dysfunction syndrome.

Reference:

1. Rajendran R., Sivapathasundharam B.: Shafer's Text Book of Oral Pathology.6th Ed.New Delhi: Elsevier; 2009-2010.

Aphthous Ulcers

Dr. Diksha Singh, Asst. Prof., Dept. of Oral Pathology

A 28 years old patient reported with multiple strong painful ulcers on ventral surface of tongue. Patient gives history of similar type of ulcers few weeks back. On clinical examination several (1-5) no. of oval ulcer less than 0.5cm in diameter, covered by yellow fibrinous membrane and surrounded by an erythematous halo was seen.

1. Canker sores is also known as:
   (A) Recurrent apthous ulcers
   (B) Recurrent herpetic gingivitis
   (C) ANUG
   (D) Recurrent herpes labialis

2. Apthous like ulcers are seen in
   (A) Bechet's syndrome
   (B) Sweet syndrome
   (C) PFAPA(periodic fever acute pharyngitis apthous stomatitis)
   (D) all of the above

3. Oral ulcers which occurs in groups, persists for about 6 weeks and leaves scars on healing are:
   (A) Recurrent apthous major
   (B) Recurrent apthous minor
   (C) Recurrent herpetiform ulcers
   (D) Acute herpetic gingivostomatitis

4. Crohn's disease:
   (A) has oral ulcerations similar to major apthous ulcerations
   (B) is a self-limiting lesion
   (C) is commonly seen among Indian populations
   (D) is usually treated with erythromycin

Answers:

1. A

   common name for Apthous ulcer.

2. D

   Apthous ulcer clinically present in all the diseases given in option.

3. A

   Major Apthous ulcers present as large deep irregular ulceration with extensive scarring.

4. A

   Crohn's Disease is autoimmune disease so it will manifest oral lesions in the form of apthous ulcers.

Reference:

1. Regezi JA, Sciubba JJ, Jordan RCK; Oral Pathology Clinical Pathologic Correlations; 4th Edition; 38-42

Drug Allergy

Dr. Diksha Singh, Asst. Prof., Dept. of Oral Pathology

A 30 years old patient reported with widespread ulcers on tongue and palate accompanied by rashes and erythema all over body after taking analgesic

1. Lichenoid drug reaction is associated with

    (A) Erosive lichen planus
    (B) reticular lichen planus
    (C) Atrophiclichen planus
    (D) Bullous lichen planus

Answers:

1. A

    Drug allergy may cause erosion of oral mucosa

Reference:

1. Regezi JA, Sciubba JJ, Jordan RCK; Oral Pathology Clinical Pathologic Correlations; 4th Edition; 46-48

Periapical Granuloma

Dr. Diksha Singh, Asst. Prof., Dept. of Oral Pathology

A 35 year old patient reported with the pain in right maxillary 1st molar on mastication. Patient gives previous history of pain in the same tooth which subsided thereafter. On clinical examination tooth was non-vital and it didn't respond on electric and thermal pulp.

1. Periapical granuloma is clinically and radiographically indistinguishable from:
    (A) Radicular cyst
    (B) Residual cyst
    (C) Odontogenickeratocyst
    (D) Dentigerous cyst

2. Following is not a possible source of epithelium in the periapical granuloma
    (A) Epithelial rests of malassez
    (B) Gastric Epithelium
    (C) Epithelial cell rests of serres
    (D) Odontogenic epithelium

3. First change in radiographic features of periapical lesions are:
    (A) Thickening of periodontal ligament at the root apex results in periapical radiolucency
    (B) Bone resorption
    (C) Root resorption
    (D) Increased radiopacity around the periphery of the root

Answers:

1. A

   Granulomas can transform into cystswithout significant radiographic change

2. B

   Gastric epithelium cannot be a source of periapical granuloma

Acute Suppurative Osteomyelitis

Dr. Diksha Singh, Asst. Prof., Dept. of Oral Pathology

A 32 year old patient reported with severe throbbing, deep seated pain & diffuse large swelling in right lower back region of jaw. Patient also complained of reduced mouth opening & excessive salivation. On clinical examination it was found that teeth are mobile & overlying gingiva is swollen & tender with pus discharging sinus

1. Clinical feature of this form of this infection arises as a result of
    (A) Fracture
    (B) Gunshot wound
    (C) Dentalinfection
    (D) Both a,b,c

2. The inflammatory exudates in the Acute Suppurative Osteomyelitis include
    (A) PMNls
    (B) Lymphocytes
    (C) Plasma cells
    (D) PMNls, lymphocyte, plasma cells

3. Osteoclastic activity leads to formation
    (A) Sequestrum
    (B) Involucrum
    (C) Lacunae
    (D) Marrow Spaces

4. Necrosis of bony tissue that takes place in Acute suppurative osteomyelitis
    (A) Liquifactive
    (B) Coagulative
    (C) Fatty
    (D) Ischemic

Answers:

1. D

   fracture, gunshot wound, dental infection are the most common etiology of acute suppurative osteomyelitis

2. D

   lymphocytes, plasma cells and Pmnls are the inflammatory cells

3. A

   sequestrum is a dead chronic necrotic bone

4. A

   liquifective necrosis is characterized by chronic inflammatory cells and degeneration of bone

Reference:

1. Rajendran R., Sivapathasundharam B.: Shafer's Text Book of Oral Pathology.6th Ed.New Delhi: Elsevier; 2009-2010.

Chronic Pulpitis

Dr. Diksha Singh, Asst. Prof., Dept. of Oral Pathology

A 30 year old patient reported to department of conservative and endodontics with cavity in right mandibular first molar with intermittent dull and throbbing pain. Tooth is less sensitive to hot and cold stimuli.

1. Which of the following is the most difficult pulpal or periapical pathology to diagnose:

    (A) Necrotic pulp

    (B) Chronic pulpitis

    (C) Internal resorption

    (D) Acute alveolar abscess

2. Most common causes of pulp pathology is

    (A) Microbes

    (B) Trauma

    (C) Leakage from filling materials

    (D) Pressure sensation from condensation of filling materials

3. Which of the following fibers are responsible for carrying pain impulse

    (A) Alpha

    (B) Beta

    (C) Delta

    (D) Gamma

4. Normal intrapulpal pressure is:

    (A) 10 mm Hg

    (B) 5mm Hg

    (C) 7mm Hg

    (D) 15mm Hg

Answers:

1. B

    pulpal inflammation cannotdetected in radiographs

2. A

    microbes can damage the pulp through toxins or directly after extension from caries or transportation via the vasculature

3. C

    delta fibers are sensory fibers carrying pain and pressure

4. A

    during inflammation pulpal pressure is increased

Reference:

1. Rajendran R., Sivapathasundharam B.: Shafer's Text Book of Oral Pathology.6th Ed.New Delhi:Elsevier; 2009-2010.

Garre's Osteomyelitis

Dr. Diksha Singh, Asst. Prof., Dept. of Oral Pathology

A 16 year old patient reported with swelling in right mandibular posterior region. On clinical examination it was found that right mandibular first molar was grossly carious & non vital &swelling is bony hard with no pain and no pus discharge.

1. Garre's osteomyelitis is also called as
   (A) chronic diffuse osteomyelitis
   (B) chronic focal osteomyelitis
   (C) chronic osteomyelitis with proliferative periostitis
   (D) florid osseous dysplasia

2. Dead bone in osteomyelitis are named as
   (A) involucrum
   (B) sequestrum
   (C) marble bone
   (D) dysplastic bone

3. Garres osteomyelitis can be investigated through
   (A) peripical radiograph
   (B) occlusal radiograph
   (C) OPG
   (D) Any of the above

Answers:

1. C

    It Is a type of chronic osteomyelitis, also called chronic osteomyelitis with proliferative periostitis.

2. B

    In Osteomyelitis infection in bone leads to increase intramedullary pressure due to inflammatory exudates which results in stripping of periosteum from osteum leading to vascular thrombosis followed by bone necrosis(due to lack of blood supply) and so sequestrum or dead bone is formed.

3. D

    All the above radiographic aids reveal bone resorption due to infection.

Reference:

1. Rajendran R., Sivapathasundharam B.: Shafer's Text Book of Oral Pathology.6th Ed.New Delhi:Elsevier; 2009-2010.

Acute Pulpitis

Dr. Diksha Singh, Asst. Prof., Dept. of Oral Pathology

A 28 year old patient reported with severe throbbing pain in left maxillary 2nd molar which is aggravated on taking hot or cold beverages and during sleep.

1. Acute reversible pulpitis is treated by

    (A) Sedative filling wait and watch
    (B) Pulpectomy
    (C) Pulpotomy
    (D) Pulp capping

2. Pain due to acute irreversible pulpitis is

    (A) Spontaneous
    (B) Sharp
    (C) Lasting for short time
    (D) a) and b)

3. In acute pulpitis pain is elicited by because of

    (A) percussion
    (B) thermal changes
    (C) Invasion of microrganisms
    (D) walking

4. The pulpitis may be painless if

    (A) Tooth is in occlusion
    (B) Tooth is out of occlusion
    (C) Pulp chamber is closed
    (D) Pulp chamber is open

Answers:

1. A

   Sedative filling wait and watch because sedatives will ease the acute pain. In reversible pulpitis pulp may become affected irreversibly.

2. D

   Acute reversible pulpitis exhibits spontaneous mild to moderate pain(pulpagia) of short duration.

3. B

   Tooth responds mostly to cold stimuli and may be initiated by heat.

4. D

   Essential feature of reversible pulpitis is that pain ceases as soon as there is access opening of pulp chamber, as it helps in e drainage of abscess.

Reference:

1. Rajendran R., Sivapathasundharam B.: Shafer's Text Book of Oral Pathology.6th Ed.New Delhi: Elsevier; 2009-2010.

Erythema Multiforme

Dr. Diksha Singh, Asst. Prof., Dept. of Oral Pathology

A 30 years old patient reported with painful ulcers on lips and palate accompanied by fever & headache. On clinical examination multiple superficial widespread ulcers were seen

1. Erythema multiforme is

   (A) An acute, self-limiting disease of skin & oral mucous membrane
   (B) Painless vesicular self-limiting disease
   (C) A viral disease
   (D) Bacterial infection

2. Target lesions are observed in case of

   (A) Erythema multiforme
   (B) Lichen planus
   (C) Pemphigus vulgaris
   (D) Psoriasis

3. Oral, ocular & genital lesions are seen in

   (A) Erythema multiforme
   (B) Stevens- Johnson's syndrome
   (C) SLE
   (D) None of the above

4. Stevens –Johnson's syndrome involves

   (A) Type 1 hypersensitivity
   (B) Type 2 hypersensitivity
   (C) Type 3 hypersensitivity
   (D) Type 4 hypersensitivity

Answers:

1. A

   Disease mediated by deposition of immune complex(IgM)and is aself-limiting disease of skin & oral mucous membrane.

2. A

   Target lesion is typical lesion of EM in which a vesicle is surrounded by often hemorrhagic maculopapule.

3. B

   Stevens- Johnson's syndrome is a form of toxic epidermal necrolysis occurring due to hypersensitivity reaction and affects skin as well as mucous membrane.

4. C

   Caused due to type III hypersensitivity reaction which is immune complex mediated. T cells recognize and respond to foreign antigens.

Reference:

1. Rajendran R., Sivapathasundharam B.: Shafer's Text Book of Oral Pathology.6th Ed.New Delhi:Elsevier; 2009-2010.

Nursing Bottle Caries

Dr. Diksha Singh, Asst. Prof., Dept. of Oral Pathology

A 3 year old patient reported with the caries in upper anterior teeth. There is no involvement of mandibular anteriors. Parents give history of feeding bottled milk with sugar for longer duration.

1. Which age group is usually not affected by Nursing bottle caries
   (A) 1 – 2 years
   (B) 2 – 3 years
   (C) Birth to six months
   (D) More than 3 years of age

2. All are true for nursing bottle caries except

   (A) Maxillary incisors are most effected
   (B) Mandibular incisors are not effected
   (C) Pacifying sugar solutions are the cause
   (D) Breast milk does not cause the condition vm,g

3. The bacteria responsible for causing nursing bottle caries are

   (A) Lactobacillus only
   (B) Streptococcus and lactobacillus
   (C) Streptococcus, lactobacillus & veilonella
   (D) Streptococcus, lactobacillus & neisseria

4. The primary reason for replacing teeth destroyed due to nursing bottle syndrome is

   (A) Speech and esthetics
   (B) Form and function
   (C) Incising and mastication
   (D) Arch perimeter requirements in the transitional dentition

Answers:

1. C

    nursing bottle caries is due to bottle feeding in infants and contact of food for long time causes tooth decay.

2. D

    maxillary central incisors are most common tooth involve in nursing bottle caries.

3. B

    streptococcus sp. are mostly associated with dental caries

4. A

    tooth loss due to caries becomes the main cause for malocclusion in a child.

Reference:

1. Rajendran R., Sivapathasundharam B.: Shafer's Text Book of Oral Pathology.6th Ed.New Delhi: Elsevier; 2009-2010.

Chronic Suppurative Osteomyelitis

Dr. Diksha Singh, Asst. Prof., Dept. of Oral Pathology

A 30 year old patient reported with mild & dull vague pain in left lower back region of jaw since 2 months. On clinical examination swelling was present with sequestrum protuding from ulcerated skin.

1. Suppuration in Chronic Suppurative Osteomyelitis leads to
    (A) formation of Sinuses and Fistulas
    (B) bleeding
    (C) fracture
    (D) fibrosis

2. Radiographic appearance of chronic diffuse osteomyelitis is
    (A) Cotton wool appearance
    (B) radiopaque lesion
    (C) radiolucency
    (D) Hazy appearance

3. Repeated resorption and deposition leads to histological appearance of
    (A) Mosaic pattern
    (B) Chinese letter pattern
    (C) Fish net pattern
    (D) Orange peel pattern

4. Chronic suppurative osteomyelitis is not a sequel of
    (A) Infection
    (B) Cyst
    (C) Periapical granuloma
    (D) irradiation

Answers:

1. A

   sinus and fistulas are the body's defense mechanism to reduce the load of infection by draining it out.

2. A

   diffuse radiopacity without any corticated borders is associated with osteomyelitis.

3. A

   areas of resorption and deposition are separated by reversal lines making mosaic pattern.

4. D

   irradiation of bone causes osteoradionecrosis, due to reduced vascularity.

Reference:

1. Rajendran R., Sivapathasundharam B.: Shafer's Text Book of Oral Pathology.6th Ed.New Delhi:Elsevier; 2009-2010

Ludwig's Angina

Dr. Diksha Singh, Asst. Prof., Dept. of Oral Pathology

A 35 year old patient reported with complain of swelling in neck since 4 days. He also complained of fever, sore throat & reduced mouth opening. On clinical examination it was found that swelling was bilateral large diffuse board like with brawny induration.

1. Cellulitis is usually associated with streptococcus because
   (A) It is a common organism causing dental caries
   (B) It releases hyaluronidase, which cleaves intercellular substances
   (C) Streptococcus never cause cellulitis
   (D) Both a) and b) are correct

2. Ludwig's angina is
   (A) Acute toxic cellulitis
   (B) Chronic cellulitis
   (C) Subacute cellulitis
   (D) Periapical infection

3. Death due to Ludwig's angina is most commonly caused by
   (A) Severe bacteremia
   (B) Septicemia
   (C) Edema of the glottis causing suffocation
   (D) Pain

4. Board like swelling in the floor of the mouth, elevation of the tongue is a feature of:
   (A) Cavernous sinus thrombosis
   (B) Ludwig's angina
   (C) Submandibular abscess
   (D) Peril apical abscess

Answers:

1. D

   production of hyaluronidase is responsible for diffuse spread of infection through ground substance of connective tissue.

2. A

   Ludwig's angina is an acute cellulitis involving submental, sub lingual and submandibular spaces.

3. C

   elevated floor of mouth causes airway blockage and causes death.

4. B

   Ludwig's angina is associated with elevation of floor of mouth and board like swelling

Reference:

1. Rajendran R., Sivapathasundharam B.: Shafer's Text Book of Oral Pathology.6th Ed.New Delhi:Elsevier; 2009-2010.

Pulp Polyp

Dr. Diksha Singh, Asst. Prof., Dept. of Oral Pathology

An 18 year old patient reported with large open carious cavity in right maxillary 1st molar with no pain. On clinical examination pinkish red lobulated mass was found which filled up the carious cavity. The lesion bleeds profusely on provocation.

1. Pulp polyp is also known as
   (A) Chronic hyperplastic pulpitis
   (B) Acute reversible pulpitis
   (C) Pulp hyperemia
   (D) Pink tooth

2. Possibility of epithelial implantation in pulp polyp are except
   (A) Gingival epithelium
   (B) Buccal mucosa
   (C) Shredded epithelium from oral mucosa
   (D) Respiratory epithelium

3. Teeth most commonly involved by pulp polyp are
   (A) 3rd molar
   (B) 2nd molar and deciduous molar
   (C) deciduous molar and 1st permanent molar
   (D) incisors

4. Foam cells are
   (A) Lipid laden macrophages
   (B) Plasma cells
   (C) Osteoclasts
   (D) Mast cells

Answers:

1. A

    pulp polyp is the form of chronic hyperplastic pulpitis mostly seen in young individuals

2. D

    epithelization of pulpal tissue in case of chronic hyperplastic pulpitis can never be from respiratory epithelium.

3. C

    deciduous molars and first permanent molars are the teeth most commonly associated with hyper plastic response of pulp.

4. A

    macrophages after engulfment of an adipocyte appears foamy cells with clear cytoplasm on H&E staining.

Reference:

1. Rajendran R., Sivapathasundharam B.: Shafer's Text Book of Oral Pathology.6th Ed.New Delhi:Elsevier; 2009-2010.

Herpessimplex And Herpes Zoster

Dr. Fahad M. Samadi, Asst. Prof., Dept. of Oral Pathology

A 50 years old patient reported to oral medicine department with rashes &ulcers on right side of the trunk and the lips. Rashes were accompanied by fever, tingling burning and pain at site of the lesion. On clinical examination the lesion was ulcerative and unilateral with vesicles on vermilion and surrounding skin.

1. The feature that distinguishes herpes zoster from other vesiculo bullous eruption is:
   (A) Unilateraloccurrence
   (B) Severe burning pain
   (C) Prominent crusting vesicles
   (D) Sub epidermal bullous formation

2. Herpes simplex is seen in:
   (A) <10yrs of age
   (B) 12-15yrs of age
   (C) 25-30yrs of age
   (D) 55-60yrs of age

3. Intra nuclear inclusions defected during the course of herpes simplex viral infection are called:
   (A) Bacteriophages
   (B) Lipchitz bodies
   (C) Negri bodies
   (D) Donavan bodies

4. Inflammation of dorsal root ganglion and vesicular eruption of the skin and mucous membrane in area supplied by a sensory nerve that is affected is characteristic of:
   (A) Herpes zoster
   (B) Herpes simplex
   (C) Uveparotid fever
   (D) Aphthous stomatitis

Answers:

1. A

    herpes zoster is a vesiculobullous lesion characterize by distribution of nerve root.

2. A

    primary herpes occurs before age 10 years in two forms subclinical and clinical forms.

3. B

    koilocytes are the cells infected by virus proteins.

4. A

    herpes zoster has characteristic distribution according to nerve ganglion

Reference:

1. Rajendran R., Sivapathasundharam B.: Shafer's Text Book of Oral Pathology.6th Ed.New Delhi: Elsevier; 2009-2010.

Candidiasis

Dr. Fahad M. Samadi, Asst. Prof., Dept. of Oral Pathology

A 12-year-old female patient reported with bilaterally white curd like lesions scattered all over dorsal surface of tongue with loss of papillae and prominent central groove, The hands and feet showed scaly lesions with involvement of intertriginous area and nails. Nails were markedly thickened, fragmented and discolored with significant edema. Erythema of the surrounding periungal tissue simulating clubbing was also present. Scrapping from the lesion revealed the presence of Candida albicans.

1. White patch seen on the buccal mucosa consisting of pseudomycelium and chalamydospors with desquamated epithelium adjacent to it, the patient. is suffering from:

    (A) Histoplasmosis
    (B) Cryptococcosis
    (C) Candidiasis
    (D) Coccidiomycosis

2. ID reaction is associated with:

    (A) Apthous ulcer
    (B) Herpetic stomatitis
    (C) Syphilis
    (D) Candidiasis

3. The microorganism most commonly cultured from a chronic bilateral ulcer at d corner of the mouth:

    (A) Mucor
    (B) Candida
    (C) Treponema
    (D) Aspergillus

4. Drug used to treat oral thrush:

    (A) Clobetasol
    (B) Cotrimoxazole
    (C) Miconazole
    (D) Penicillin

5. Prolonged use of antibiotics in children result in:
   (A) NUG
   (B) Candidiasis
   (C) Actinomycosis
   (D) Apthous ulcer

Answers:

1. C

   All other mycotic infections except candidiasis present different clinical presentation and are prevalent to other sites than oral mucosa.

2. D

   Candidiasis presents 1 D reaction in oral lesions.

3. B

   Angular Chelitis is a type of oral candidiasis.

4. C

   Imidazole derived antifungal drug, shows good efficacy and absorption.

5. D

   Prolong use of antibiotics destroys symbiotic microorganisms and suppressesimmunity.

Reference:

1. Rajendran R., Sivapathasundharam B.: Shafer's Text Book of Oral Pathology.6th Ed.New Delhi:Elsevier; 2009-2010.

Measles

Dr. Fahad M. Samadi, Asst. Prof., Dept. of Oral Pathology

A 10 years old patient reported with severe headache, skin rash, high fever, malaise and cough. On clinical examination cluster of white yellow pin point papules on inflamed background was seen on labial mucosa, buccal mucosa and soft palate.

1. Koplik's Spots
   (A) First manifestation of measles
   (B) Rarely seen in measles
   (C) Are seen 2-3 days after cutaneous rashes
   (D) Is first manifestation but seldom seen

2. Measles are caused by:
   (A) Epstein-barr virus
   (B) varicella zoster virus
   (C) Paramyxo virus
   (D) Coxsackie virus

3. Rubeola refers to:
   (A) German measles
   (B) Measles
   (C) Small pox
   (D) Chicken pox

4. Which of the following is false regarding measles:
   (A) Koplik's spot
   (B) Maculo papular skin rash
   (C) Fever and malaise
   (D) Nikolsky's sign

Answers:

1. D

    koplik pots are seen in buccal mucosa and soft palate so rarely noticed.

2. C

    paramyxovirus group is considered as etiologic agent for measles

3. B

    rubeola is measles and rubella is Germanmeasles.

4. D

    nikolsky's sign is the formation of bullae on normal skin on firm lateral pressure.

Reference:

1. Rajendran R., Sivapathasundharam B.: Shafer's Text Book of Oral Pathology.6th Ed.New Delhi: Elsevier; 2009-2010.

Pemphigus And Pemphigoid

Dr. Fahad M. Samadi, Asst. Prof., Dept. of Oral Pathology

A 50 years old patient reported with painful ulcers at lower lip. On clinical examination general traction on unaffected mucosa produced stripping of epithelium.

1. the most common form of pemphigus involving oral mucosa is
   - (A) Pemphigus vulgaris
   - (B) Pemphigus vegetans
   - (C) Pemphigus erythematosus
   - (D) Pemphigus foliaceous

2. Immunofluorescence is seen at the basement membrane as patchy distribution in
   - (A) Lichen planus
   - (B) Pemphigus
   - (C) Pemphigoid
   - (D) Lupuserythematosus

3. Bullae formation after striking an intact skin/mucosal surface is known as
   - (A) tinel's sign
   - (B) bablnski's sign
   - (C) nikolsky's sign
   - (D) chovstek's sign

4. Intra epithelial bulla are found in
   - (A) Pemphigus
   - (B) Bullous pemphigoid
   - (C) Bullous lichen planus
   - (D) Pemphigoid

Answers:

1. A

   pemphigus vulgaris is most common form present in the oral mucosa.

2. C

   in pemphigoid immunofluorescent dye is deposited in the basement membrane showing patchy linear pattern.

3. C

   nikolsky's sign is the formation of bullae on normal skin on firm lateral pressure,

4. A

   supra basilar split is associated with pemphigus.

Reference:

1. Neville BW, Damn DD, Allen CM, Bouquot JE.Oral & Maxillofacial Pathology, 2nd Ed.New Delhi:Elsevier:2005.

Syphilitic Ulcer

Dr. Fahad M. Samadi, Asst. Prof., Dept. of Oral Pathology

A 32 years old patient reported with painless ulcers on lip and palate. On clinical examination indurated ulcer with rolled margin without exudate was seen. Regional lymphadenopathy with firm and painless swelling was also present.

1. Which of the following is not characteristics of congenital syphilis

   (A) Ghon complex
   (B) Interstitial keratitis
   (C) Mulberry molars
   (D) Notched incisors

2. Syphilis becomes seropositive in

   (A) Chancre (primary syphilis)
   (B) Mucopatches (secondary syphilis)
   (C) Gumma (tertiary syphilis)
   (D) Congenital syphilis

3. Oral lesions of secondary syphilis include all except

   (A) Snail track ulcers
   (B) Mucous patches
   (C) Chancre of tongue
   (D) Hutchinson's wart

4. Gumma occurs in

   (A) Primary stage of syphilis
   (B) Secondary stage of syphilis
   (C) Tertiary stage of syphilis
   (D) Primary tuberculosis

Answers:

1. A

   Hutchinson's triad is associated with syphilis.

2. B

   mucopatches are only painful ulcer in syphilis and associated with second stage of syphilis.

3. C

   chancre is associated with primary syphilis.

4. C

   gumma is associated with tertiary syphilis which is followed by multi organ involvement such as neurosyphilis.

Reference:

1. Rajendran R., Sivapathasundharam B.: Shafer's Text Book of Oral Pathology.6th Ed.New Delhi: Elsevier; 2009-2010.

Tubercular Ulcer

Dr. Fahad M. Samadi, Asst. Prof., Dept. of Oral Pathology

A 50 year old patient reported with low grade fever, night sweats, malaise & weight loss accompanied by cough, hemoptysis & chest pain. Patient also complains of non-healing painless ulcers on tongue and palate. On clinical examination ulcers were multiple and indurated

1. Tuberculous ulcer of oral cavity is usually

    (A) Painless
    (B) Painful
    (C) Itching
    (D) Asymptomatic

2. Most common site of tuberculous lesion in the oral cavity is

    (A) Buccal mucosa
    (B) Lips
    (C) Tongue
    (D) Palate

3. Lesions of tuberculosis are associated with all of the following except

    (A) Central caseation
    (B) Hyaline degeneration
    (C) Giant cells in the center
    (D) Presence of epithelioid cells

4. Drug combination for tuberculosis are often used for

    (A) 5 months
    (B) 3 years
    (C) 4 months
    (D) 1 year

Answers:

1. A

    Tubercular ulcer is caused by mild pathogenic mycobacterium and clinically present as Apple jelly nodule without any symptom.

2. C

    The most vulnerable areas include gingiva extraction sockets, buccal folds and tongue

3. B

    Hyaline degeneration is not seen in granulomatous lesions like tuberculosis.

4. D

    Studies show drug efficacy and resultant eradication of disease in 1 year duration.

Reference:

1. Neville BW, Damn DD, Allen CM, Bouquot JE.Oral & Maxillofacial Pathology, 2nd Ed.New Delhi:Elsevier:2005.

ungal Ulcer

Dr. Fahad M. Samadi, Asst. Prof., Dept. of Oral Pathology

A 45 year old patient reported with fever, cough, weight loss and ulcers on tongue and palate. On clinical examinations multiple non healing persistent ulcers were seen.

1. Vascular involvement and thrombosis is seen in

   (A) Coccidiomycosis
   (B) Aspergillosis
   (C) Mucormycosis
   (D) Histoplasmosis

2. Darling disease is

   (A) Histoplasmosis
   (B) Phycomycosis
   (C) Actinomycosis
   (D) Bleomycosis

3. Non septate hyphae with a tendency to branch at 90 degree angle is characteristic of

   (A) Mucor
   (B) Aspergillosis
   (C) Cryptococcus neoformans
   (D) Coccidioides immitis

4. The yeast which shows thick gelatinous capsule and positive for mucicarmine is

   (A) Cryptococcus neoformans
   (B) Histoplasmosis
   (C) Blastomycosis
   (D) Paracoccidiomycosis

Answers:

1. C

This disease is often characterized by hyphae growing in and around blood vessels.

2. A

Histoplasmosis (also known as "cave disease,"[1] "Darling's disease,", Ohio valley disease, reticuloendotheliosis, spelunker's lung" and "caver's disease"is a disease caused by the fungus Histoplasma capsulatum'.

3. A

classification if fungi based on hyphae formation; Mucor shows branching at 90* angle.

4. A

For identification in tissue, mucicarmine stain provides specific staining of polysaccharide cell wall in C. neoformans.

Reference:

1. Regezi JA, Sciubba JJ, Jorrdan RCK; Oral Pathology Clinical Pathologic Correlations; 4th Edition; 35-38

Tetracycline Staining of Tooth

Dr. Fahad M. Samadi, Asst. Prof., Dept. of Oral Pathology

Patient reports with discolored teeth bearing brown stains. The teeth glow fluorescent in UV light.

1. The most likely diagnosis of above is:

   (A) Porphyria
   (B) Amelogenesic imperfecta
   (C) Hutchinson's teeth
   (D) Tetracycline staining of teeth

2. Yellowish discolouration of teeth is seen in children fed on:

   (A) High protein diet
   (B) Tetracycline
   (C) Penicillins
   (D) erythromycin

3. tetracycline stains appear as

   (A) yellow and brown stains in enamel & dentin
   (B) yellow & brown stains only in enamel
   (C) yellow & brown stains only in dentin
   (D) only yellow stain in enamel

4. pigmentation of the permanent teeth may develop if tetracyclines are given between the ages of

   (A) 5 & 7 years
   (B) 0.2 & 5 years
   (C) 6 & 10 years
   (D) 10 & 12 years

Answers:

1. D

   Tetracycline staining of teeth in brown in colour and teeth glow in flouresent UV light.

2. B

   Tetracycline will bind to calcium in the teeth

3. 3.A

   yellow and brown stains in enamel & dentin caused by tetracycline

4. B

   because it is developing stage of tooth

Reference:

1. Rajendran R., Sivapathasundharam B.: Shafer's Text Book of Oral Pathology.6th Ed.New Delhi: Elsevier; 2009-2010.

Pg 56- onwaeds

Pigmented Lesion Of Oral Cavity: Nevus

Prof. Shaleen Chandra, Dept. of Oral Pathology & Microbiology

A ten year boy came to OPD with complain of a blueish dot over the palate. He noticed it suddenly when he trying to pull out the meat fiber lodged in between his teeth. He does not have any problem with it. He also does not have any other spot like this in his entire oral region

1. Nevi can be categorized as
   (A) Teratoma
   (B) Noma
   (C) Hamartoma
   (D) Low grade malignant tumor

2. Which is not a type of nevi
   (A) Junctional nevi
   (B) Compound nevi
   (C) Intradermal nevi
   (D) Complex nevi

3. Which is the correct sequence of maturation of nevi
   (A) Compound -> junctional -> intramucosal
   (B) Junctional -> compound -> intra mucosal
   (C) Intramucosal -> Compound -> junctional
   (D) Compound = junctional = intramucosal

4. compound nevus composed of two elements
   (A) Blue nevus and overlying epithelium
   (B) Intra dermal nevus and overlying junctional nevus
   (C) Junctional nevus and garment nevi
   (D) None of the above

5. which is not histologic variant of acquired nevi
   (A) Neural cells
   (B) spindle cell
   (C) Baloon cell
   (D) Halo nevi

Answers:

1. C

   hamartoma is the proliferation of the cells native to that region.

2. D

   intradermal nevi inside the oral cavity refer to as intramucosal nevi

3. B

   nevus cells proliferate deep into the mucosa so Junctional nevus changed to compound and finally to intra mucosal

4. B

   Intra dermal nevus and overlying junctional nevus are the two main components of nevi.

5. B

   acquired nevi are appears after birth. Also called as neural cell, balloon cells and halo nevi

Reference:

1. Rajendran R., Sivapathasundharam B.: Shafer's Text Book of Oral Pathology.6th Ed.New Delhi:Elsevier; 2009-2010.

Ulcerated Lesion Of Oral Cavity

Prof. Shaleen Chandra, Dept. of Oral Pathology & Microbiology

Twenty five-year-old white male with the complaint of intense pain associated to a tongue lesion, with duration of two months. He reported a reddish spot for ten years in the location where afterwards the current lesion developed. Upon physical examination, an extensive ulceration was observed, with largest diameter of 2.5 cm, irregular borders, surrounded by an erythematous atrophic area, located at dorsum and left lateral border of the tongue Whitish areas could be observed in the periphery of the ulceration. There was hardening of borders and surrounding areas, indicating large infiltration. A cervical lymph node was detected on the left, fix and not painful.

1. Most common ulcerative malignant lesion of oral cavity

    (A) Basal cell carcinoma
    (B) Small cell carcinoma
    (C) Squamous cell carcinoma
    (D) Round cell carcinoma

2. Most common site for oral squamous cell carcinoma In India due to tobacco

    (A) Floor of mouth
    (B) Buccal mucosa
    (C) Tongue
    (D) Lip

3. Most common site for metastasis of primary oral squamous cell carcinoma

    (A) Lung
    (B) Liver
    (C) Breast
    (D) Regional lymph nodes

4. Fate of well differentiated squamous cell carcinoma if not treated for long term it will turn into

    (A) Moderately differentiated squamous cell carcinoma
    (B) Poorly differentiated squamous cell carcinoma
    (C) Remain well differentiated squamous cell carcinoma
    (D) Anaplastic carcinoma

5. Characteristic feature of oral squamous cell carcinoma histologically
   (A) Drop shaped bulbous rete pegs
   (B) Intraepithelial keratin pearl formation
   (C) Invasion of dysplastic cells into connective tissue
   (D) prominent and distinct basement membrane

Answers:

1. C

   squamous cell carcinoma accounts for more than 90 percent of oral malignancies.

2. B

   tobacco chewing is the most common form so placement of tobacco in the buccal vestibule is the most preferred place to keep the quid.

3. D

   submaxillary lymph nodes are the primary metastatic site for metastasis.

4. C

   malignant tumors can be monoclonal or polyclonal so dysplastic cells remain proliferating in the same pace and start invading into deeper tissue.

5. C
   Invasion of dysplastic cells into connective tissue is the most striking finding for malignancy

Reference:

1. Rajendran R., Sivapathasundharam B.: Shafer's Text Book of Oral Pathology.6th Ed.New Delhi:Elsevier; 2009-2010.

Oral Submucous Fibrosis

Prof. Shaleen Chandra, Dept. of Oral Pathology & Microbiology

A 43-year-old man presented with a complaint of reduced mouth opening over the past 2 years. He had a longstanding habit of chewing fresh areca nut (4–5 pouches a day for 20–25 years). Extra oral examination revealed that his lips were thin and mouth opening was limited to about 26 mm (average normal opening is 40 mm). There was erosion at the corners of his mouth. The entire oral mucosa was pale, with focal blanched areas. The tongue was devoid of papillae and extensive fibrosis had occurred on its ventral surface and the floor of the mouth. The patient could not touch the hard palate with the tip of his tongue. Thick fibrotic bands were palpable bilaterally on the buccal mucosa. Intraoral examination was problematic as it was difficult to retract the patient's fibrotic cheeks. During examination the mirror often stuck to the oral mucosa, suggesting dry mouth. When the patient was asked to blow out air with closed lips, the usual puffed cheek appearance was not seen, suggesting loss of cheek elasticity. General examination was normal.

1. What is the stage of condition based on presented case?

    (A) Moderately advance stage
    (B) Advance stage
    (C) Early stage
    (D) Late stage

2. Mostaccepted etiology of OSMF?

    (A) Immunological diseases
    (B) Prolonged deficiency to iron and vitamins in the diet
    (C) Extreme climatic conditions
    (D) Betel quid with areca nut

3. Most commonly known irritant to be associated with OSMF?

    (A) Tobacco specific nitrosamines
    (B) Polyphenols
    (C) Alkaloids and copper
    (D) Tannins

4. What are the most studied molecule associated with OSMF?

    (A) O 6 -methyl guanine DNA methyl transferase (MGMT)
    (B) Cystatin C mRNA (CST3)
    (C) HLA-A10, -B7 and DR3
    (D) COL1A2, COL3A1, COL6A1, COL6A3, and COL7A1

5. What is the rate of malignant transformation of OSMF?

 (A) 6-8%

 (B) 3-6%

 (C) 3-19%

 (D) More than 25%

Answers:

1. A.

Moderately advanced stage was made based on the characteristic oral features: generalized blanching of mucosa, extensive fibrosis and limited mouth opening.[1]

2. D

The strongest risk factor for OSMF is the chewing of betel quid containing areca nut. The amount of areca nut in betel quid and the frequency and duration of chewing betel quid are clearly related to the development of OSMF.[2]

3. C

The direct contact of the quid mixture with oral tissues results in their continuous irritation by various components including; biologically active alkaloids (arecoline, arecaidine, arecolidine, guvacoline, guvacine, flavonoids (tannins and catechins) and copper.[2]

4. C

Raised frequencies of HLA-A10, -B7 and DR3 are found in OSF patients compared to normal subjects. Further HLA typing done by use of PCR also demonstrates significantly increased frequencies of HLA A24, DDRB I-I I and DRB3 0202/3 antigens in 21 OSF patients when compared with the English controls.[3]

5. C

Epidemiological studies have shown that the rate of malignant transformation ranges from 3 to 19%. [4]

References:

1. Rajendran R. Oral submucous fibrosis. J Oral MaxillofacPathol 2003;7:1-4

2. Rajalalitha P, Vali S. Molecular pathogenesis of oral submucous fibrosis- a collagen metabolic disorder. J Oral Pathol Med 2005; 34(6):321–8.

3. Saeed, B, Haue, MF, Meghji, S, Harris, M (1997) HLA typing in oral submucous fibrosis. J Dent Res 76: pp. 1024

4. Chen HM, Hsieh RP, Yang H, Kuo YS, Kuo MY, Chiang CP. HLA typing in Taiwanese patients with oral sub mucous fibrosis. J Oral Pathol Med 2004;33:191-9

Malignant Tumors Of Melanocytes: Melanoma

Prof. Shaleen Chandra, Dept. of Oral Pathology & Microbiology

A 32-year-old Asian woman reported for consultation regarding a rapidly growing pigmented mass in the maxillary anterior region. Three months earlier, she had developed an asymptomatic bluish-black patch on her anterior maxillary gingiva. On palpation, there was no tenderness, bleeding or regional lymphadenopathy

1. Melanoma is:

    (A) Benign neoplasm of melanocytes
    (B) Malignant neoplasm of melanocytes
    (C) Hamartomatous growth of melanocytes
    (D) All of the above.

2. Metastasis of oral melanoma is possible when it is in

    (A) Radial phase
    (B) Superficial phase
    (C) Vertical phase
    (D) All of the above

3. Melanoma can be suspected if any nevi shows

    (A) Uniformly dark pigmentation
    (B) Uniformly light pigmentation
    (C) Irregular Blue pigmentation
    (D) All of the above

4. Melanoma is

    (A) Twice more common in male
    (B) Thrice more common in male
    (C) Equal in male and female
    (D) More common in female

5. Which is not a clinical type of oral melanoma

    (A) Nodular melanoma
    (B) Lentigo maligna melanoma
    (C) Acral lentiginous melanoma
    (D) melasma

Answers:

1. B

   Melanoma is a malignant neoplasm of melanocytes.

2. C

   Metastasis in melanoma occurs only in the vertical growth phase

3. C

   Irregular pigmentation is a sign of melanoma out of the five signs described in Clark's rule

4. A

   Melanoma affects males twice more commonly than females

5. D

   Melasma is pigmentation present during pregnancy

Reference:

1. Rajendran R., Sivapathasundharam B.: Shafer's Text Book of Oral Pathology.6th Ed.New Delhi:Elsevier; 2009-2010.

Papilloma

Prof. Shaleen Chandra, Dept. of Oral Pathology & Microbiology

An 11 year old female patient reported, with the chief complaint of a growth on the right side of the palate since 7-8 months and attained the present size with 4-5 moths. She also gave the history of same type of growth on the palate 3 years back and which she got it excised in a private clinic. A thorough clinical examination revealed a pedunculated cauliflower like growth on the hard palate of size around 8 X 10 mm. 12- 15 pink finger like projections was noticed

1. Papilloma share the common etiology with

   (A) Skin warts
   (B) Nevi
   (C) Fever blisters
   (D) Noma

2. Squamous papilloma is associated with

   (A) HPV 11 & 18
   (B) HPV 6 & 11
   (C) HPV 9 & 10
   (D) HPV 19 only

3. Papilloma is clinically presented as

   (A) Smooth surface
   (B) Rough patch
   (C) Fingerlike projection
   (D) Hairy projection

4. Histologically squamous papilloma presents as

   (A) Dens keratin layer
   (B) Proliferation of spinous cells in papillary pattern
   (C) Epithelial projection with connective tissue core
   (D) All of the above

5. Human papilloma virus altered epithelial cells are known as

   (A) Keratinocytes
   (B) Oligodendrocytes
   (C) Koilocytes
   (D) Karyocytes

Answers:

1. A

   Both may be caused by HPV virus

2. B

   HPV 6 & 11 is frequently associated with squamous papilloma

3. C

   Finger like papillary surface is present

4. D

   All are features of papilloma

5. C

   Koilocytes is the term used for cells with viral inclusion bodies

Reference:

1. Rajendran R., Sivapathasundharam B.: Shafer's Text Book of Oral Pathology.6th Ed.New Delhi: Elsevier; 2009-2010.

Fibroma

Prof. Shaleen Chandra, Dept. Of Oral Pathology & Microbiology

A 29 year old male patient presented with complaint of a solitary painless well-defined broad base growth in right buccal mucosa along the occlusal plane of maxillary & mandibular teeth since four months. The lesion was in whitish red color, measuring about 10x8 mm of size in longest diameter and extending from the buccal surfaces of 33 and 3The superficial surface of lesion was keratinized with well-defined margin. Growth was firm in consistency but compressible, it wasnon tender and does not bleed on pressure. An excisional biopsy was performed and on histopathological examination, a stratified squamous parakeratinised epithelium without rete-ridges was seen covering a dense connective tissue stroma. The collagen bundles were numerous and densely packed along with few fibroblasts. Moderate amount of lymphocytes and plasma cells infiltration was also noted. Postoperative healing was uneventful. No recurrence was reported on follow-up.

1. What is the diagnosis of the presented case?
    (A) Lipoma
    (B) Schwannoma
    (C) Neurofibroma
    (D) Irritation fibroma

2. What is the most common site of fibroma?
    (A) Buccal mucosa
    (B) Lip
    (C) Gingiva
    (D) Tongue
    (E) Palate

3. What are the majority of localized overgrowths of the oral mucosa considered as?
    (A) Neoplastic growth
    (B) Reactive hyperplasia
    (C) Benign growth
    (D) None

4. What is the etiology of fibroma?
    (A) Chronic and constant irritation
    (B) Viral infection
    (C) Fungal infection
    (D) All the above

5. What makes the overlying epithelium to stretch?

   (A) Destruction of basement membrane

   (B) Collagen accumulation causing tension on epithelium

   (C) Atrophy of epithelium and Loss of rete ridges

   (D) b and c

Answers:

1. D

   This a case of irritation fibroma or "Focal fibrous hyperplasia" (FFH). Lesions generally presents as a solitary painless, sessile, round or ovoid, broad based growth that is lighter in colour than surrounding tissue due to a reduced vascularity.[1]

2. A

   The most common location is the buccal mucosa along the bite line.[1]

3. B

   The great majority of localized overgrowths of the oral mucosa are considered to be reactive inflammatory hyperplasia rather than neoplastic in nature.[2]

4. A

   It is usually due to chronic and constant irritation such as; cheek or lip biting, rubbing from a rough tooth, dentures or other dental prostheses.[3]

5. D

   fibroma consist of dense collagen fibers, the accumulation of collagen fibers creates tension on surrounding epithelium. This causes epithelium to stretch, resulting in epithelial atrophy. There is also blunt or no reteridges.[4]

Reference:

1. Regezi JA, Sciubba J. Oral Pathology: Clinical Pathologic Correlations.2nd ed.Philadelphia, Pa: WB Saunders. 1997.

2. Toida M et al. Irritation fibroma of the oral mucosa: A clinicopathological study of 129lesions in 124 cases. Oral Med Pathol2001;6:91-94

3. Gonsalves WC, Chi AA, Neville BW. Common oral lesions: Part II. Masses and neoplasia. Am Fam Physician 2007;75: 509-12.

Lichen Planus

Prof. Shaleen Chandra, Dept. Of Oral Pathology & Microbiology

A 17-year-old male presented with burning sensation in his gums, difficulty in eating, discomfort and sensitivity in the gingiva on consumption of acidic or spicy food and drinks and swallowing for 6 months. No cutaneous lesions were visible. Intraoral examination revealed peeling of the underlying gingival epithelium, where red erosion of the connective tissue involving the entire maxillary and mandibular buccal and lingual/palatal surfaces was observed.

1. Grinspan syndrome is associated with-
   (A) Hypertension, diabetes, O.L.P
   (B) Oral, ocular, genital lesions
   (C) Hypertension with oral lesions
   (D) Pemphigus, CHF, diabetes

2. Lichen planus:
   (A) Can undergo malignant change
   (B) Treated only by medication
   (C) Must be excised
   (D) Is an idiosyncrasy reaction

3. Wickham'sstriae are seen in:
   (A) Lichen planus
   (B) Leukoplakia
   (C) Leukoedema
   (D) Psoriasis

4. White radiating lines can be observed in case of lesions of:
   (A) lichen planus
   (B) leukoplakia
   (C) pemphigus
   (D) erythema multiforme

5. Primary skin lesions In lichen planus is:
   (A) macule
   (B) papule
   (C) vesicle
   (D) bulla

Answers:

1. A

   Grinspan syndrome is associated withHypertension, diabetes, O.L.P

2. A

   Lichen Planus is a premalignant condition

3. A

   Lichen Planus is characterized by presence of Wickham's striae.

4. A

   These lines are the Wickham's striae

5. B

   Skin lesions in Lichen Planus appears are papules

Reference:

1. Neville BW, Damn DD, Allen CM, Bouquot JE.Oral & Maxillofacial Pathology, 2nd Ed.New Delhi:Elsevier:2005.

Leukoplakia

Prof. Shaleen Chandra, Dept. of Oral Pathology & Microbiology

A white-colored, even area within the left maxillary mucolabial sulcus, of uncertain duration, is noted by a dental practitioner in a 64-year-old woman who denies smoking and alcohol consumption. The surrounding mucosa is clinically normal. The intra-oral and head and neck examination is otherwise unremarkable.

1. The most common pre-cancerous lesion for oral malignancy is:

    (A) Chronic hypertrophic candidiasis
    (B) Leukoplakia
    (C) Dental ulcer
    (D) Atrophic glossitis

2. Acanthosis with intraepitilialvacuolation and hyper parakeratosis is seen in:

    (A) Hairy tongue
    (B) Hyperplastic candidiasis
    (C) Speckled leukoplakia
    (D) Desquamative gingivitis

3. Leukoplakia with the worst prognosis is seen on the:

    (A) Dorsum of tongue
    (B) Floor of mouth
    (C) Buccal mucosa
    (D) Palate

4. Most common site of oral leukoplakia is:

    (A) angle of mouth
    (B) cheek mucosa
    (C) soft palate
    (D) gingiva

5. Iincreased incidence of carcinoma is observed with:

    (A) homogenous leukoplakia
    (B) verrucous leukoplakia
    (C) nodular leukoplakia
    (D) none of the above

Answers:

1. B

    Leukoplakia is the most common oral premalignant lesion

2. C

    Speckled leukoplakia is characterized by, acanthosis with intraepitilialvacuolation and hyper parakeratosis

3. B

    Lesions present on floor of mouth have the highest rate of malignant transformation

4. B

    Buccal mucosa is the most common site of Leukoplakia

5. C

    Nodular leukoplakia has higher incidence of malignant transformation

Reference:

1. Neville BW, Damn DD, Allen CM, Bouquot JE.Oral & Maxillofacial Pathology, 2nd Ed.New Delhi:Elsevier:2005.

Keratoacanthoma

Prof. Shaleen Chandra, Dept. of Oral Pathology & Microbiology

A 40-year-old farmer was referred to us with a 7-month complaint of lower lip ulceration. There was no description of previous local trauma, as well as 20 years of smoking. Her medical history was otherwise unremarkable. Facial examination revealed a 1.5-cm nodule on the vermillion border of lower lip. It was asymptomatic, sessile, flat and well-defined. Its surface was erythematous and ulcerated, partially recovered by a brown and adherent crust. The margins of the lesion were indurated and apparently infiltrative.

1. What can be the provisional diagnosis for the case described above

    (A) Basal cell carcinoma
    (B) Squamous cell carcinoma
    (C) keratoacanthoma
    (D) Verrucous carcinoma

2. Keratoacanthoma is a ....malignancy originated in ....cells

    (A) High grade, epithelial
    (B) Low grade, pilosebaceous gland
    (C) High grade, salivary gland
    (D) Low grade, spinous layer of epithelial

3. Keratoacanthoma is also called as

    (A) Self-healing carcinoma
    (B) Molluscum sebaceum
    (C) Verrucoma
    (D) All of above

4. which is the characteristic of keratoacanthoma histologically

    (A) Cellular atypia with central crater
    (B) Cellular Dysplasia with central crater
    (C) Gradual change of normal epithelium into hyperplastic acanthotic epithelium with central crater
    (D) Abrupt change of normal epithelium into hyperplastic acanthotic epithelium with central crater

5. Treatment of choice for self-healing carcinoma is

    (A) Wait and watch
    (B) Surgical excision
    (C) Modified radical neck dissection
    (D) Topical steroid application

351

Answers:

1. C

   lower lip is the most common site for actinic chelitis, keratoacanthoma, and squamous cell carcinoma

2. B

   Keratoacanthoma or self-healing ulcer is a low grade malignancy of pilosebaceous glands.

3. D

   Dkeratoacanthoma or self-healing ulcer is a low grade malignancy of pilosebaceous glands.

4. D

   Abrupt change of normal epithelium into hyperplastic acanthotic epithelium with central crater.

5. B

   Usually this lesion heals by its own, but surgical excision is the treatment of choice.

Reference:

1.   Rajendran R., Sivapathasundharam B.: Shafer's Text Book of Oral Pathology.6th Ed.New Delhi:Elsevier; 2009-2010.

Chapter - 6

Periodontology

Gingival Enlargement

Dr. RameshwariSinghal, Assistant Professor, Departmentof Periodontology

A 29 year old female presented to the outpatient department of Periodontology with the chief complaint of painless, localised swelling in her gums. On taking history the patient was found to be three months pregnant without any other contributory medical history. Her clinical oral examination revealed poor oral hygiene with inflammatory changes in the gingiva. The clinical presentation of the pedunculated swelling is displayed in the picture below. As the treating dentist analyse the case with the following questions:

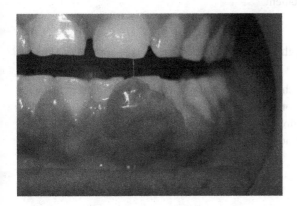

1. What would be the most likely clinical diagnosis

    (A) (A) Pregnancy epulis
    (B) Drug induced gingivitis
    (C) Plasma cell gingivitis
    (D) Leukemic gingivitis

2. The confirmation of diagnosis is based on:

    (A) Clinical presentation of the lesion alone
    (B) Clinical presentation of the lesion and clinical condition of the patient
    (C) Clinical presentation, clinical condition of patient and biopsy of the lesion
    (D) None of the above

3. The above enlargement is

    (A) Induced by hormonal changes alone
    (B) Induced by inflammation due to plaque alone
    (C) Induced due to exaggerated response of plaque on gingival tissue due to pregnancy
    (D) Induce due to trauma from occlusion.

4. Which bacteria are mostly associated with this kind of enlargement
   (A) Streptoccoccusmitis
   (B) Aggregatibacteractinomycetemcomitans
   (C) Porphyromanasgingivalis
   (D) Prevotellaintermedia

5. The present case could resemble pregnancy induced gingival enlargement due to the following features
   (A) Dusky red or magenta in colour
   (B) Deep red pinpoint markings on a smooth shining glistening surface
   (C) Mushroom like enlargement
   (D) All of the above

6. The treatment of choice for this lesion would be
   (A) SRP alone
   (B) Conservative (SRP) with excision of enlargement as it is interferring with occlusion and mastication.
   (C) Excision of the lesion alone
   (D) Conservative with excision and reinforced oral hygiene measures.

Answers:

1. A

   Pregnancy epulis.

   It may be a conditioned enlargement associated with the hormonal changes in the patient inducing exaggerated plaque response on the gingival tissues. [1]

2. C

   Clinical presentation, clinical condition of patient and biopsy of the lesion.

   Altough clinical presentation and ptient's clinical condition are enough diagnostic parameters, biosy confirmation is required to rule out other causes of gingival enlargement. [1]

3. C

   Induced due to exaggerated response of plaque on gingival tissue due to pregnancy.

   It is a conditioned enlargement. [1]

4. D

   Prevotellaintermedia

   This bacterial species utilises estradiol and progesterone (hormones increased in pregnancy) as their essential growth factors. [1]

5. D

   All of the above

   The clinical presentation of pregnancy tumour is a discrete, mushroom like, pedunculated or sessile spherical mass protruding from the interproximal space. It is mostly magenta or dusky red in colour and has a smooth, glistening surface with numerous pinpoint deep red markings. [1]

6. D

   Conservative with excision and reinforced oral hygiene measures.

   Treatment includes thorough scaling and root planing with excision of the lesion. However, it tends to reoccur if meticulous oral hygiene measures are not followed. Therefore, reinforcement of oral hygiene measures are of utmost importance in treatment planning. [1]

Reference:

1. Newman GM, Takei HH, Klokkevold PR, Carranza FA. Carranza's Clinical Periodontology. 10th ed. Missouri: Saunders; 2006. p. 373- 87.

Endo- Perio Lesion

Dr. RameshwariSinghal, Assistant Professor, Department of Periodontology

A 17 year old female presented to the presented to the outpatient department of Periodontology with the chief complaint of pain in her right upper molar region with swelling. Patient also complained of on and off salty discharge in her right side posterior region. On clinical examination, a deep carious lesion was present in relation to tooth no. 16. The patient had very poor oral hygiene. The calculus was seen covering the occlusal surfaces on the right sided posterior dentition. A sinus tract was also observed on the overlying gingiva of 16. Probing measurements of the tooth were not possible due to heavy band of calculus circumscribing the tooth. The clinical case may be evaluated as:

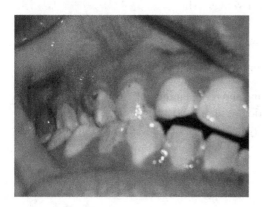

1. The present sinus opening may be due to:

   (A) Periodontal lateral abscess
   (B) Endodontic apical abscess
   (C) Gingival abscess
   (D) Combined perioendo lesion.

2. The occlusal surface on right side is covered by calculus. This indicates

   (A) Bilateral chewing by the patient
   (B) Unilateral chewing on the left side by the patient
   (C) Unilateral chewing on the right side by the patient
   (D) No relation with mastication.

3. The confirmation regarding the origin of sinus tract may be done utilising

   (A) Intraoral periapical radiograph
   (B) Panaromic radiograph

    (C) Intraoral periapical radiograph with guttaperchamanoevoured through the sinus opening

    (D) Intraoral periapical radiograph with guttaperchamanoevoured through the gingival sulcus

4.   Assuming that the lesion is primary endodontic lesion with no periodontal attachment loss, the treatment that would suffice for sinus resolution is

    (A) Scaling root planing alone

    (B) Endodontic and conservative periodontal treatment.

    (C) Periodontal surgery and curettage.

    (D) Combined periradicular and periodontal surgery.

5.   The treatment sequence for the following case would be:

    (A) SRP→ Endodontic opening→ completion of endodontic treatment → periodontal surgery→ endodontic surgery→ maintenance therapy→ prosthodontic tooth rehabilitation

    (B) Endodontic opening→ SRP→ completion of endodontic treatment → endodontic surgery→ periodontal surgery→ prosthodontic tooth rehabilitation→ maintenance therapy

    (C) Endodontic opening→ SRP→ completion of endodontic treatment → endodontic and periodontal surgery (if required both or any one) → prosthodontic tooth rehabilitation→ maintenance therapy

    (D) SRP → Endodontic opening→ completion of endodontic treatment → endodontic and periodontal surgery (if required both or any one) → prosthodontic tooth rehabilitation→ maintenance therapy

Answers:

1.   D

Combined perioendo lesion.

Since we are not able to assess the periodontal status and are aware of just the endodontic status; we will have to presume it to be a periodontal as well as endodontic lesion until proved otherwise. [1,2]

2.   B

Unilateral chewing on the left side by the patient.

The occlusal surface on the right side is covered with calculus indicating that this side is not used for chewing. The mastication process has a cleansing action on the tooth nad it prevents calculus deposition. [1]

3. C

    Intraoral periapical radiograph with gutta-percha manoevoured through the sinus opening. It may also be manoevoured through the gingival sulcus but since the band of calculus has prevented the probing measurements, the GP entry was also not possible. [1,2]

4. B

    Endodontic and conservative periodontal treatment.

    Main treatment requirement is endodontic. However SRP is required for resolution of gingival inflammation, esthetics and infection control. [1,2]

5. C

    Endodontic opening→ SRP→ completion of endodontic treatment → endodontic and periodontal surgery (if required both or any one) → prosthodontic tooth rehabilitation→ maintenance therapy

    Treatment sequence is emergency opening of root canal for pain relief and drainage establishment through the tooth followed by phase I therapy i.e. SRP.

    The Root canal therapy is completed and resolution of sinus analysed. If required endodontic surgery for sinus resolution is done and surgical periodontal therapy for pocket resolution if required is planned. Occlusal rehabilitation for proper mastication on right side is established and patient put on maintenance periodic recall program. [1, 2]

References:

1. Newman GM, Takei HH, Klokkevold PR, Carranza FA. Carranza's Clinical Periodontology. 10th ed. Missouri: Saunders; 2006.

2. Cohen S, Burns RC. Pathways of the pulp. 6th ed. St Louis: Mosby; 2008.

Gingival Recession

Dr. Rameshwari Singhal, Assistant Professor, Department of Periodontology

An 18 year old male patient presented to the outpatient department of Periodontology with the chief complaint of sensitivity to cold in his lower anterior teeth. On taking history, he reported to have got his oral prophylaxis done one week earlier due to the problem of bleeding from gums and bad breath. On examination exposed root in relation to tooth no. 41 was observed. Tooth no. 31 and 41 were also found to be Grade I mobile with shallow pockets mesially and distally. Fremitus test was positive (+) for anterior teeth. The case may be evaluated as:

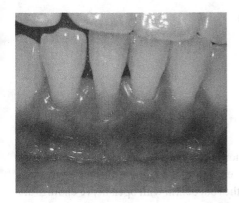

1. What would be the most likely cause of cold sensitivity in this case:

    (A) Exposed root surface
    (B) Post scaling exposure of root surface
    (C) Reduction in gingival inflammation
    (D) Trauma to the tooth

2. The most likely reason for gingival recession in this case may be:

    (A) Gingival inflammation
    (B) Trauma from occlusion
    (C) Faulty toothbrushing
    (D) Tooth malposition

3. What kind of gingival recession is present in tooth no. 41:

    (A) Miller's class I
    (B) Miller's class II
    (C) Miller's class III
    (D) Miller's class IV

4. Tooth mobility in tooth no. 31 & 41 may be due to:

   (A) Gingival inflammation
   (B) Trauma from occlusion
   (C) Both A+B
   (D) None of the above

5. Treatment for sensitivity in this case would be:

   (A) Desensitising paste
   (B) SRP+ splinting+ root coverage with increase in width of attached gingiva
   (C) SRP + relief of trauma+ splinting+ root coverage with increase in width of attached gingiva
   (D) SRP + relief of trauma+ splinting

Answers:

1. B

   Post scaling exposure of root surface.

   The patient had different complaint prior to scaling. The oral prophylaxis in itself leads to tooth sensitivity. In this case, exposure of recession further aggravated the condition. The dentinal tubules in the root dentin with open nerve endings are exposed leading to cold sensation. [1]

2. A

   Gingival inflammation.

   The mechanism of trauma from occlusion in causing recession is not demonstrated. No abrasion is observed in the picture ruling out abrasion due to toothbrush trauma. [1]

3. C

   Miller's class III

   The case mentions interproximal pockets indicating interproximal bone loss. [1]

4. C

   Gingival inflammation + Trauma from occlusion.

   Since fremitus test is positive TFO cannot be ruled out in causing tooth mobility. [1]

5. C

SRP + relief of trauma+ splinting+ root coverage with increase in width of attached gingiva.[1]

Reference:

1. Newman GM, Takei HH, Klokkevold PR, Carranza FA. Carranza's Clinical Periodontology. 10th ed. Missouri: Saunders; 2006.

Periodontal Abscess

Dr. Rosy Bansal, JR III, Dr. Pavitra Rastogi, Associate
Professor, Department of Periodontology

A 62 year old female presented with asymptomatic discharging sinus in buccal sulcus between the apical areas of upper lateral incisor and canine. Radiograph taken of 22, 23, and 24 revealed a radiolucency associated with 23 and 2A further radiograph taken with gutta purcha point inserted into sinus revealed a pear shaped radiolucency between 22and 23.

1. What is the diagnosis of this lesion between 22 and 23:

    (A) Periapical abscess.
    (B) Periodontal abscess.
    (C) Pericoronal abscess.
    (D) Gingival abscess.

2. How the periodontal abscess formed:

    (A) Incomplete removal of calculus during treatment of periodontal pocket.
    (B) Trauma to the tooth.
    (C) Perforation of the lateral wall of the root during endodontic therapy.
    (D) All of the above

3. Periodontal abscess may be:

    (A) Abscess in the supporting periodontal tissue along the lateral aspect of the root.
    (B) Abscess in the soft tissue wall of the deep periodontal pocket.
    (C) Abscess is the localized accumulation of viable and nonviable PMNs within the periodontal pocket wall.
    (D) All of the above.

4. What is the treatment of chronic periodontal abscess:

    (A) Drainage through the periodontal pocket.
    (B) Drainage through the external incision on the most prominent part of abscess.
    (C) Antibiotic coverage
    (D) All of above.

<u>Answers:</u>

1. B

    Periodontal abscess is localized accumulation of pus in the gingival wall of the periodontal pocket. [1]

2. D

    All of above. [1]

3. D

    All of above. [1]

4. D

    All of above. The treatment of periodontal abscess is incision and drainage with systemic antibiotics. [1]

<u>Reference:</u>

1. Newman GM, Takei HH, Klokkevold PR, Carranza FA. Carranza's Clinical Periodontology. 10th ed. Missouri: Saunders; 2006

Periodontal Pathology

Dr. Surendra Singh, JR. III, Dr. Pavitra Rastogi, Associate
Professor, Department of Periodontology

A 26 years old female patient reported to the department of Periodontology with chief complaint of pain, bad breath and spontaneous gingival bleeding. On clinical examination, erythematous gingival tissues with punched out crater like depression at the crest of interdental papillae were seen. No evidence of clinical attachment loss was observed.

1. The most likely diagnosis of the above case described

    (A) NUP
    (B) NUG
    (C) Desquamative gingivitis
    (D) Pregnancy gingivitis

2. Most common bacteria associated with the above case described

    (A) Gram positive aerobic
    (B) Gram positive anaerobic
    (C) Gram positive anaerobic
    (D) Gram negative anaerobic

3. The condition in which pocket formation does not occur

    (A) Periodontal abscess
    (B) NUG
    (C) Pyogenic granuloma
    (D) Chronic periodontitis

4. Clinical feature of above mention case

    (A) Punched-out crater like depressions at the crest of the interdental papillae
    (B) Erythematous and ulcerated interdental papillae
    (C) Magenta red gingiva
    (D) Widened periodontal ligament

Answers:

1. B

   Necrotizing Ulcerative gingivitis [1]

2. D

   Microorganisms that morphologically resemble cocci, fusiform bacilli, and spirochetes. [1]

3. B

   NUG or NUP does not usually lead to periodontal pocket formation because the necrotic changes involve the marginal gingiva causing recession rather than pocket formation. [1]

4. A

   Characteristic of NUG is Punched-out crater like depressions at the crest of the interdental papillae. [1]

Reference:

1. Newman GM, Takei HH, Klokkevold PR, Carranza FA. Carranza's Clinical Periodontology. 10th ed. Missouri: Saunders; 2006

Periodontal Abscess

Dr. Surendra Singh, JR III, Dr. Pavitra Rastogi, Associate Professor,
Department of Periodontology

A 25 year old female patient reported to the department of periodontology with a chief complaint of dull pain and swelling in lower right back region. On clinical examination there was swelling, pocket and mobility in relation to right mandibular 1st molar. On gentle digital pressure there was pus discharge from gingival sulcus:

1. Most likely diagnosis for the above case

    (A) Pulpal abscess
    (B) Periodontal abscess
    (C) Gingival abscess
    (D) Pericoronal abscess

2. Periodontal abscess is differentiated from periapical abscess

    (A) Pocket depth
    (B) Vitality of tooth
    (C) Radiograph
    (D) Periapical radiolucency

3. Gold standard treatment of abscess is

    (A) Incision and drainage
    (B) Scaling and root planning
    (C) Curettage
    (D) Gingivectomy

4. On pulp vitality test the tooth presents

    (A) Vital
    (B) Non-vital
    (C) Radiolucent
    (D) Radioopaque

Answers:

1. B

   Periodontal abscess [1]

2. B

   In periodontal abscess the tooth is vital. [1]

3. A

   Incision and drainage. [1]

4. A

   Tooth is vital in periodontal abscess on pulp vitality test. [1]

Reference:

1. Newman GM, Takei HH, Klokkevold PR, Carranza FA. Carranza's Clinical Periodontology. 10th ed. Missouri: Saunders; 2006

Oral And Periodontal Manifestations In HIV Patient

Dr. Surendra Singh, JR III, Dr Jaya Dixit, Professor, Dr. Pavitra
Rastogi, Associate Professor, Department of Periodontology

A 42 year old HIV infected male patient reported to the clinic with a white lesion on the lateral border of tongue in his mouth from the last 6 month and no discomfort during mastication. He was diagnosed with HIV infection in 2007, and on ART medications till now. Recent laboratory findings showed a CD4 count of 284cells/mm³ and intraoral examination presents a nonmovable, corrugated or "hairy" white lesion on the lateral margins of the tongue:

1. What would be the most likely clinical diagnosis?

    (A) Candidiasis
    (B) Plasma cell gingivitis
    (C) Oral hairy leukoplakia
    (D) Kapsosis sarcoma

2. Which Organism is mainly associated with above diagnosis

    (A) Cytomegalovirus
    (B) E.B Virus
    (C) Papillomavirus
    (D) Herpes Simplex Virus

3. Most Common site for above lesion

    (A) Base of Tongue
    (B) Lateral Border of Tongue
    (C) Dorsum of Tongue
    (D) Buccal Mucosa

4. Clinical Characteristic of above lesion

    (A) Hairy, Shaggy, Horizontal striations
    (B) Hairy, Shaggy, Vertical striations
    (C) Hairy, Shaggy, No striations
    (D) None of the above

5. According to the CDC Surveillance Case Classification (1993), above lesion categorize in

    (A) Category A
    (B) Category B
    (C) Category C
    (D) Category D

Answers:

1. C

   Oral Hairy Leukoplakia primarily occurs with HIV infections found on lateral border of tongue. [1]

2. B

   Epstein-Barr Virus(EBV) is associated with OHL [1]

3. B

   OHL is found exclusively on the lateral borders of Tongue [1]

4. B

   Clinical characteristic of OHL, Vertical striations, Corrugated appearance, Shaggy and appear HAIRY when dried. [1]

5. B

   According to the CDC Surveillance Case Classification (1993), OHL lesion categorize In Category B [1]

Reference:

1. Newman GM, Takei HH, Klokkevold PR, Carranza FA. Carranza's Clinical Periodontology. 10th ed. Missouri: Saunders; 2006.

Oral and Periodontal Manifestations in HIV Patient

Dr. Surendra Singh, JR III, Dr Jaya Dixit, Professor, Dr.PavitraRastogi,
Associate Professor, Department of Periodontology

A 35year old HIV infected female patient reported to the clinic with 1 month history of a redness in upper anterior region of gingiva with mild burning sensation in his mouth that is accentuated when eating acidic or spicy foods. She was diagnosed with HIV infection in 2014, and on ART medication till now. Recent laboratory finding showed a CD4 count of 87 cells/mm^3 and intraoral examination shows erythema of the marginal gingiva in maxillary anteriors.

1. What would be the most likely clinical diagnosis

   (A) Gingivitis
   (B) Linear Gingival Erythema
   (C) Bacillary angiomatosis
   (D) OHL

2. Which Organism are mostly associated with above lesion

   (A) Candida albicans
   (B) Candida dubliniensis
   (C) CMV
   (D) EBV

3. Site for above Lesion

   (A) Marginal gingiva
   (B) Attached gingiva
   (C) Alveolar mucosa
   (D) All of the above

4. Clinicalcharacteristic of above Lesion

   (A) Erythematous, linear, marginal gingiva
   (B) Erythematous, diffuse, marginal gingiva
   (C) Erythematous, linear, attached gingiva
   (D) Erythematous, diffuse, attachedgingva

5. Treatmentof choice for above lesion

   (A) Amoxicillin
   (B) Fluconazole
   (C) Erythromycin
   (D) Clindamycin

Answers:

1. B

   Linear Gingival Erythema (LGE) [1]

2. B

   Candida dubliniensis are mostly associated with LGE. [1]

3. D

   Limited to marginal gingiva, extend to Attached gingivaand alveolar bone.[1]

4. A

   Clinical characteristic of LGE. Erythematous, linear, marginal gingiva. [1]

5. B

   Treatment of choice for LGE is Antifungal agent –Fluconazole. [1]

Reference:

1. Newman GM, Takei HH, Klokkevold PR, Carranza FA. Carranza's Clinical Periodontology. 10th ed. Missouri: Saunders; 2006.

Acute Gingival Infections

Dr. Manisha Dixit, JR II, Dr. Pavitra Rastogi, Associate
Professor, Department of Periodontology

A 12 year old boy suffers from vesiculating painful ulcers., Oral temperature of 103 degree Fahrenheit since 3 days and lymphadenopathy is present. On oral examination gingiva appears to be shiny and erythematous with varying degrees of edema and gingival bleeding. Ulcers were painful with a red elevated halo- like margin and depressed yellowish or grayish white central portion

1. The most likely diagnosis is

    (A) Herpes zoster
    (B) Acute herpetic gingivostomatitis
    (C) Major apthae
    (D) Recurrent apthae

2. The disease usually occurs

    (A) Prior to age 10
    (B) Between 13 to 30
    (C) At the onset of puberty
    (D) During menopause

3. Treatment of this condition include

    (A) Corticosteroids to reduce inflammation
    (B) Penicillin
    (C) Local antibiotic application
    (D) Antiviral drugs

4. The causative agent of this disease is

    (A) Streptococcus viridians
    (B) HSV-1
    (C) EBV
    (D) None of the above

5. Histological examination will reveal presence of which type of cell

    (A) Tzanck cell
    (B) Lacunar cell
    (C) Giant cell
    (D) Popcorn cell

Answers:

1. B

   All the clinical features are suggestive of acute herpetic gingivostomatitis. [1]

2. A

   It occurs in infants and children of younger age group only. [1]

3. D

   Antiviral drugs can dramatically alter the course of the disease as it is a viral disease. [1]

4. B

   HSV-1 is responsible for infections occurring above the waist. [1]

5. A

   Virus targets epithelial cells, which show ballooning degeneration these cells are called tzanck cells. [1]

Reference:

1. Newman GM, Takei HH, Klokkevold PR, Carranza FA. Carranza's Clinical Periodontology. 10th ed. Missouri: Saunders; 2006

Conditioned Gingival Enlargement

Dr. Manisha Dixit, JR. II, Dr. Pavitra Rastogi, Associate
Professor, Department of Periodontology

A 13 year old girl presented with gingival enlargement that greatly exceeds than that usually seen in association with comparable local factors but it is limited to margins and is characterized by bulbous interproximal papillae

1. The most likely diagnosis is

    (A) Chronic inflammatory gingival enlargement
    (B) Acute inflammatory gingival enlargement
    (C) Pubertal gingival enlargement
    (D) Allergic gingival enlargement

2. This comes under which type of enlargement

    (A) Conditioned GE
    (B) Systemic disease causing GE
    (C) Nonspecific conditioned enlargement
    (D) False enlargement

3. The surface least commonly involved is

    (A) Facial
    (B) Lingual
    (C) Mesial
    (D) distal

4. The distinguishing feature of this disease

    (A) Massive recurrence in the presence of relatively scant plaque deposits
    (B) Excessive amount of supragingival deposits
    (C) Excessive amount of subgingival deposits
    (D) Ulceration present with the enlargement

5. The microorganism responsible for its initiation

    (A) Capnocytophaga
    (B) Prevotellaintermedia
    (C) Porphyromonasgingivalis
    (D) Aggregati bacteria ctinomycetamcomitans

6. The treatment involves
    (A) Scaling root planing and gingivectomy
    (B) Antibiotics
    (C) Open flap debridement
    (D) Only SRP to remove local deposits

Answers:

1. C

    As the enlargement is associated with minimal calculus which is not a feature of inflammatory enlargement and the patient's age is clearly an indication of its nature. [1]

2. A

    Pubertal enlargement comes under conditioned enlargment in which systemic condition of the patient exaggerates or distorts the usual gingival response to dental plaque. [1]

3. B

    Lingual surface is protected by mechanical action of tongue. [1]

4. A

    Pubertal enlargement has a strong tendency to recur even in the absence of calculus. [1]

5. A

    Capnocytophaga is responsible for its initiation. [1]

6. D

    SRP is done to remove local irritants as the disease undergoes spontaneous reduction after puberty. [1]

Reference:

1. Newman GM, Takei HH, Klokkevold PR, Carranza FA. Carranza's Clinical Periodontology. 10th ed. Missouri: Saunders; 2006.

Trauma from Occlusion

Dr.Uzma Ansari, JR II, Dr.PavitraRastogi, Associate
Professor, Department of Periodontology

35 year old female patient reported to the department of periodontology with chief complaint of mobility of teeth and pain on chewing. On clinical examination mandibular anteriors were found to be grade II mobile with wear facets in the absence of any gingival inflammation and pockets in otherwise healthy dentition.

1. What likely diagnosis can be made by above clinical features

    (A) Primary trauma from occlusion
    (B) Secondary trauma from occlusion
    (C) Both of the above
    (D) None of the above

2. What will be the radiographic finding in trauma for occlusion

    (A) Widened periodontal space
    (B) Bone loss (Angular)
    (C) Root resorption
    (D) All of the above

3. Which periodontal structure remain unaffected in trauma from occlusion

    (A) Marginal gingival
    (B) Bone
    (C) Periodontal ligament
    (D) Cementum

4. What treatment must be considered to treat trauma from occlusion

    (A) Occlusal adjustment
    (B) Management of parafunctional habits
    (C) Orthodontic tooth movement
    (D) All of the above

5. Which of the following is not a feature of chronic trauma from occlusion

    (A) Tooth wear
    (B) Drifting movement
    (C) Extrusion of teeth
    (D) Tooth pain

Answers:

1. A

   Primary trauma from occlusion

2. D

   All of the above

3. A

   Marginal gingival

4. D

   All of the above

5. D

   Tooth pain

Reference:

1. Newman GM, Takei HH, Klokkevold PR, Carranza FA. Carranza's Clinical Periodontology. 10th ed. Missouri: Saunders; 2006

Acute Necrotizing Ulcerative Gingivitis

Dr.Uzma Ansari, JR. II, Dr. Pavitra Rastogi, Associate
Professor, Department of Periodontology

A 40 years old male reported to the department of Periodontology with the chief complaint of ulcers on the gums, bad breath and pain on chewing. On general examination headache, fever and malaise was observed. On intra oral examination sharply punched out crater like lesions of the interdental papillae with pseudomembrane were noted.

1. What likely diagnosis can be made

   (A) ANUG
   (B) Pericornitis
   (C) Aute herpetic gingivitis
   (D) Desquamative gingivitis

2. In the first visit these patient should be treated with

   (A) Antifungal drugs.
   (B) Deep scaling and root planing
   (C) Superficial scaling debridement and chlorhexidine mouth wash.
   (D) Mucogingival surgery

3. Most common microorganisms involved in ANUG are

   (A) Actinobacillusactinomycetemcomitans
   (B) Streptococcus viridians
   (C) Fusiform bacilli and spirochetes
   (D) None of the above

4. Most commonly affected site is

   (A) Interdental papillae and marginal gingival
   (B) Attached gingival
   (C) Buccal mucosa and lips
   (D) Diffuse gingival involvement

Answers:

1. A

   ANUG: Punched out crater like erosions of the interdental papillae a characteristic features of ANUG [1]

2. C

   Superficial scaling debridement and chlorhexidine mouth wash. Lesion are painful so only symptomatic treatment is given in the first visit. [1]

3. C

   Fusiform bacilli and spirochetes. [1]

4. A

   Interdental papillae and marginal gingiva. [1]

Reference:

1. Newman GM, Takei HH, Klokkevold PR, Carranza FA. Carranza's Clinical Periodontology. 10th ed. Missouri: Saunders; 2006.

Necrotising Gingival Diseases

Dr. Shalini Kaushal, Associate Professor, Dr.Vaibhav Sheel, JR.
III, Dr. Umesh Patel, JR II, Department of Periodontology

A 30 year old male reported to the department of Periodontology with the chief complaint of ulceration of the gums and on general examination fever, headache and malaise was seen. On oral examination sharply punched out crater like erosion of the interdental papillae of sudden onset were observed.

Patient also complains of metallic taste and halitosis.

1. Identify the condition

    (A) Pericoronitis

    (B) ANUG

    (C) Chediak Higashi syndrome

    (D) Desquamative gingivitis

2. In the first appointment, the patient should be treated with

    (A) Deep scaling and curettage

    (B) Superficial scaling and chlorhexidine mouthwash

    (C) Antifungal drugs

    (D) All of the above

3. The microbiota associated with ANUG is

    (A) Actinomycetumcomitans

    (B) Borrelia and Fusobacterium

    (C) Streptococcus mutans

    (D) Candida albicans

4. ANUG affects mainly

    (A) Attached gingival

    (B) Interdental papilla

    (C) Marginal gingival

    (D) Alveolar mucosa

5. Stage V of ANUG is characterised by

    (A) Necrosis exposing alveolar bone

    (B) Necrosis perforating cheek

    (C) Necrosis extending to attach gingival

    (D) Necrosis extending into buccal mucosa

Answers:

1. B

   ANUG [1]

2. B

   Treatment of NUP includes local debridement of lesions with scaling and root planning.[1]

3. B

   Light microscopy shows that the exudate on the surface of the necrotic lesions contains microorganisms that morphologically resemble cocci, fusiform bacilli, and spirochetes. [1]

4. B

   Characteristic lesions are punched-out, craterlike depressions at the crest of the interdental papillae. [1]

5. D

   Horning and cohen extended the staging of these oral necrotising diseases, Stage V: necrosis extend into buccal or labial mucosa. [1]

Reference:

1. Newman GM, Takei HH, Klokkevold PR, Carranza FA. Carranza's Clinical Periodontology. 10th ed. Missouri: Saunders; 2006.

Localised Aggressive Periodontitis

Dr. Shalini Kaushal, Associate Professor, Dr.Vaibhav Sheel, JR.
III, Dr. Umesh Patel, JR. II, Department of Periodontology

A 16 year old female reported to the department of periodontology with the chief complaint of spacing between the teeth. Her OPG revealed vertical bone defects in the 1st molar and incisor region and clinically minimal amounts of supragingivalplaque was present.

1. The condition referred to is

    (A) Generalised juvenile periodontitis
    (B) Localised juvenile periodontitis
    (C) Desquamative gingivitis
    (D) Chronic periodontitis

2. The bacteria associated with above condition is

    (A) Gram positive aerobic cocci
    (B) Gram negative aerobic cocci
    (C) Gram positive anaerobic cocci
    (D) Gram negative anaerobic rods

3. Term juvenile periodontitis was coined by

    (A) Chaput and Butler
    (B) Gottlieb and Orban
    (C) Gustafson et al
    (D) Socransky

4. Antibiotic of choice in juvenile periodontitis

    (A) Tetracycline
    (B) Penicillin
    (C) Metronidazole
    (D) Amoxycillin

Answers:

1. B

   In 1989 the world workshop in clinical periodontics categorized this disease as"localized juvenile periodontitis" (LJP). [1]

2. B

   Actinomycetemcomitans is found in high frequency (approximately 90%) in lesions characteristic of LAP. [1]

3. A

   Chaput and colleagues in 1967 and by Butler in 1969. [1]

4. A

   Systemic tetracycline (250 mg of tetracycline hydrochloride four times daily for atleast 1 week) should be given in conjunction with local mechanical therapy. [1]

Reference:

1. Newman GM, Takei HH, Klokkevold PR, Carranza FA. Carranza's Clinical Periodontology. 10th ed. Missouri: Saunders; 2006.

Gingival Changes in Childhood

Dr. Shalini Kaushal, Associate Professor, Dr. Vaibhav Sheel, JR III, Dr. Umesh Patel, JR II, Department of Periodontology

A 13 year old female reported to the department of Periodontology with inflammation of marginal gingiva along with crowding of teeth. She also gave the history of frequent consumption of sweets between the meals

1. The most prevalent type of gingival disease in childhood

   (A) Primary herpetic gingivostomatitis
   (B) ANUG
   (C) Chronic marginal gingivitis
   (D) Chronic Periodontitis

2. The primary cause of gingivitis in children is

   (A) High fever
   (B) Oral habits
   (C) Malocclusion
   (D) Poor oral hygiene

3. Increased calculus formation in children is associated with which of the following

   (A) AIDS
   (B) Papillion LeFevre syndrome
   (C) Cystic fibrosis
   (D) All of the above

4. The incidence of marginal gingivitis in children is maximum at

   (A) 4-5 yrs of age
   (B) 11-13 yrs of age
   (C) At the eruption of all teeth
   (D) None of the above

Answers:

1. C

   The most prevalent type of gingival disease in childhood is chronic marginal gingivitis. [1]

2. D

   In children, as in adults, the primary cause of gingivitis is dental plaque, which is favoured by poor oral hygiene. [1]

3. C

   In children with cystic fibrosis the incidence of dental calculus is much higher and the deposits are greater this may be caused by increased calcium and phosphate concentrations in saliva. [1]

4. B

   The incidence of marginal gingivitis peaks at 11to 13 years of age, then decreases slightly after puberty. [1]

Reference:

1. Newman GM, Takei HH, Klokkevold PR, Carranza FA. Carranza's Clinical Periodontology. 10th ed. Missouri: Saunders; 2006.

Gingival Enlargement

Dr. ShaliniKaushal, Associate Professor, Dr. VaibhavSheel, JR
II, Dr. Umesh Patel, JR II, Department of Periodontology

A 23 year old pregnant female reported with the chief complaint of over growth of gum in upper front teeth since 5 months. On clinical examination oral hygiene status was fair and gingiva appeared reddish, ulcerated, soft and friable and was associated with bleeding on slight provocation. Radiographically no changes in bone seen.

1. The most likely diagnosis of the case described

   (A) Pregnancy gingivitis
   (B) Drug induced enlargement
   (C) Chronic marginal gingivitis
   (D) Idiopathic drug enlagement

2. Most causative agent associated with pregnancy gingivitis

   (A) Prevotellaintermedia
   (B) Fusobacterium
   (C) T.forsythia
   (D) P.gingivalis

3. The microorganisms associated with pregnancy belongs to which complex

   (A) Red
   (B) Orange
   (C) Green
   (D) Yellow

4. Gingivitis in pregnangy is called as

   (A) Pyogenic granuloma
   (B) Angiogranuloma
   (C) Wegener's granulomatosis
   (D) Sarcoidosis

5. The histopathological picture of pregnangy gingivitis

   (A) Localized areas of necrosis
   (B) Replacement of the fatty marrow by fibrous tissue
   (C) Chronic inflammatory infiltrate with varying degrees of edema
   (D) Spongiosis and infiltration with inflammatory cells

Answers:

1. A

    Enlargement during pregnancy may be marginal and generalized or may occur as single or multiple tumor-like masses. [1]

2. A

    The subgingivalmicrobiota may also undergoes changes, including an increase in prevotellaintermedia. [1]

3. B

    The orange complex includes fusobacterium, prevotella, and campylobacter species. [1]

4. B

    Gingival enlargement in pregnangy is called angiogranuloma. [1]

5. C

    Engorged capillaries lined by cuboid endothelial cells, as well as amoderately fibrous stroma with varying degrees of edema and chronic inflammatory infiltrate. [1]

Reference:

1. Newman GM, Takei HH, Klokkevold PR, Carranza FA. Carranza's Clinical Periodontology. 10th ed. Missouri: Saunders; 2006.

Influence of Systemic Disorders on Periodontium

Dr. Shalini Kaushal, Associate Professor, Dr. Vaibhav Sheel, JR
II, Dr. Umesh Patel, JR II, Department of Periodontology

A 35 year old female suffering from advanced kidney disease reported to the department of Periodontolgy and her periapical radiograph shows ground glass appearance of bone and loss of lamina dura.

1. The condition referred to is

   (A) Hyperparathyroidism
   (B) Hypoparathyroidism
   (C) Hypothyroidism
   (D) Hyperthyroidism

2. Hyperparathyroidism is also known as

   (A) Von Recklinghausen disease of bones
   (B) Von Recklinghausen disease of skin
   (C) both of above.
   (D) none of above

3. Pseudocysts or brown tumours are a characteristic feature of

   (A) osteitisdeformans
   (B) fibrous dysplasia
   (C) osteitisfibrosacystica
   (D) osteomalacia

4. Radiographic signs of hyperparathyroid bone disease is/are

   (A) widening of periodontal ligament
   (B) absence of lamina dura
   (C) giant cell tumours
   (D) all of the above

Answers:

1. A

    Hyperparathyroidism. [1]

2. A

    The disease is called osteitisfibrosacystica, or von recklinghausen's bone diseases. [1]

3. C

    Bone cysts become filled with fibrous tissue with abundant hemosiderinladen macrophages and giant cells. these cysts have been called brown tumors. [1]

4. D

    Radiographic evidence of alveolar osteoporosis with closely meshed trabeculae, widening of the periodontal liagament, absence of lamina dura, and radiolucent cystic spaces. [1]

Reference:

1. Newman GM, Takei HH, Klokkevold PR, Carranza FA. Carranza's Clinical Periodontology. 10th ed. Missouri: Saunders; 2006.

Gingival Recession

Dr. Rosy Bansal, JR II, Dr. Pavitra Rastogi, Associate
Professor, Department of Periodontology

A 20 year old male patient reported to the department of periodontology with chief complaint of receding gums in lower anterior region. On intraoral examination, an isolated gingival recession on the labial surface of lower right central incisor (#41) with inter-proximal soft tissue loss and presence of trauma from occlusion.

1. The most likely cause of gingival recession in this case may be:

   (A) Class I
   (B) Class II
   (C) Class III
   (D) Class IV

2. What type of recession in lower left canine?

   (A) Gingival inflammation
   (B) Trauma from occlusion
   (C) Faulty tooth brushing
   (D) Tooth mal-position

3. Clinical feature of trauma from occlusion:

   (A) Gingival recession
   (B) Mobility
   (C) Wear facets
   (D) Widening of periodontal ligament space
   (E) All of above

4. What type of recession in lower right incisor

   (A) Class I
   (B) Class II
   (C) Class III
   (D) Class IV

Answers:

1. B

    The most common cause of gingival recession is faulty tooth brushing but in this case recession is due to trauma from occlusion. [1]

2. E

    Excessive occlusal forces causes painful spasm, injure the TMJ, produce excessive tooth wear, widening of ligament space, tooth mobility and gingival recession. [1]

3. C

    Miller's class III type of recession because there is marginal tissue recession extends beyond the mucogingival junction with inter-proximal bone and soft tissue loss. [1]

4. B

    Miller's class II because of buccal gingival recession extend to or beyond the mucco-gingival junction without inter-proximal bone loss. [1]

References:

1. Newman GM, Takei HH, Klokkevold PR, Carranza FA. Carranza's Clinical Periodontology. 10th ed. Missouri: Saunders; 2006.

Advanced Implant Surgery

Dr.Umesh PratapVerma, Associate Professor, Department of Periodontology

A 24 year old female was referred to Department of Periodontology. She had lost her tooth due to endodontic failure a year ago. She was interested for best treatment modality to replace her missing tooth. On Clinical examination a concavity at facial aspect of maxillary left lateral incisor region. Radiological analysis consisted of Intra-Oral Peri apical X-rays, OPG, Dentascan of Maxilla. Initially, Phase I Therapy and subsequently 3.3x10mm Threaded Implant (US-FDA Certified) was placed, resulting in the visibility of 5 to 6 threads due to peri-implant defects. Bio-oss with resorbable barrier membrane (BioMesh) were placed to cover the defect. 6 months later during second stage surgery, re-entry was performed.

Clinically, the defect was restored by the GBR. The patient was satisfied with her treatment after more than 18 months. Thus, the use of Bio-Oss and BioMesh is effective in guided bone regeneration procedure for restoration of an unintentionally occurring facial peri-implant defects associated with the placement of implant.

1. The exposures of the implant's axial surface that do not include the coronal aspect of the implant is called as-

   (A) Fenestration defects
   (B) Dehiscence defects
   (C) Horizontal defects
   (D) Vertical defects

2. When a part of the implant's axial surface expose, including the coronal aspect of the implant, while maintaining sufficient bone volume around all remaining implant surfaces is known as

   (A) Fenestration defects
   (B) Dehiscence defects
   (C) Horizontal defects
   (D) Vertical defects

3. Which of the following is best treatment modality of dehiscence and fenestration defects during placement of implants

   (A) Guided bone regeneration
   (B) Autogenous bone graft
   (C) Cancellous bone graft
   (D) Collagen membrane

4. Which of the following is resorbable membrane used in guided bone regeneration
   (A) Titanium reinforced
   (B) Biomesh
   (C) PTFE
   (D) ePTFE

5. Which of the following type of flap is best for regenerative procedures.
   (A) Modified widman flap
   (B) Conventional flap
   (C) Papilla preservation flap
   (D) Displaced flap

Answers:

1. A

   Most common type of defects can be seen during simultaneous placement of implants in alveolar deficient patients. [1]

2. B

   When bucco-lingual width of alveolar crest is minimal and clinically soft tissue concavity can be seen in such kind of alveolar deficient patients. [1]

3. A

   The main aim of the guided bone regeneration is to regenerate the alveolar bone by using membrane with osseous graft. [1]

4. B

   It contains PGA and PLA which is biodegradable by hydrolysis. [1]

5. C

   It provides the complete coverage of the interdental area. [1]

Reference:

1. Newman GM, Takei HH, Klokkevold PR, Carranza FA. Carranza's Clinical Periodontology. 11th ed. Missouri: Saunders; 2011.

Periimplantitis

Dr.UmeshPratapVerma, Associate Professor, Department of Periodontology

A 35 year old patients reported to the department of Periodontology with chief complain of slight mobility of his artificial tooth in right mandibular posterior region. His dental history revealed that his missing tooth was restored with dental implant about 12months back. Clinical examination showed inflamed red gingiva with 1° mobility in that tooth. Deep periodontal pocket was observed on mesial, distal, and buccal surfaces of 4Radiologically, periapical radiolucency was depicted which extended to apical portion of Implant.

1. Which of the following is a diagnosis of the above periapical lesion?

    (A) Periodontitis
    (B) Periimplantitis
    (C) Pericoronitis
    (D) Mucositis

2. Which of the following is a best method to diagnose a compromised implant site?

    (A) Periodontal probing
    (B) Clinical evaluation
    (C) Radiological
    (D) Biochemical

3. The following are the risk indicators for periimplantitis EXCEPT.

    (A) Diabetes
    (B) Smoking
    (C) Implant surface
    (D) Keratin ized gingival

4. Which of the following is best treatment modality of alveolar bone augmentation in Periimplantitis?

    (A) Guided bone regeneration
    (B) Debridement
    (C) Detoxification
    (D) CHX irrigation

Answers:

1. B

   Inflammatory process affecting the tissue around osseointegrated implants. [1]

2. C

   Standardized radiographic techniques have been well documented and found to be useful in evaluating periimplant bone level. [1]

3. D

   Keratinized tissue forms strong seal around the implant and provides better functional and esthetic results for implant restoration. [1]

4. A

   This procedure is well documented for the regeneration of bone. [1]

Reference:

1. Newman GM, Takei HH, Klokkevold PR, Carranza FA. Carranza's Clinical Periodontology. 11th ed. Missouri: Saunders; 2011.

Interdisciplinary Dentistry

Dr.Umesh Pratap Verma, Associate Professor, Department of Periodontology

A 17 year old girl reported to the Department of Periodontology. The patient was in excellent general health with no known allergies, no medications and denied use of tobacco. The patient was presented with spacing and flaring of upper and lowers anterior teeth with poor oral hygiene. The patient had grade I gingival recession present on all surfaces of 31, 32, 41 and 42 and Angle's class I type 2 malocclusion. The spacing was contributed by pressure of tongue on the teeth with reduced periodontal support. The soft tissue of the patient was also unhealthy due to undesirable air flow from mouth (mouth breathing, incompetent lips and large intralabial gaps). This case was successfully managed with collaboration to Department of Orthodontics.

1. What are the adjunctive roles of orthodontic treatment in the management of this case

    (A) Aligning crowded teeth
    (B) Improve the osseous defects
    (C) Aligning the gingival margin
    (D) Corrected the open gingival embrasure

2. What is the importance of initial periodontal therapy during orthodontic treatment in patients

    (A) Control crowding of teeth
    (B) Helps in movement of teeth
    (C) Control periodontal inflammation
    (D) Helps in proper diagnosis

3. In which of the following periodontal conditions require orthodontic treatment for better results.

    (A) Crown lengthening
    (B) Furcation involvment
    (C) Mobile teeth
    (D) Horizontal defect

4. Which of the following factor determined the positon of orthodontic brackets in a periodontally healthy individuals.

    (A) Margin of gingiva
    (B) Anatomy of the crowns of teeth
    (C) Diastema
    (D) Crowding

Answers:

1. D

   In the present case the open gingival embrasure is corrected by the orthodontic treatment to regain lost papilla. [1]

2. C

   It is essential that all calculus is removed and plaque is minimized. Failure to control these factors can lead to gingivitis and even bone loss. [1]

3. A

   Orthodontic extrusion may be used to move tooth correctly in selected patients needing crown lengthening. [1]

4. B

   In periodontally healthy individuals, the position of brackets usually determind by anatomy of the crown. Anterior brackets should be positioned relative to incisal edges and posterior band/brackets are positioned relative to the marginal ridges. [1]

References:

1. Newman GM, Takei HH, Klokkevold PR, Carranza FA. Carranza's Clinical Periodontology. 11th ed. Missouri: Saunders; 2011.

Periodontal Medicine

Dr. Rameshwari Singhal, Assistant Professor and Prof. Nandlal, Professor,
Department of Periodontology

A 45 year old male patient presented with chief complaint of stickiness of mouth. Oral examination revealed severe gingival inflammation, suppuration and deep pockets. Medical history revealed uncontrolled diabetic status.

1. Periodontal disease exacerbation is

   (A) Related to diabetic status of the patient
   (B) Independent of diabetic status of the patient
   (C) The relationship is bidirectional
   (D) the relationship is unidirectional.

2. American diabetes association has termed Periodontal disease as the

   (A) Risk factor for diabetes
   (B) Complication of diabetes
   (C) Sign of diabetes
   (D) Sequence in diabetes development

3. Exacerbation of periodontal disease occurs due to

   (A) Altered leukocyte response
   (B) Change in microbiology
   (C) Formation of altered collagen metabolism
   (D) All of the above.

Answers:

1. C

    Periodontal disease and diabetes relationship is bidirectional with one causing the other factor to exacerbate. [1]

2. B

    Periodontal Disease is the sixth complication of Diabetes.[1]

3. D [1]

Reference:

1. Newman GM, Takei HH, Klokkevold PR, Carranza FA. Carranza's Clinical Periodontology. 10th ed. Missouri: Saunders; 2006.

Furcation Involvement

Dr. Anjani Kumar Pathak, Assistant Professor, Department of Periodontology

A patient reported to the department with pain in the mandibular right first molar. The tooth is sensitive to both thermal stimuli and biting. Also clinical examination reveals a bifurcation involvement with 4-5 mm pockets adjacent to both the roots and the involved tooth was tender on percussion. The remaining dentition was found periodontally sound. The intensity of pain was mild and increased during mastication.

1. The ideal treatment for the above mentioned case would be

    (A) Periodontal scaling and curettage
    (B) Periodontal scaling, curettage and surgery
    (C) Endodontic treatment combined with periodontal therapy
    (D) Endodontic therapy only

2. What surgical procedure is indicated most frequently following endodontic therapy on a mandibular molar having both periodontal bifurcation involvement and extensive bifurcation caries

    (A) Hemisection
    (B) Root Amputation
    (C) Fenestration
    (D) Apical curettage

3. Which of the following perforations has the poorest prognosis

    (A) Perforation near the apex
    (B) Perforation into the furcation
    (C) Perforation through the crown
    (D) Perforation at the cemento enamel junction

4. Most common preferred tooth for hemisection is

    (A) Mandibular 1st molar
    (B) Maxillary 1st molar
    (C) Maxillary premolar
    (D) Mandibular premolar

Answers:

1. C

   The periapical, pulpal and periodontal lesion can be healed through combined endodontic and periodontal therapy.[1]

2. A

   Hemisection obliterates furcation area and makes it self cleansing. [1]

3. B

   Furcation area has poor blood supply and its accessibility is limited. [1]

4. A [1]

Reference:

1. Newman GM, Takei HH, Klokkevold PR, Carranza FA. Carranza's Clinical Periodontology. 10th ed. Missouri: Saunders; 2006.

Pericoronitis

Dr. Anjani Kumar Pathak Assistant Professor, VaibhavSheel
JR III, Department of Periodontology

An 18 yr old female patient reported with the chief complaint of pain and swelling in the lower left jaw and mild difficulty in opening his mouth since last 3-4 days. Her general examination revealed increased pulse rate and fever. Intraoral examination showed signs off inflammation around the gingiva of the partially impacted third molar. Clinical examination revealed that the involved tooth was not completely visible in the oral cavity and was covered by bone distally on radiographic interpretation.

1. The most likely diagnosis is

   (A) OSMF
   (B) Pericoronitis
   (C) Localised Aggressive periodontitis
   (D) Herpetic gingivostomatitis

2. The microorganisms most commonly associated with this condition are

   (A) E.coli
   (B) T. Denticola
   (C) Anaerobic bacteria and streptococci
   (D) Actinomycosis

3. Ideal management of this condition is

   (A) Operculectomy
   (B) Analgesics, antibiotics and irrigation
   (C) Extraction of partially erupted 3rd molar under local anaesthesia
   (D) No treatment, Leave as such

Answers:

1. B

    OSMF and LAP are not associated with fever and herpetic gingivostomatitis is usually seen in infants and children < 6years. [1]

2. B [1]

3. 3 C

    Third molar is a vestigial tooth with no functional importance and associated with lots of complications. [1]

Reference:

1. Newman GM, Takei HH, Klokkevold PR, Carranza FA. Carranza's Clinical Periodontology. 10th ed. Missouri: Saunders; 2006.

Fenestration Defect

Dr. Anjani Kumar Pathak Assistant Professor, Department of Periodontology

The patient was a 22-year-old boy who reported with chief complaint of exposed root of lower left central incisor below the gingiva for the past $2^{1/2}$ to 3 years. The patient was well until 3 years back when he had pain in the concerned tooth which was subsequently discoloured. The patient sought treatment from a local doctor who prescribed medications whereafter the pain subsided. A few weeks later there was pus discharge, for which he again took medications. Thereafter he started loosing the gum over that tooth, for which he visited many dentists, all of whom advised extraction. The patient was apprehensive and continued to live with the problem and seeking alternative treatment and any possibility to save the tooth. He came to OPD of the department of periodontology KGMU for the treatment. The patient was systemically healthy. There was no history of drug intake. He did not smoke or drink alcohol and no habit of tobacco chewing. On clinical examination approximately 10mm long defect was present on non vital lower left central incisor with exposed root apex of tooth along with intact marginal gingiva and a approximately 3mm band of attached gingiva. Periapical radiographic examination revealed a small radiolucent area around the apex of that tooth. A routine haematological examination was advised which revealed no abnormality.

1. The possible diagnosis is

   (A) Dehiscence
   (B) Fenestration
   (C) Apical periodontitis
   (D) Periapical cyst

2. The possible etiology is

   (A) Trauma
   (B) Caries
   (C) Trauma from occlusion
   (D) Periodontal diseases

3. The correct treatment for the defect will be

   (A) Endodontic treatment
   (B) Endodontic treatment with periapical curettage
   (C) Endodontic treatment, periapical curettage followed by bone grafting
   (D) Endodontic treatment, periapical curettage, bone grafting along with soft tissue grafting.

Answers:

1. B

   Isolated areas in which the root is denuded of bone and root surface is covered only by periosteum and overlying gingiva; with marginal bone intact, are termed fenesteration. [1]

2. C

   Trauma from occlusion, prominent root contours and labial protrusion of root with thin bony plates are predisposing factors.[1]

3. D [1]

Reference:

1. Pathak AK, Dixit J, Lal N, Verma UP. Single step perio plastic surgical procedures for combined mucogingivalperiapical and fenesteration defects. J Ind Dent Assoc 2011; 5 (9): 982-984.

Idiopathic Gingival Enlargement

Dr. Anjani Kumar Pathak, Assistant professor, DrUzma
Ansari, JR-II, Department of Periodontology

A 13 year old male patient reported to the Department of Periodontology with a chief complaint of swollen gums involving all his teeth, since last 3 years, preventing proper speech and mastication and causing poor esthetics. She did not give any history of drug intake nor was having any physical and mental disorder, also familial and postnatal history was not contributory. An intraoral examination revealed generalized, diffuse, nodular enlargement of the gingiva involving the upper and lower arches, which were pink in color and had firm and fibrous consistency. Enlarged gingiva covers the incisal / occlusal 3rd of all teeth.

Histological examination shows bulbous increase in connective tissue that is avascular and consist densely arranged collagen bundles and numerous fibroblasts.

1. What likely diagnosis can be made on medical and familial history and by histological and clinical findings?

    (A) Drug induced gingival enlargement.
    (B) Idiopathic gingival enlargement
    (C) Leukemic gingival enlargement
    (D) Pubertal gingival enlargement

2. What is the treatment plan for this patient

    (A) Phase-I therapy followed by gingivectomy.
    (B) Immediate excision of the gingiva
    (C) Antibiotic and anti-inflammatory only
    (D) No treatment can be given

3. Fibrous enlargement of the gingiva is generally attributed to hereditary factors. The mode of transmission is mainly

    (A) Autosomal dominant
    (B) Autosomal recessive
    (C) X-linked recessive
    (D) X-linked dominant

4. Gingival enlargement has been seen in Tuberous Sclerosis, which is an inherited condition characterized by a triad of

    (A) Mental retardation, intestinal polyps and angiofibroma
    (B) Neurological deficits, Deafness and osteofibroma
    (C) Epilepsy, mental retardation and cutaneous angiofibroma
    (D) None of the above

Answers:

1. B

   The condition is associated with no family history, no drug history, nohistopathological correlation. [1]

2. A

   Phase I therapy and Gingivectomy. [1]

3. A

   Autosomal Dominant [1]

4. C

Reference:

1. Newman GM, Takei HH, Klokkevold PR, Carranza FA. Carranza's Clinical Periodontology. 10th ed. Missouri: Saunders; 2006.

Gingival Recession

Dr. Anjani Kumar Pathak, Assistant Professor, DrUmesh
Patel, JR-II, Department of Periodontology

A 25 year old female patient came to the department of periodontology with the chief complaint of hypersensitivity and esthetic concerns. On clinical examination the oral hygiene was satisfactory but the margin of gingiva in mandibular incisors were inflamed and apically displaced. There was insufficient width of attached gingiva with significant root prominence and exposure. Radiographic examination reveals severe interproximal bone loss.

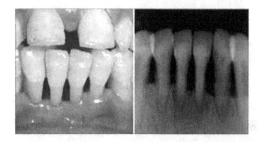

1. The most likely diagnosis for the case described

    (A) Gingival recession
    (B) Root caries
    (C) Gingivitis
    (D) Periodontal pocket

2. Type of recession present according to miller's classification

    (A) Class I
    (B) Class II
    (C) Class III
    (D) Class IV

3. Most probable etiology

    (A) Faulty toothbrushing
    (B) Trauma from occlusion
    (C) Bacterial plaque
    (D) Tooth malpositioning

4. Prognosis for class IV miller's recession

    (A) Excellent prognosis
    (B) Good prognosis

(C) Poor prognosis

(D) Hopeless prognosis

5. Most appropriate treatment for class IV miller's recession

   (A) Coronal repositioning

   (B) Free gingivalraft

   (C) Connective tissue graft

   (D) Vestibular deepening

Answers:

1. A

Marginal tissue recession extends to or beyond mucogingival junction. [1]

2. D

Marginal tissue recession to or beyond mucogingival junction. There is severe bone and soft tissue loss interdentallyor severe tooth malposition.

3. A

The most common cause of the defects described is abrasive and traumatic toothbrushing habits. Teeth positioned buccally tend to have greater recession. [1]

4. 4 C

The prognosis for class I & II is good to excellent; whereas for class III, only partial coverage can be expected. Class IV has a very poor prognosis with current techniques. [1]

5. B

Some of the techniques used for widening the attached gingiva apical to the area of recession can also be used for root coverage. Both the free gingival and the connective tissue autograft used for apical widening can be used for coronal augmentation by incorporating some modifications. [1]

Reference:

1. Newman GM, Takei HH, Klokkevold PR, Carranza FA. Carranza's Clinical Periodontology. 10th ed. Missouri: Saunders; 2006.

Halitosis

Dr. Anjani Kumar Pathak, Assistant Professor, Dr. Amitesh
Bhargava, JR-II, Department of Periodontology

A 40 year old male patient came to the department of periodontology with complains of bad breath from past three years. He regularly received periodontal treatment but his malodour did not reduce. He even uses lemon and vinegar to mask his breath odour and he has not been suffering from any systemic disease. Clinical examination revealed fair oral hygiene and a periodontal pocket on maxillary Ist molar with overhang restoration. On application of compressed air we can sense some malodour from this tooth. On intra oral periapical radiograph of this tooth no periapical and periodontal changes are seen.

1. Most probable cause for the bad breath is

   (A) Microbiota of subgingival areas.
   (B) Microbiota beneath overhang restoration.
   (C) Microbiota of supragingival areas.
   (D) Systemic disorder

2. Halitosis is primarily due to

   (A) Volatile sulphur compounds
   (B) Alkaline phosphatase
   (C) Trypsin like enzyme
   (D) Collagenase

3. Gold standard test for the examination of bad breath

   (A) Organoleptic assessment
   (B) Gas chromatography(Oral Chroma)
   (C) Saliva incubation test
   (D) Sulphide monitor(Halimeter)

4. Best treatment for bad breath in the above case is

   (A) Removal of overhang restoration and SRP
   (B) Mouth rinses
   (C) Masking the malodour
   (D) SRP

Answers:

1. B

   Since the patient gave no history of systemic disorder and was receiving regular periodontal care so microbiota from subgingival and supragingival areas may not be the cause. He has an overhanging restoration which harbours volatile gases producing microbiota and are difficult to clean areas, it may be the most probable cause. [1]

2. A

   VSC' s are hydogen sulfide, methyl mercaptan and dimethyl sulfides. [1]

3. A

   It is done on an organoleptic scale of Rosenberg and McCulloch by a trained judge.[1]

4. A [1]

Reference:

1. Newman GM, Takei HH, Klokkevold PR, Carranza FA. Carranza's Clinical Periodontology. 10th ed. Missouri: Saunders; 2006.

Refractory Periodontitis

Dr. Abhaya Gupta, Senior Resident, Dr. Rameshwari Singhal, Assistant Professor
Department of Periodontology

A 42 year old male came with the presentation of low plaque scores, continual loss of periodontal attachment & bone despite well executed therapeutic and patient efforts to stop the progression of disease. Patient gave a history of previous long term low dose antibiotic therapy. Microbial analysis confirmed the presence of *Prevotellaintermedia, Porphyromonasgingivalis, Tannerella forsythia, Aggregati bacteractinomycetemcomitans* and spirochetes. The hematology showed elevated CD8 + T cells count.

1. Most likely diagnosis?

    (A) Aggressive Periodontitis
    (B) Periodontitis refractory to treatment
    (C) Necrotising ulcerative periodontitis
    (D) Chronic Periodontitis

2. Characterization of the above mentioned condition can be done in which of the following forms of periodontal diseases?

    (A) Chronic Periodontitis
    (B) Aggressive Periodontitis
    (C) Both a & b
    (D) None

3. Which of the following systemic antibiotic therapy offers greater promise as an adjunct to scaling and root planning for the treatment of above mentioned condition?

    (A) Clindamycin
    (B) Amoxicillin-clavulanate potassium
    (C) Azithromycin
    (D) All of the above

4. Rapid microbial susceptibility analysis is done for the selection of antibiotics utilizing which of the following diagnostic techniques?

    (A) Dark field / Phase contrast microscopy
    (B) Bacterial culturing
    (C) Immunofluorescent assay
    (D) None

5. The diagnosis of above mentioned case as a separate entity has been eliminated from the AAP International workshop for the classification of periodontal diseases, 1999 due to:

    (A) Non-prevalence of the above mentioned condition nowadays.
    (B) Diversity of clinical conditions and treatments under which periodontal therapy fails to arrest the progression of periodontitis.
    (C) Non-availability of diagnostic aids to detect such condition at present.
    (D) All of the above

Answers:

1. B

    Continual periodontal attachment and bone loss despite well-executed treatment in a patient with good oral hygiene and no other infections or etiologic factors is suggestive of Refractory Periodontitis. [1,2]

2. C

    A patient with periodontitis that is refractory to treatment often does not have any distinguishing clinical characteristics on initial examination compared with cases of periodontitis that respond normally. Therefore it is possible to characterize any form of periodontal diseases as refractory to treatment (e.g aggressive refractory periodontitis & chronic refractory periodontitis). [1,2]

3. B

    The rationale behind the use of combined antibiotic therapy is based on the diversity of putative submicrobial periodontal pathogens. Further combinations broaden the antimicrobial range beyond that attained by single antibiotic and provide synergy against targeted organisms. It also prevents emergence of bacterial resistance. [1,2]

4. C

    Since the main putative periopathogens like *Aa, Pg, Tf, Ec* are nonmotile, Dark field microscopy seems an unlikely candidate as a diagnostic test. Although bacterial culturing is the gold standard amongst tests for microbial analysis but it is relatively time consuming. Immunodiagnostic tests are rapid and employ antibodies that recognize specific bacterial antigens to detect target microorganisms. [1,2]

5. B

Refractory periodontitis is heterogeneous group of periodontal diseases that refers to instances in which there is a continuing progression of periodontitis in spite of excellent patient compliance and the provision of periodontal therapy that succeeds in most patients. [1,2]

References:

1. Newman GM, Takei HH, Klokkevold PR, Carranza FA. Carranza's Clinical Periodontology. 10th ed. Missouri: Saunders; 2006.p.693-705.

2. Armitage GC. Development of a classification system for periodontal diseases and conditions. Ann Periodontol 1999; 4(1):1-6.

Primary Herpetic Gingivostomatitis

Dr. Rebecca Chowdhry, Senior Resident, Dr. Rameshwari Singhal,
Assistant Professor, Department of Periodontology

A 14 year old boy presented to the Outpatient Department of Periodontology with the chief complaint of vesiculating painful ulcers and high temperature of 102 degree Fahrenheit since 4 days. Oral soreness and difficulty in eating and drinking were also reported. On oral examination gingiva appeared to be shiny and erythematous with varying degrees of edema and gingival bleeding. Ulcers were painful with a red elevated halo- like margin and depressed yellowish or grayish white central portion.

1. What would be the most likely diagnosis:

    (A) ANUG
    (B) Primary Herpetic Gingivostomatitis
    (C) Desquamative Gingivitis
    (D) Lichen Planus

2. Which Organism is mainly associated with above diagnosis

    (A) Cytomegalovirus
    (B) (B) Epstein Barr Virus
    (C) (C) Papillomavirus
    (D) Herpes Simplex Virus

3. Most commonly affected site:

    (A) Interdental papillae and marginal gingival
    (B) Soft palate
    (C) Buccal mucosa and Labial Mucosa
    (D) All of the above

4. Clinical feature of above mention case:

    (A) Punched-out crater like depressions at the crest of the interdental papillae
    (B) Erythematous and ulcerated interdental papillae
    (C) Diffuse, erythematous, shiny discolouration of gingiva
    (D) Widened periodontal ligament

5. Histological examination will reveal presence of which type of cell

    (A) Tzanck cell
    (B) Lacunar cell
    (C) Giant cell
    (D) Popcorn cell

Answers:

1. B

    All the clinical features are suggestive of acute herpetic gingivostomatitis. [1]

2. D

    HSV-1 is responsible for Primary herpetic gingivostomatitis. [1]

3. D

    It is characterized by the presence of discrete, spherical gray vesicles, which may occur on the gingiva, labial and buccal mucosa, soft palate, pharynx sublingual mucosa and tongue. [1]

4. C

    Clinically the condition appears as a diffuse, erythematous, shiny involvement of the gingiva and adjacent oral mucosa with varying degrees of edema and gingival bleeding. [1]

5. A

    Virus targets epithelial cells, which show ballooning degeneration these cells are called tzanck cells. [1]

Reference:

1. Newman GM, Takei HH, Klokkevold PR, Carranza FA. Carranza's Clinical Periodontology. 10ᵗʰ ed. Missouri: Saunders; 2006.

Gingival Inflammation

Dr. Neetu Rani, Senior Resident, Prof. M. A. Khan, Professor, Dr. Rameshwari Singhal, Assistant Professor, Department of Periodontology

Forty years old woman reported with complain of bleeding gums and swelling in relation to maxillary and mandibular teeth since 8 months. The patient gave no history of taking medication associated with gingival enlargement. On intra-oral examination poor oral hygiene and gingival enlargement was observed in relation to maxillary and mandibular anterior teeth. Generalized gingival bleeding on probing and periodontal pockets of more than 5 mm was also recorded.

1. What are the causes of gingival inflammation?

    (A) Plaque
    (B) Calculus
    (C) Oral Hygiene
    (D) All the above

2. Bleeding on probing is first observed in which stage of gingival inflammation?

    (A) Stage I: Initial lesion
    (B) Stage II: Early lesion
    (C) Stage III: Established lesion
    (D) All the above

3. The swelling in the present case is

    (A) Drug induced gingival enlargement
    (B) Inflammatory gingival enlargement
    (C) Idiopathic gingival enlargement
    (D) Puberty associated gingival enlargement

4. Neutrophills are predominately found in which stage of gingivitis?

    (A) Initial lesion
    (B) Early lesion
    (C) Advanced lesion
    (D) Established lesion

5. Which stage is known as subclinical gingivitis:

    (A) Initial lesion
    (B) Early lesion
    (C) Advanced lesion
    (D) Established lesion

Answers:

1. D

    All are etiological factors of gingival inflammation. [1]

2. B

    Proliferation of capillaries occurs with increased formation of capillary loop between the rete pegs. [1]

3. B

    Poor oral hygiene may be the most probable cause of gingival enlargement. [1]

4. A

    Neutrophils are the markers of acute inflammation. They leave the capillary through the phenomenon of diapedesis. Increase in concentration of neutrophils is seen at the site of inflammation. [1]

5. A

    The initial response of gingiva to bacterial plaque is not apparent at this stage. [1]

Reference:

1. Newman GM, Takei HH, Klokkevold PR, Carranza FA. Carranza's Clinical Periodontology. 10th ed. Missouri: Saunders; 2006.

Chapter - 7

Pediatrics & Preventive Dentistry

Delayed Exfoliation of Primary Teeth

Dr. Richa Khanna, Assistant Professor, Department
of Paediatric and Preventive Dentistry

A male child, 9 years of age, presented with the chief complaint of pain in teeth in the lower right posterior region. The intraoral photograph of the region is shown below. On clinical examination it was found that FDI* tooth number 84 was mobile. The parents also complained of irregular teeth in the upper arch. Tooth number 21 (FDI)* was erupting palatally and 61 was firm in position.

1. What is the etiology of irregular teeth in both maxillary and mandibular arches in the case presented?

   (A) Delayed eruption of permanent teeth
   (B) Delayed exfoliation of primary teeth.
   (C) Improper restorations in primary teeth
   (D) Poor oral hygiene

2. What is the treatment of choice in maxillary arch?

   (A) Extraction of retained primary tooth
   (B) Extraction of erupting permanent tooth
   (C) Wait for normal exfoliation of retained primary tooth
   (D) Extract all primary teeth present

3. What is the treatment of choice in mandibular arch?

   (A) Extraction of retained primary tooth
   (B) Extraction of erupting permanent tooth
   (C) Wait for normal exfoliation of retained primary tooth
   (D) Extract all primary teeth present

4. Retained deciduous tooth when results in changed/altered path of eruption of permanent successor, the clinical condition is termed as:

   (A) Early eruption
   (B) Failure of eruption
   (C) Ectopic eruption
   (D) Normal eruption

5. Which of the dental arches in the presented case, show signs of ectopic eruption?

   (A) Maxillary arch
   (B) Mandibular arch
   (C) Both maxillary and mandibular arches
   (D) None of the arches.

*= Fédération Dentaire Internationale

Answers:

1. B

   [2]

2. A

   Extraction of primary teeth is needed if its delayed exfoliation has led to ectopic eruption. [1, 2]

3. A

   In case of mobile primary teeth near exfoliation, waiting for normal exfoliation can be done. In the present case, however, the mobile primary tooth may interfere in normal eating, hence should be extracted [1, 2]

4. C

   [1, 2]

5. A

   [1, 2]

References:

1. Tandon S. Text book of Pedodontics. 2nd ed. India: Paras Medical Publisher; 2009

2. McDonald RE, Avery DR, Dean JA. Dentistry for the Child and Adolescent. 9th ed. Missouri: Mosby; 2011.

Assessment of Affective Domain for Patient Dental Patient Management

Dr. Richa Khanna, Assistant Professor, Department
of Paediatric and Preventive Dentistry

A seven year old paediatric dental patient reports in a dental office with a history of spontaneous pain during night in mandibular right posterior region. Radiographic examination reveals carious exposure of pulp in FDI* tooth number 7The involved tooth required pulpectomy, but the child was very uncooperative and anxious.

1. Which of the following factors present in the dental office would help in reducing the anxiety of the child?

   (A) Strict attitude of the staff
   (B) A calm and pleasant environment simulating home
   (C) A dark, dull atmosphere in the dental office
   (D) Long waiting period during appointment.

2. The dental surgeon treating the child patient described the procedure to be done in brief to him. The explanation was simple and in a language well understood by the child. What was the dentist actually doing?

   (A) Structuring
   (B) Modelling
   (C) Distraction
   (D) Externalisation

3. While administering local anesthesia, the dentist asked the child to count from one to ten in his mind. He was actually:

   (A) structuring the situation
   (B) distracting the child
   (C) involving the child
   (D) tell-show-do

4. The dentist described local anesthesia as sleep medicine to the child. This is an example of:

   (A) Tell-show-do
   (B) Desensitization
   (C) Euphemisms
   (D) Non verbal communication

Answers:

1. B

   A calm and pleasant environment in the dental office simulating home reduces anxiety of the child [1].

2. A

   Structuring refers to guidelines established by the dentist and his team to the child so that the child knows what to expect and how to treat. By these guidelines, the dentist prepares the child for each phase of treatment in advance [1].

3. B

   By distraction, the child's focus is shifted away from the procedure [1].

4. C

   Euphemisms are substitute words for technical terms used by the dentist. These help in reducing anxiety of the child [1,2].

*= Fédération Dentaire Internationale

References:

1. Tandon S. Text book of Pedodontics. 2nd ed. India: Paras Medical Publisher; 2009

2. McDonald RE, Avery DR, Dean JA. Dentistry for the Child and Adolescent. 9th ed. Missouri: Mosby; 2011.

Premature Loss of Primary Anterior Teeth

Dr. Richa Khanna, Assistant Professor, Department
of Paediatric and Preventive Dentistry

Parents of five year old female patient reported with the chief complaint of teeth loss due to trauma in the upper front region few hours back. The parents had brought the avulsed incisors with them in normal saline. The parents were worried for the poor esthetics after avulsion. Following is the clinical intraoral photograph at the time of presentation.

1.   What advice should be given to the parents concerning esthetics?

(A) esthetics can be restored by reimplanting natural teeth

(B) esthetics can be restored by prosthetic replacement for natural teeth

(C) esthetics need not be restored.

(D) esthetics cannot be restored

2.   While planning for restoring esthetics for the child, what should be done for the space created by loss of both primary central incisors?

(A) Tanaka Johnston mixed dentition model analysis.

(B) Moyer's radiographic mixed dentition analysis.

(C) Calculation of space deficiency

(D) No space management for lost incisors is needed.

3.   What would be the primary concern of the dentist for this patient?

1.   to restore esthetics and guide the parents regarding potential of developing   ·
deleterious oral habits

(E) to maintain space for the lost incisors.

(F) both to restore esthetics and maintain space for lost incisors.

(G) to convince the parents that restoring esthetics is not needed.

2.   Which of the following treatment options can be used to restore esthetics for the lost primary incisors?

(A) Nance palatal arch

(B) Removable partial denture

(C) Transpalatal arch

(D) Lingual holding arch

3. What would have been the choice of treatment if incisors in mandibular anterior region are lost due to trauma before primary canine stabilization?

    (A) restoration of esthetics, space maintainence and advise regarding potential of developing deleterious oral habits
    (B) to maintain space for the lost incisors only
    (C) No treatment needed
    (D) restoration of esthetics only

Answers:

1. A

    Primary teeth are not reimplanted as they might damage the permanent tooth bud and also may get ankylosed causing difficulty in normal exfoliation [1]

2. D

    Premature loss of maxillary primary incisors does not generally result in decreased upper intracanine dimensions if the incisor loss occurs after the primary canines have erupted into occlusion at approximately 2 years of age [2]

3. A

    The major consequence of early loss of maxillary primary incisors is most likely delayed eruption timing of the permanent successors as reparative bone and dense connective tissue covers the site. In addition, unattractive appearance and potential development of deleterious habits (e.g., tongue-thrust swallow, forward resting posture of the tongue, improper pronunciation of fricative sounds—"s," "f") may be of concern following premature loss of primary maxillary incisors [2].

4. B

    An anterior appliance incorporating artificial primary teeth may be considered to satisfy esthetic and functional needs. Acrylic partial dentures have been successful in the replacement of single and multiple maxillary primary incisors [2].

5. A

    Early loss of lower primary incisors is generally due to ectopic eruption of the permanent incisors in reflecting excessive incisor liability. Given the potential for increased intracanine width during permanent incisor eruption, the clinician should monitor development in the lower incisor area and generally not intervene. Individual circumstances may indicate extraction of the antimere primary incisor to enhance incisor positioning and midline symmetry. The loss of lower incisors in other circumstances such as trauma, advanced caries, or extraction of a neonatal tooth may result in anterior space loss if it occurs before primary canine stabilization is realized.[2]

References:

1. Tandon S. Text book of Pedodontics. 2nd ed. India: Paras Medical Publisher; 2009

2. McDonald RE, Avery DR, Dean JA. Dentistry for the Child and Adolescent. 9th ed. Missouri: Mosby; 2011.

Crowding In Permanent Incisors In Mixed Dentition Period

Dr.Richa Khanna, Assistant Professor, Department
of Paediatric and Preventive Dentistry

A female child patient, eight years of age, presented with the chief complaint of irregular teeth in mandibular anterior region. On intraoral examination, it was found that the patient had Angle's Class I molar relation. Overjet was 2 millimetres and overbite 75%. All the permanent incisors and first permanent molars were present along with deciduous canines and molars in all the four quadrants. The intraoral clinical photograph of the mandibular arch at the time of presentation is as follows:

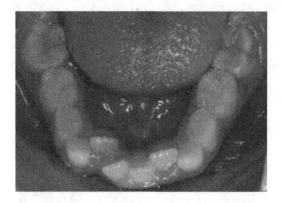

1. What is the preferred treatment approach for the present case?

    (A) Send the patient with a follow-up appointment without any investigation and intervention.
    (B) Take clinical photographs and send the patient with a follow-up appointment
    (C) Perform proximal stripping and send the patient with a follow-up appointment
    (D) Take impressions, prepare models for both dental arches and perform model analysis, decide on the intervention.

2. Which mixed dentition analysis can be done in the present situation if radiographs are not present?

    (A) Tanaka-Johnston
    (B) Carey's
    (C) Bolton's
    (D) Moyer's

3. A space deficiency of 0.8 mm per quadrant was found in the mandible as a result of mixed dentition analysis. What management should now be done?

    (A) No management.
    (B) Lingual holding arch with regular follow up.
    (C) Disking of primary canines with lingual holding arch
    (D) Extraction of primary canines.

4. What should be done if in the present situation moderate space deficiency (2-3 millimetres per quadrant) is calculated?

    (A) No management.
    (B) Lingual holding arch with regular follow up.
    (C) Disking of primary canines with lingual holding arch
    (D) Extraction of primary canines with no space maintenance.

5. If lingual arch is not given with extraction of primary canines in case of moderate-severe space deficiency, what would be the consequence?

    (A) Lower arch collapse
    (B) Upper arch collapse
    (C) Gingival recession
    (D) Gingival inflammation

Answers:

1. D

Space analysis combined with evaluation of the impact of compensating factors on dental arch status is the means by which overall space requirements for the lower arch can be determined during the mixed dentition phase [1]. This should be performed in cases of lower incisor crowding on the study models.

2. A

Out of these Moyer's and Tanaka-Johnston are only employed in mixed dentition. Out of these two, Moyer's analysis requires intraoral periapical radiographs [1].

3. B

If analysis indicates a positive arch length or deficiency of less than 1 to 2 mm per quadrant, the use of a space maintainer to hold tooth positions may be considered potentially beneficial. If the space is not held, the total arch length may be further decreased and lead to possible premolar extractions requirements. Disking of primary canines and extraction of primary canines are done in case of moderate and severe space deficiencies respectively, each with a lingual holding arch given [1].

4. C

If the arch length deficiency is 2 to 3 mm per quadrant or more, a significant discrepancy exists where space regaining, serial extraction, and/or comprehensive orthodontic treatment may be indicated. If there is no question that permanent teeth will have to be removed to obtain a favorable occlusion, space maintenance may not be desirable as the space would need to be closed during orthodontic treatment anyway. In less obvious extraction cases, holding the space to allow teeth to erupt and prevent impactions can be a valuable service. Bilateral disking can provide up to 2 to 3 mm of space for unraveling" of lingual displaced incisors. [1].

5. C

If disking of the canines is not an option due to the level of crowding or positioning of the incisors, elective extraction of the primary canines to maintain arch symmetry, coincident midlines, and incisor integrity may be considered. Such intervention becomes more viable when the incisor liability and crowding is greater than 4 mm in the anterior segment. However, the clinician must remember early loss of lower primary canines will likely result in significant lower arch collapse. Therefore the extraction of primary canines should not be undertaken without parental understanding of the consequences and, ideally, orthodontic consultation. Given the long-term implications, such intervention goes beyond a first step in guidance of eruption and actually represents the start of either a phased early treatment program or a serial extraction program [1].

Reference:

1. Mc Donald RE, Avery DR, Dean JA. Dentistry for the Child and Adolescent. 9th ed. Missouri: Mosby; 2011

Premature Loss of Primary Posterior Teeth

Dr. Richa Khanna (Assistant Professor), Dr. Afroz Alam Ansari (Assistant Professor) Department of Paediatric and Preventive Dentistry

A female patient age five years, presented with grossly carious primary first molars in all the four quadrants. On clinical and radiographic examination, it was decided to extract all the four first primary molars. None of the permanent teeth was found to be erupted/erupting on clinical examination. Space management needed to be planned before extractions. Following diagrams can be used as a representation for both maxillary and mandibular arches after extractions. The spaces shown represent extraction sites for first primary molars.

1. What is the choice of space maintainer for maxillary arch?

   (A) Lingual holding arch
   (B) Nance palatal arch
   (C) Distal shoe space maintainer
   (D) Bilateral band and loop

2. What is the choice of space maintainer for mandibular arch?

   (A) Lingual holding arch
   (B) Nance palatal arch
   (C) Distal shoe space maintainer
   (D) Bilateral band and loop

3. What is the choice of space maintainer for maxillary arch if permanent first molars and permanent incisors are also present?

   (A) Lingual holding arch
   (B) Nance palatal arch
   (C) Distal shoe space maintainer
   (D) Bilateral band and loop

4. What is the choice of space maintainer for mandibular arch if permanent first molars and permanent incisors are also present?

   (A) Lingual holding arch
   (B) Nance palatal arch
   (C) Distal shoe space maintainer
   (D) Bilateral band and loop

Answers:

1. B

   When permanent first molars and incisors are not fully erupted, Nance palatal arch is preferred for bilateral loss of primary first molars in maxillary arch [1]

2. D

   When permanent first molars and incisors are not fully erupted, bilateral band and loop is preferred for bilateral loss of primary first molars in mandibular arch [1]

3. D

   Even when permanent first molars and incisors are fully erupted, Nance palatal arch is preferred for multiple loss of primary teeth in maxillary arch [1]

4. A

   When permanent first molars and incisors are fully erupted, Lingual holding arch is preferred for multiple loss of primary teeth in mandibular arch [1]

Reference:

1.   Tandon S. Text book of Pedodontics. 2nd ed. India: Paras Medical Publisher; 2009

Eruption Problems - Delayed Eruption Of Permanent Teeth

Dr. Richa Khanna (Assistant Professor), Dr. Afroz Alam Ansari (Assistant Professor) Department of Paediatric and Preventive Dentistry

Following are two clinical intraoral photographs of two different paediatric dental patients, about 11 years of age, reporting with the same chief complaint but with different etiology and clinical presentation.

1. What would have been the chief complaint of both the patients?

    (A) Pain in erupted teeth
    (B) Food impaction in posterior teeth
    (C) Delayed eruption of teeth
    (D) Unesthetic appearance

2. What is the etiology of delayed eruption in the first photograph?

    (A) Gingival fibromatosis
    (B) Ankylosis of primary teeth
    (C) Hypothyroidism
    (D) Cleidocranial dysplasia

3. Which of the following factors does **not** affect eruption of teeth locally?

    (A) Early Loss of Primary teeth
    (B) Delayed Loss of Primary teeth
    (C) Hormonal balance
    (D) Space Available

4. A patient with increased vertical dimension due to excessive eruption of posterior teeth can be best treated by:

    (A) An intraoral appliance for early morning wearing
    (B) An intraoral appliance for full day wearing
    (C) An intraoral appliance for night wearing
    (D) An intraoral appliance for night and early morning wearing.

5. Which of the following is an example of early eruption of teeth?

    (A) Natal tooth
    (B) Turner's tooth
    (C) Ankylosed tooth
    (D) Carious tooth

Answers:

1. C

    Both the clinical photographs demonstrate delayed eruption of permanent teeth correlating with the chronological age [2].

2. A

    Gingival fibromatosis may be associated with multiple retained and non-erupted primary teeth as well as absence of eruption of permanent teeth. Ankylosis should be considered an interruption in the rhythm of eruption. The mandibular primary molars are the teeth most often observed to be ankylosed. Ankylosed tooth is in a state of static retention, whereas in the adjacent areas eruption and alveolar growth continue. The tooth may appear to be submerging into the mandible or maxilla [2].

3. C

    Hormonal balance is a systemic factor affecting eruption of teeth. Rest all factors are local [2].

4. D

    Excessive eruption of posterior teeth is a characteristic of long face. Since teeth erupt primarily at night and early morning it is possible that wearing an appliance during this time would be helpful [1].

References:

1. Tandon S. Text book of Pedodontics. 2nd ed. India: Paras Medical Publisher; 2009

2. McDonald RE, Avery DR, Dean JA. Dentistry for the Child and Adolescent. 9th ed. Missouri: Mosby; 2011

Traumatic Dental Injury, Permanent Tooth Avulsion

Dr. Rajeev Kumar Singh (Assistant Professor), Dr. P. Gayathri (Ex-Junior Resident), Department of Paediatric and Preventive Dentistry

A 10-year-old patient reported to a dentist within 30 minutes of a traumatic dental injury. The patient came with the avulsed tooth placed in the milk. On clinical and radiological examination, no alveolar fracture was found. Following is the intraoral photograph of the patient.

1. What is the preferred treatment in this case:
    (A) Reimplantation without splinting
    (B) Reimplantation with splinting
    (C) Placement of a bridge
    (D) No treatment but to wait for healing

2. What is the effect of time interval between avulsion and reimplantation on the long term prognosis of the reimplanted tooth?
    (A) Less the time interval, better the prognosis
    (B) Less the time interval, poor the prognosis
    (C) More the time interval, better the prognosis
    (D) No effect of time interval on prognosis

3. Which of the following is considered as preferable storage media for avulsed tooth?
    (A) Normal saline
    (B) Milk
    (C) Tap water
    (D) Hank's Balanced Salt Solution

4. Which of the following is true regarding traumatic dental injuries between girls and boys in their first decade of life?
    (A) Girls are affected more commonly than boys
    (B) Girls are affected less commonly than boys
    (C) Both girls and boys are affected equally
    (D) Incidence may vary in primary and permanent dentitions

5. Ellis and Davey classified tooth avulsion in which of the following class:
    (A) Class II
    (B) Class III
    (C) Class IV
    (D) Class V

6. Which of the following is an expected outcome of reimplantation, when extraoral dry time exceeds 60 minutes?

   (A) Ankylosis of implanted tooth
   (B) Supra eruption of reimplanted tooth
   (C) Good long term prognosis
   (D) It can't be pre-determined

Answers:

1. B

   The tooth should be reimplanted and a flexible splint should be applied for up to 2 weeks[1].

2. A

   Prognosis is excellent, when the tooth is reimplanted immediately. As the time interval between avulsion and reimplantation increases, more PDL cells are damaged and long term prognosis becomes poor [1].

3. D

   Hank's Balanced Salt Solution is considered the best storage media for avulsed teeth [2].

4. B

   Boys are affected almost twice as often as girls in both the primary and permanent dentitions[1].

5. D [1].

6. A

   Delayed reimplantation has a poor long-term prognosis. The periodontal ligament will be necrotic and can not be expected to heal. The expected eventual outcome is ankylosis and resorption of the root and the tooth will be lost eventually[2].

References:

1. Tandon S. Text book of Pedodontics. 2nd ed. India: Paras Medical Publisher; 2009

2. Guidelines for the Management of Traumatic Dental Injuries: Avulsion of Permanent Teeth. Originating Group International Association of Dental Traumatology, Endorsed by the American Academy of Pediatric Dentistry 201Reference manual 14/15; 36(6): 328-35.

Developmental Aspects Of Dentition, Natal / Neonatal Teeth

Dr. Rajeev Kumar Singh, Assistant Professor, Department
of Paediatric and Preventive Dentistry

A 2 days old newborn reported to the dentist with the presence of a teeth in lower anterior region. The newborn was born with the tooth.

1. The tooth in the above patient is known as?

    (A) Neonatal tooth
    (B) Natal tooth
    (C) Ectopic tooth
    (D) Supplemental tooth

2. The tooth which is not present at birth but erupts within 30 days of birth is called?

    (A) Neonatal tooth
    (B) Natal tooth
    (C) Ectopic tooth
    (D) Supplemental tooth

3. The preferable approach to treat a natal tooth, which is firm and without any complication, is?

    (A) Extract the tooth
    (B) Leave the tooth in place
    (C) Selective grinding of the tooth
    (D) Root canal treatment of the tooth

4. The preferable approach to treat a neonatal tooth, which is mobile and cause difficulty in feeding, is?

    (A) Selective grinding of the tooth
    (B) Leave the tooth in place
    (C) Extract the tooth
    (D) Root canal treatment of the tooth

5. Ulceration of the sublingual area in an infant due to natal tooth is also known as?

    (A) Cardarelli Boyd disease
    (B) Medley Stanley disease
    (C) King Lee disease
    (D) Riga Fede disease

6.   Natal teeth are present more often than neonatal teeth in an approximate ration of?
    (A) 1:2
    (B) 2:1
    (C) 1:3
    (D) 3:1

Answers:

1.   B

Teeth present at birth are known as natal teeth [1].

2.   A

Teeth that erupt within 30 days of birth are called neonatal teeth [1].

3.   B

It is desirable to preserve the asymptomatic tooth because of their importance in growth of the jaw [1].

4.   C

Such teeth should be extracted because of danger of aspiration [1].

5.   D

Riga and Fede described the lesion histologically [1]

6.   D

    (A) [1]

Reference:

Marwah N. Text book of Pediatric Dentistry, Third 3rd ed. India: Jaypee brothers Medical publishers; 2014

Traumatic Dental Injury, Root Fracture

Dr. Rajeev Kumar Singh, Assistant Professor, Department
of Paediatric and Preventive Dentistry

A 12-year-old patient reported to the Department of Paediatric and Preventive Dentistry with the chief complaint of pain in upper anterior region. Patient had a history of traumatic injury to his left permanent central incisor (FDI* tooth number) one month back. On clinical examination, the tooth had pain on percussion. Radiological examination revealed root fracture as seen in the radiograph.

1. What is this class of fracture according to Ellis and Davey's classification?
   (A) Class 4
   (B) Class 5
   (C) Class 6
   (D) Class 7

2. What is the treatment of choice when fracture is present in middle third of the root?
   (A) Extraction of the entire tooth
   (B) Obturation till the possible working length and apical surgery to remove the fragment
   (C) Orthodontic or surgical extrusion of the fragment followed by immobilization
   (D) No treatment required

3. What is the treatment of choice when fracture is present in apical third of the root?
   (A) Extraction of the entire tooth
   (B) Orthodontic or surgical extrusion of the fragment followed by immobilization
   (C) Obturation till the possible working length and apical surgery to remove the fragment
   (D) No treatment required

4. What is the treatment of choice when fracture is present near to gingival margin?
   (A) Obturation till the possible working length and apical surgery to remove the fragment
   (B) Extraction of the entire tooth
   (C) Removal of coronal fragment and orthodontic or surgical extrusion of the apical fragment followed by immobilization and crown fabrication
   (D) No treatment required

5. Cracked tooth syndrome is:
    (A) Horizontal middle third root fracture
    (B) Horizontal apical third root fracture
    (C) Horizontal gingival third root fracture
    (D) Vertical root fracture

Answers:

1. C [1]

2. A

    (A) Prognosis of middle third root fracture remains poor [1].

3. C [1]

4. C

    (A) Proximity of the fracture to gingival crevice makes pulpal infection more probable [1].

5. D

    (A) It is vertical root fracture in which the fracture extends lengthwise from crown towards the apex [1].

Reference:

1. Marwah N. Text book of Pediatric Dentistry, Third 3rd ed. India: Jaypee brothers Medical publishers; 2014

Traumatic Dental Injury, Pulp Exposure, Apexogenesis

Dr. Rajeev Kumar Singh, Assistant Professor, Department
of Paediatric and Preventive Dentistry.

An 8-year-old patient reported to the Department of Paediatric & Preventive Dentistry with the fracture of his permanent right central incisor 6 hours before presentation. Clinical examination revealed a large pulp exposure. Radiographic examination revealed blunderbuss canal of the fractured tooth:

1. What is the treatment of choice in this case?

    (A) Indirect pulp capping
    (B) Direct pulp capping
    (C) Pulpotomy
    (D) Root canal treatment

2. Which is the preferred medicament to be placed in such cases?

    (A) Calcium hydroxide
    (B) Formocresol
    (C) Zinc oxide eugenol
    (D) Glutaraldehyde

3. What is a blunderbuss canal?

    (A) Mature root with closed apex
    (B) Immature root with open apex
    (C) Immature roots with closed apex
    (D) Mature root with narrow canal

4. What is the type of the fracture in the picture shown?

    (A) Ellis class 1
    (B) Ellis class 2
    (C) Ellis class 3
    (D) Ellis class 4

5. What will be the treatment of choice if the above patient reports after 7 days?

    (A) Direct pulp capping
    (B) Pulpotomy
    (C) Root canal treatment
    (D) Apexification

6. What will be the treatment of choice in another patient who is 13 years old and reports after 7 days with the same type of fracture?
    (A) Direct pulp capping
    (B) Pulpotomy
    (C) Root canal treatment
    (D) Apexification

Answers:

1. C

This patient has a class 3 fracture with pulpal involvement. The exposure is large with moderate hemorrhage and the patient is seen within 24 hours. Pulpotomy is the treatment of choice in such cases [1].

2. A

Calcium hydroxide is the preferred Pulpotomy medicament in permanent teeth [1].

3. B

A blunderbuss canal indicates divergent and flaring root canal walls in which apex is funnel shaped and typically wider than the coronal aspect of the canal [1].

4. C

[1].

5. D

In this case, the pulp tissue will be nonvital. In such cases, where pulp is nonvital and root apex is open, apexification procedure is done to induce root apex closure [1].

6. C

In a 13 year old child, the root apex of permanent central incisor is closed, but because the patient reported after 7 days, the pulp is nonvital. So we can do the conventional root canal treatment [1].

Reference:

1. Tandon S. Text book of Pedodontics. 2nd ed. India: Paras Medical Publisher; 2009

Oral Habits

Prof. (Dr.) Rakesh Kumar Chak, Dr. Anamika Jain (Ex-resident),
Department of Paediatric and Preventive Dentistry.

A 9 year old male child patient reported with the complaint of proclined upper front teeth and spacing between upper and lower teeth on closing. He had flaccid lips with upper lip being short along with high palatal vault. He had slit external nares with a narrow nose.

1. Which of the following oral habit can be associated as the etiology of this clinical presentation?

    (A) Mouth breathing
    (B) Tongue thrusting
    (C) Thumb sucking
    (D) Nail biting

2. What is the skeletal pattern of such patients?

    (A) Dolicocephalic
    (B) Brachycephalic
    (C) Mesocephalic
    (D) Ectocephalic

3. Clinical tests that help in diagnosis of the habit are:

    (A) Mirror test
    (B) Butterfly test
    (C) Water holding test
    (D) All

4. Most reliable method for determining the mode of respiratory function in patients is:

    (A) Water holding test
    (B) CBCT
    (C) Plethysmography
    (D) Myography

5. All of the following dental effects are associated with the habit except:

    (A) Narrow palatal width
    (B) Posterior open bite
    (C) Increase in vertical overlap of anterior teeth
    (D) Flaring of incisors

6. Typical appearance of long narrow face, with narrow nose and nasal passages, along with flaccid lips are seen in these patients. This facial appearance is known as:
   (A) Flat face
   (B) Elderman's appearance
   (C) Adenoid facies
   (D) Angleman's facies

Answers:

1. A
   (A) [1]

2. A

   The patients with this habit present with increased facial height, long narrow face with dolicocephalic skeletal pattern. [1]

3. D

   All of these tests are used to test breathing by nose and differentiate from normal nasal breathing. [1]

4. C

   Inductive Plethysmography helps in quantifying the extent of mouth breathing. It helps in establishing quantity of air going through nose and through mouth separately. [1]

5. C

   Posterior openbite is not seen associated with habit of mouth breathing. [1]

6. C

   The presented feature are together characteristic of the facial form called as 'Adenoid facies'. [1]

Reference:

1. Tandon S. Text book of Pedodontics. 2nd ed. India: Paras Medical Publisher; 2009

Oral Habits

Prof. (Dr.) Rakesh Kumar Chak, Dr. Anamika Jain (Ex-resident),
Department of Paediatric and Preventive Dentistry.

A 7.5 year old patient presented with proclined maxillary anteriors and habit of placing one or more fingers in various depths into the mouth. The intraoral photograph for the developing dentition is presented below:

1. Which of the following oral habit is the patient having?

    (A) Tongue thrusting
    (B) Digit sucking
    (C) Mouth breathing
    (D) Nail biting

2. This habit is considered normal and the need of intervention is questionable till the age group of:

    (A) 4 years
    (B) 6 years
    (C) 9 years
    (D) 12 years

3. The effects of the persisting habit as seen on maxilla are all of the following except:

    (A) Increased proclination of anteriors with diastema
    (B) Increased mandibular anterior teeth retroclination
    (C) Anterior deep bite
    (D) Constriction of maxillary arch

4. Various theories given for thumb sucking are all except:

    (A) Classical Freudian theory
    (B) Oral drive theory of Sear's and Wise
    (C) Chemicoparasitic theory
    (D) Benjamin's rooting reflex

5. Typical appearance of digits associated with the habit is known as:

    (A) Calculus
    (B) Callus
    (C) Wallus
    (D) Crusting

6. Correction of the habit can be done with:

    (A) Reminder therapy –extraoral approach
    (B) Reminder therapy-intraoral approach
    (C) Quad helix for maxillary constriction
    (D) All

Answers:

1. B

    [1]

2. A

    Persistent digit-sucking habits extending into the incisor transition period can cause a malocclusion or aggravate an already existing one. Therefore, if the intensity of the habit persists or increases and adverse dental and skeletal changes are noted beyond age 4 years, corrective measures may be needed to avoid undesirable occlusion problems. Additionally, the understanding of the child complicates cooperation with any of the intervention options. [2]

3. C

    Pressure generated from the habit can produce changes in the anterior segments of the dental arches with labial flaring and protrusive spacing of maxillary anterior teeth and increased overjet. Remodelling of the maxillary alveolar process and vertical displacement of the maxillary anterior teeth can result in an open-bite relationship. In addition, the digit positioning can interfere with eruption of the lower incisors to exaggerate the open-bite appearance in the incisor segment. Intense patterns of habit may contribute to pronounced lingual inclination of the mandibular incisors that further increases the overjet situation. [1,2]

4. C

    Chemicoparasitic theory is given for etiology of dental caries.[1]

5. B

    Fibrous roughened 'Callus' may be seen in the digit involved in sucking habit.[1]

6. D

All these modalities together or individually help in treatment. Extraoral approaches involve-Bandages on digits, long sleeve nightware, etc. Intraoral approaches involve-Palatal cribs, rakes etc. [1]

References:

1. Tandon S. Text book of Pedodontics. 2nd ed. India: Paras Medical Publisher; 2009

2. McDonald RE, Avery DR, Dean JA. Dentistry for the Child and Adolescent. 9th ed. Missouri: Mosby; 2011

Preventive Resin Restorations And Pit And Fissure Sealants

Prof. (Dr.) Rakesh Kumar Chak, Dr. Pritika Rai (Ex-resident),
Department of Paediatric and Preventive Dentistry

A 7 year old girl visits a dental clinic with her mother, with the chief complaint of visible stains in her newly erupted teeth. The mother gives a history of decay and multiple restorations in the child's mouth when only her milk teeth were present. Extreme care and oral hygiene practises were followed by the mother for her child and was worried about any fresh decay in the teeth newly erupted. Clinical examination and radiographs revealed superficial caries restricted to enamel only in the mesial fissures and deeply stained pits and fissures in the rest of the occlusal surface of permanent first molars.

1. The treatment that should be given for the child is:

    (A) Removal of caries and amalgam restoration
    (B) Composite Restoration without removal of caries
    (C) Pit and fissure sealants
    (D) Preventive resin restorations

2. The concentration of phosphoric acid used for acid etching in permanent teeth is usually:

    (A) 30-50% acid solution or gel
    (B) 10-20% acid solution or gel
    (C) 70-80% acid solution or gel
    (D) less than 10%

3. When the caries in fissure is definite and requires considerable preparation, which type of Preventive Resin Restoration will be done?

    (A) Type A
    (B) Type B
    (C) Type C
    (D) all of the above

4. The disadvantage of using a clear resin for a sealant is:

    (A) Aesthetically unpleasant
    (B) Low strength
    (C) Poor retention
    (D) Difficult to detect on recall examinations

Answers:

1. D

   The preventive resin restoration is an alternative procedure for restoring young permanent teeth that require only minimal tooth preparation for caries removal but also have adjacent susceptible fissures. [2]

2. A

   The cavity for PRR and the enamel beside the susceptible grooves are etched. A gel or liquid form of 37% phosphoric acid is commonly used for 20 seconds.[2]

3. C

   In Type C PRR, carious lesion requires considerable preparation. A large size bur may be used for preparation. [1]

4. D

   Clear sealants have better flow characteristics than tinted sealants, but they are difficult to detect at recalls. [1]

References:

1. Tandon S. Text book of Pedodontics. 2nd ed. India: Paras Medical Publisher; 2009

1. McDonald RE, Avery DR, Dean JA. Dentistry for the Child and Adolescent. 9th ed. Missouri: Mosby; 2011

Enamel Hypoplasia (Molar – Incisor Hypoplasia)

Prof. (Dr.) Rakesh Kumar Chak, Dr. Pritika Rai (Ex-resident),
Department of Paediatric and Preventive Dentistry

An 8 year old child visited a dental clinic with the chief complaint of pain in the upper right and left posterior regions and unsightly creamy yellow discolouration in the anterior teeth. Clinical observation revealed carious enamel breakdown in all of the first permanent molars. Radiographically the carious involvement of dentin was also seen.

1. The provisional diagnosis of the following case can be:

   (A) Turners tooth
   (B) Flourosis
   (C) Tetracycline staining
   (D) Molar incisor hypomineralization (MIH)

2. The clinical picture of Molar incisor hypomineralization can include:

   (A) Presence of demarcated opacities
   (B) Posteruptive enamel breakdown
   (C) Atypical restorations and caries involvement in the affected teeth
   (D) All of the above

3. The enamel breakdown seen on the posterior molars occurs:

   (A) Prior to eruption due to insufficient enamel formation
   (B) Prior to eruption due to defective enamel formation
   (C) Post eruptive due to occlusal load on the molars
   (D) All of the above

4. Hypomineralization of a single permanent tooth due to localized infection in the corresponding primary tooth is called:

   (A) Turners tooth
   (B) Taurodontism
   (C) Dens evaginautus
   (D) Mulberry molar

Answers:

1. D

   Turners tooth is the enamel hypoplasia or hypomineralization of a single permanent tooth due to localized infection/trauma in the corresponding primary tooth. Fluorosis and tetracycline staining involves all the teeth. Only MIH presents in permanent incisors and first permanent molars [1, 2].

2. D

   All of these clinical features may be present in MIH, depending on the severity of defective enamel [1].

3. D

   Depending on the severity of defective enamel, breakdown may occur at any point of time [1, 2].

4. A

   [1]

References:

1. Tandon S. Text book of Pedodontics. 2nd ed. India: Paras Medical Publisher; 2009

2. McDonald RE, Avery DR, Dean JA. Dentistry for the Child and Adolescent. 9th ed. Missouri: Mosby; 2011

Common Gingival Cysts

Prof. (Dr.) Rakesh Kumar Chak, Dr. Suvidha Seth (Ex-resident),
Department of Paediatric and Preventive Dentistry.

A mother of a 15 days old child reported, complaining of yellowish white swelling of gums in upper back region of mouth. The child was born full term and his mother gave history of presence of lesion since birth with no contributory findings in medical history. Intraoral examination of child revealed small yellowish-white nodular papules over left side alveolar ridge of posterior maxilla. The size of the papules varied from 4-6 millimetres. On intraoral examination, no other abnormality or relevant findings were found in mucosa, tongue, palate or floor of mouth. Mother reported no difficulty in feeding the child.

1. Based on the clinical examination and charactertics of appearance of the lesion, what provisional diagnosis can be made?

    (A) Natal or neonatal teeth

    (B) Epstein pearls

    (C) Cyst of dental lamina

    (D) Bohn's nodules

2. Gingival cysts of newborn that usually appear along buccal and lingual aspects of the dental ridges and on the palate away from the raphe are:

    (A) Epstein pearls

    (B) Eruption cyst

    (C) ohn's nodules

    (D) Dental lamina cysts

3. Epstein's pearls seen in a newborn are considered as:

    (A) Remnants of mucous gland tissue‎

    (B) Remnants of dental lamina

    (C) Cysts derived from developing salivary glands

    (D) Remnants of epithelial tissue trapped along the raphe as the fetus grows

4. Which of the following is not true about gingival cysts of the newborn?

    (A) They are usually symptomatic

    (B) They usually continue to increase in size

    (C) Commonly seen in relation to the mandibular arch

    (D) Commonly seen in relation to the maxillary arch

5. Which of the following represents true microscopic picture of dental lamina cysts?

    (A) hin flattened parakeratotic epithelial lining with empty lumen
    (B) Cyst with no epithelial lining
    (C) Keratin filled lumen with thin parakeratotic epithelium
    (D) none of the above

6. Differential diagnosis between the various gingival cysts of newborn is made on the basis of:

    (A) (A Location in the oral cavity
    (B) Histological examinations
    (C) The age of appearance of the cysts in oral cavity
    (D) Symptoms of the lesions

Answers:

1. C

    Gingival cyst of dental lamina is a variant of gingival cyst of newborn located on crest of alveolar ridges in newborns, usually asymptomatic and not more than 4-6 mm in size [1].

2. C

    Bohn's nodules are remnants of mucous glands usually scattered at junction of hard and soft palate away from mid-palatal raphe [1].

3. D

    Epstein's Pearls are gingival cysts of newborns formed away from mid palatal raphe considered as remnants of epithelial tissue entrapped along raphe as the foetus grows [1].

4. D

    Gingival cysts of newborn are more commonly seen in the maxillary arch [1].

5. C

    Dental Lamina cysts are cysts lined by thin epithelium and filled by keratin in lumen [1].

6. A

Epstein's pearls, Bohn's. Nodules and dental lamina cysts are all considered common gingival cysts of newborn, differentiated on the basis of their location in the oral cavity [1].

Reference:

1. McDonald RE, Avery DR, Dean JA. Dentistry for the Child and Adolescent. 9th ed. Missouri: Mosby; 2011

Hypodontia In Primary/Permanent Teeth

Prof. (Dr.) Rakesh Kumar Chak, Dr. Suvidha Seth (Ex-resident),
Department of Paediatric and Preventive Dentistry

A 6 year old male child, reported with the chief complaint of missing primary teeth. His parents gave a positive history of consanguineous marriage with no associated prenatal birth or medical condition. According to the mother, the child had difficulty in speaking and chewing because of absence of teeth. Growth assessment of the child by a pediatrician did not reveal any underlying systemic condition. Intra oral examination revealed presence of primary maxillary central incisors, maxillary primary first and second molars and mandibular primary first molars on both sides. Panoramic radiograph revealed presence of only permanent maxillary central incisors, maxillary left first premolar, maxillary second molars, mandibular first premolars on both sides, first molar on both sides, second molar right side.

1. Based on the clinical and radiographic findings, the case can be diagnosed as:

   (A) Oligodontia involving only primary teeth
   (B) Hypodontia involving both primary and permanent teeth
   (C) Oligodontia involving both primary and permanent teeth
   (D) Complete Anodontia

2. Which of the following is true for missing teeth?

   (A) Hypodontia implies more than five missing teeth
   (B) Oligodontia implies less than 6 missing teeth
   (C) Hypodontia is the same as oligodontia
   (D) Oligodontia implies six or more missing teeth

3. Hypodontia can occur in association with any of the following aetiologies except:

   (A) Intra uterine disturbance
   (B) Familial autosomal recessive pattern
   (C) Infection of the developing tooth bud
   (D) Radiation over does during preganancy

4. Clinical features or dental anomalies which usually may accompany hypodontia are all of the following except

   (A) Taurodontism
   (B) Premature eruption of teeth
   (C) Prolonged retention of teeth
   (D) Transposition

5. Which of the following craniofacial syndrome is not associated with hypodontia
   (A) Chondro ectodermal dysplasia
   (B) Down's syndrome
   (C) Reiger's sundrome
   (D) Van der Woude syndrome

6. Variant of ectodermal dysplasia most commonly associated with multiple congenitally missing teeth is:
   (A) Hydrotic Ectodermal dysplasia
   (B) Hypo hydotic ectodermal dysplasia
   (C) Ectrodactyly ectodermal dysplasia plus cleft lip and palate
   (D) Rapp-hodgkins dysplasia

Answers:

1. C

   Oligodontia involving both primary and permanent teeth since number of missing teeth in both primary and secondary dentition is more than five and child appears to be healthy otherwise [1].

2. D

   Missing primary or permanent teeth between 0-5 is called as hypodontia (partial anodontia) and more than 5 (6 or more) implies oligodontia [1].

3. B

   Hypodontia exhibits an auto dominant pattern of inheritance caused due to mutation in MSX 1 gene [1]

4. B

   Hypodontia is usually accompanied by delayed eruption of teeth [1].

5. D

   Syndromes associated with hypodontia are chondroectodermal dysplasia, Down's syndrome, Reiger syndrome, Gorlin-Goltz syndrome & Osteogenesis imperfect type 1 [1].

6. B

Hypohydoric ectodermal dysplasia is a variant of ecto dermal dysplasia most commonly associated missing teeth followed by hydrotic ectodermal dysplasia, ectrodactyly ectodermal dysplasia [1].

Reference:

1. McDonald RE, Avery DR, Dean JA. Dentistry for the Child and Adolescent. 9th ed. Missouri: Mosby; 2011

Space Regainers

Prof. (Dr.) Rakesh Kumar Chak, Dr. Jyoti Verma (Ex-resident),
Department of Paediatric and Preventive Dentistry.

An 11 year old male patient reported with the chief complaint of missing tooth in lower right back region of mouth. On examination it was seen that FDI* tooth number 44 was erupted and there was space loss between tooth numbers (FDI*) 44 and 46. Patient gave history of extraction of tooth number 85 (FDI*) five years back. He did not get any space maintainer at that time leading to space loss.

1. Which of the following can be used in the present case?

    (A) Open coil spring regainer
    (B) Band and loop
    (C) Nance palatal arch
    (D) Transpalatal arch

2. Which of the following is incorrect about Gerber space regainer?

    (A) It is a fixed space regainer
    (B) It requires long appointment and complex lab work
    (C) The appliance can be fabricated directly in the mouth on appointment
    (D) Push coil spring is used

3. Which of the following is correct about lip bumper:

    (A) It is used for space regaining where bilateral movements are needed
    (B) It can be used when unilateral movement is required
    (C) It is used to transfer the lip pressure on the lower anteriors
    (D) Very thin labial arch wire is used in this appliance

4. Open coil space regainer is a

    (A) passive fixed regainer
    (B) active space regainer
    (C) reciprocal active fixed regainer
    (D) reciprocal passive fixed regainer

*=Fédération Dentaire Internationale

Answers:

1. C

   All the others are space maintainers and cannot be used in the present case as space loss was evident [1].

2. C

   Gerber's space maintainer is fabricated directly in mouth and requires no lab work [1].

3. A [1]

4. C [1]

Reference:

1. Tandon S. Text book of Pedodontics. 2nd ed. India: Paras Medical Publisher; 2009

Teething and Associated Problems

Prof (Dr.) R.K. Pandey, Dr. Apurva Mishra (Senior Resident), Department
of Paediatric and Preventive Dentistry, KGMU, Lucknow

Six months old male patient reported with a chief complaint of flushed cheeks,
gnawing, poor appetite, sore and red gums, drooling saliva along with disturbed sleep.

1. Which of the following conditions can be considered as the underlying etiology
   for the present clinical signs and symptoms?

   (A) Oral ulcers
   (B) Odontiasis
   (C) Nutritional deficiency
   (D) Mumps

2. Recommended treatment for the present case is:

   (A) Antibiotics
   (B) Vitamin supplements
   (C) Teething rings
   (D) No treatment required

3. Aspirin as an analgesic is not prescribed in the present situation because:

   (A) of risk of Reye syndrome
   (B) it doesn't provide symptomatic relief to the patient
   (C) it may cause allergic reactions
   (D) it has no effect

4. Parents of the patient in the present condition would often give history of soreness
   and swelling in the gums occurring at:

   (A) 3-5 days before tooth eruption
   (B) 3-5 hours after tooth eruption
   (C) 3-5 weeks before tooth eruption
   (D) 3-5 days after tooth eruption

5. How can chin rash occurrence be prevented in children with the present condition:

   (A) By constantly wiping the drooling saliva
   (B) Barrier cream application
   (C) Avoid rubbing of chin
   (D) All of above

6. Cold temperature rings provide local relief in symptoms for the present condition by:

(A) localized vasoconstriction
(B) localized vasodilation
(C) have no effect on vascularity
(D) none of above

Answers:

1. B

Odontiasis is also known teething. The signs and symtoms with which the patient has presented are associated with 'teething'. In most children the eruption of primary teeth is preceded by increased salivation, and the child will want to put the hand and fingers into the mouth [1,2].

2. B

Teething rings are the best treatment modality offered to the parents as they help in increasing the blood circulation of the gums affected and relieve itching. [1,2]

3. A

Reye syndrome can be caused by prescription of analgesics in young children/ infants. [1,2]

4. A

5. D

All of these modalities help. [1,2]

6. A

Localized vasoconstriction is caused by the low temperature in the affected area [1,2].

References:

1. Tandon S. Text book of Pedodontics. 2nd ed. India: Paras Medical Publisher; 2009

2. Marwah N. Text book of Pediatric Dentistry, Third 3rd ed. India: Jaypee brothers Medical publishers; 2014

Early Childhood Caries-Anterior Teeth

Prof (Dr.) R.K. Pandey, Dr. Apurva Mishra (Senior Resident), Department of Paediatric and Preventive Dentistry, KGMU, Lucknow

Five years old female patient reported with a chief complaint of decay in multiple milk teeth as shown in picture below:

1. Identify the condition:

    (A) Early childhood caries

    (B) Enamel hypoplasia

    (C) Dentin dysplasia

    (D) Teething problem

2. Etiological factors for the present condition can be:

    (A) Night feeding

    (B) Feeding beyond weaning age

    (C) Improper oral hygiene

    (D) All of above

3. Major concern for early primary tooth lost in anterior segment is:

    (A) Esthetics

    (B) Space loss

    (C) Both

    (D) None

4. Primary teeth that are usually not involved in early childhood caries is:

    (A) Maxillary central incisor

    (B) Mandibular incisors

    (C) Maxillary molars

    (D) Mandibular molars

Answers:

1. A

    The American Academy of Pediatric Dentistry (AAPD) defines early childhood caries (ECC) as the presence of one or more decayed (noncavitated or cavitated), missing (as a result of caries), or filled tooth surfaces in any primary tooth in a child 71 months of age or younger [1].

2. D

    For many years it has been recognized that, after eruption of the primary teeth begins, excessively frequent bottle feedings and/or prolonged bottle or breast-feeding, especially during night, is often associated with early and rampant caries. Salivary flow is also decreased during sleep, and clearance of the liquid from the oral cavity is slowed. AAPD also discourages extended or excessive frequency of feeding times (from the breast or bottle) and encourage appropriate oral hygiene measures for infants and toddlers [1].

3. A

    Premature loss of maxillary primary incisors does not generally result in decreased upper intracanine dimensions if the incisor loss occurs after the primary canines have erupted into occlusion at approximately 2 years of age [1]. Therefore, space loss does not occur.

4. D

    There is early carious involvement of the maxillary anterior teeth, the maxillary and mandibular first primary molars, and sometimes the mandibular canines in early childhood caries. The mandibular incisors are usually unaffected. The child falls asleep, and the liquid becomes pooled around the teeth (the lower anterior teeth tend to be protected by the tongue) [1].

Reference:

1. McDonald RE, Avery DR, Dean JA. Dentistry for the Child and Adolescent. 9th ed. Missouri: Mosby; 2011

Early Childhood Caries-Posterior Teeth

Prof. (Dr.) R.K. Pandey, Dr. Apurva Mishra (Senior Resident),
Department of Paediatric and Preventive Dentistry

A 3 year boy reported with a chief complaint of multiple decayed tooth and pain in lower back regions of both sides. On radiographic examination, carious pulp exposure was found in all deciduous molars of mandibular arch.

1. The child will be diagnosed for the condition known as:

    (A) Dental caries
    (B) Milk bottle syndrome
    (C) Malformed molars
    (D) Hypoplastic molars

2. The choice of treatment for primary molars involved will be:

    (A) Pulpectomy
    (B) Pulpectomy with stainless steel crown
    (C) Extraction
    (D) Pulp capping

3. Risk based management approach is preferred for Early childhood caries. It includes:

    (A) Fluoride application
    (B) Xylitol pacifiers
    (C) Diet counseling
    (D) All of the above

4. Early childhood caries term was coined by:

    (A) Davies
    (B) Winter
    (C) Moss
    (D) Horowitz

5. ECC is also known as:

    (A) Tooth clearing neglect
    (B) Nursing bottle syndrome
    (C) Maternally derived streptococcus mutans disease
    (D) All of the above

Answers:

1. B

   'Milk bottle syndrome' is an alternative term for early childhood caries [1]

2. B

   Stainless steel crowns are indicated as restorations for pulpotomized or pulpectomized primary or young permanent teeth when there is increased danger of fracture of the remaining coronal tooth structure [2]

3. D

   It is recommended that all possible preventive measures and approaches must be considered in the hope of successfully controlling and preventing the caries process. Risk based management approach requires all these modalities mentioned depending on the grade of risk for caries development in the child [2]

4. A [1]

5. D [1]

References:

1. Tandon S. Text book of Pedodontics. 2nd ed. India: Paras Medical Publisher; 2009

2. McDonald RE, Avery DR, Dean JA. Dentistry for the Child and Adolescent. 9th ed. Missouri: Mosby; 2011

Common Gingival Problems In Children

Prof. R.K. Pandey, Dr. Garima Jindal, Department
of Paediatric and Preventive Dentistry

An 11 year old, with a history of epilepsy, presented with a painless gingival enlargement of the interproximal region, present since 3 months.

1. What is the provisional diagnosis of the above case-

    (A) Chronic marginal gingivitis.
    (B) Drug induced gingival enlargement.
    (C) Acute gingival abcess.
    (D) Congenital gingival enlargement.

2. Which of the following drug is associated with gingival enlargement-?

    (A) Prilocaine
    (B) Piroxicam
    (C) Phenytoin
    (D) Phenobarbitone

3. Which of the following is the line of treatment for the above case-?

    (A) Change the drug.
    (B) Gingivectomy
    (C) Gingivoplasty
    (D) All of the above.

4. In the above case, clinician found presence of bleeding on probing, what could be the eitiology?-

    (A) Superimposed secondary inflammation.
    (B) Traumatic bleeding.
    (C) Vitamin C deficiency.
    (D) None of the above.

5. Which of the following is false for vitamin C deficiency gingival enlargement-?

    (A) Gingiva is smooth, soft, shiny and friable.
    (B) It is a fibrotic gingival enlargement.
    (C) Spontaneous or haemorrhage on slight provocation.
    (D) Surface necrosis with pseudomembrane formation can be seen.

Answers:

1. B

   The patient is epileptic and might be on phenytoin drug. The swelling of interproximal gingiva is characteristic of phenytoin induced gingival enlargement [1]

2. B

   Amongst all the drug choices given, only phenytoin induces gingival enlargement. Other drugs that have been reported to induce gingival overgrowth in some patients include cyclosporin, calcium channel blockers, valproic acid, and Phenobarbital [2]

3. D

   All of the treatment options can be performed at different stages.[2]

4. B

   Bleeding on probing in the above case is suggestive of secondary inflammation due to local factors. It is common because of inability of the patient to perform proper oral hygiene procedures due to gingival enlargement [2]

5. B

   Vit C deficiency induced gingival enlargement is edematous type of gingival enlargement. Fibrotic gingival enlargement is seen in drug induced and congenital varieties [2]

References:

1.   Tandon S. Text book of Pedodontics. 2nd ed. India: Paras Medical Publisher; 2009

2.   McDonald RE, Avery DR, Dean JA. Dentistry for the Child and Adolescent. 9th ed. Missouri: Mosby; 2011

Common Acute Gingival Problems In Children

Prof R.K. Pandey, Dr. Garima Jindal, Department
of Paediatric and Preventive Dentistry

A 4 year old girl, presented with a complaint of oral pain and bleeding from gums since one day.

1. Which of the following is not included in the differential diagnosis of the above case?

    (A) Acute Necrotizing Ulcerative Gingivitis.
    (B) Acute herpetic gingivostomatitis.
    (C) Aphthous stomatitis.
    (D) Drug induced gingival hyperplasia.

2. In the above case, clinician found punched out ulcers of interproximal papillae, the diagnosis would be-

    (A) Apthous stomatitis.
    (B) Acute herpetic gingivostomatitis.
    (C) Acute Necrotizing Ulcerative Gingivitis.
    (D) Lichen planus.

3. Acute herpetic gingivostomatitis can be differentiated from Acute Necrotizing Ulcerative Gingivitis by presence of ulcers in the oral cavity at:

    (A) Soft palate.
    (B) Labial mucosa.
    (C) Hard palate and attached gingiva.
    (D) Buccal mucosa and floor of the mouth.

4. Which of the following condition does not predisposes a child to Acute Necrotizing Ulcerative Gingivitis?

    (A) Local factors like erupting teeth.
    (B) Nutritional deficiency.
    (C) Blood dyscrasias.
    (D) HSV infection.

5. Acute Necrotizing Ulcerative Gingivitis is also known as-

    (A) Cancrum oris
    (B) Canker sore
    (C) Cold sore
    (D) Vincent's angina

Answers:

1. D

    pain and bleeding are not found in drug induced gingival enlargement [1,2]

2. C

    punched out ulcers of interproximal papillae is a characteristic feature of Acute Necrotizing Ulcerative Gingivitis [1,2]

3. C

    the ulcers of Acute herpetic gingivostomatitis are located on rigid oral mucosa that is firmly attached to the underlying bone, that is, Hard palate and attached gingival [1,2]

4. D

    HSV is a virus and does not cause ANUG. ANUG occurs in immunocompromised and debilitating conditions [1,2]

5. D

    Vincent's angina is another name of Acute Necrotizing Ulcerative Gingivitis [1,2]

References:

1. Tandon S. Text book of Pedodontics. 2nd ed. India: Paras Medical Publisher; 2009

2. McDonald RE, Avery DR, Dean JA. Dentistry for the Child and Adolescent. 9th ed. Missouri: Mosby; 2011

Cleft Lip And Palate

Prof. R. K. Pandey, Dr. Garima Jindal, Department of Paediatric
and Preventive Dentistry, KGMU, Lucknow

A 2 month old patient presented with bilateral cleft lip and palate.

1. The criteria for deciding the appropriate time for surgical lip closure in cleft lip case includes all except:

    (A) 10 gm% haemoglobin.
    (B) 10 pounds weight.
    (C) 10 weeks age.
    (D) 10 months age.

2. Which one of the following statement is true for 2 stage surgical cleft palate repair-

    (A) Growth of midface is hampered.
    (B) Speech results are poor.
    (C) Hard palate repair is followed by soft palate repair.
    (D) First stage surgery is done at 10 weeks of age.

3. Which of the following problems is associated with cleft lip and palate-?

    (A) Difficulty in articulation.
    (B) Nasal twang in voice.
    (C) Middle ear infection.
    (D) All of the above.

4. Which of the following is not found in untreated bilateral cleft palate cases-?

    (A) Anterior open bite.
    (B) Ectopic eruption.
    (C) Anterior deep bite.
    (D) Posterior cross bite.

5. Which of the following methods of feeding does not contribute in preventing regurgitation of fluids in cleft lip and palate infant?

    (A) Keeping the child upright while feeding.
    (B) Use of obturators.
    (C) Mead Johnson feeding bottle.
    (D) Removable maxillary Hawley's appliance.

6. Surgical correction of nasal deformity with cleft lip and palate should be performed –

    (A) Before correcting cleft deformity.

(B) After correcting cleft deformity.

(C) Anytime.

(D) Nasal repair not required.

Answers:

1. D

The rule of 10 for deciding the timing of surgical repair of lip includes "10 gm% haemoglobin, 10 pounds weight, 10 weeks age" [1,2]

2. B

In two stage cleft palate repair, surgical repair of soft palate at 18 months is followed by hard palate at 4-5 years. This allows better midface growth but speech results are unacceptably poor [1,2].

3. D

Defective speech and middle ear infection are seen in cleft palate cases [1,2].

4. A

In untreated bilateral cleft palate cases, premaxilla is protuberant and upper incisors falls on gingiva of lower incisors causing complete closed overbite [1,2].

5. D

Hawley's appliance cannot be fabricated in an infant as there are no teeth present [1,2].

6. B

Surgical correction of nasal deformity with cleft lip and palate should be performed after correcting cleft deformity [1,2].

References:

1.   Tandon S. Text book of Pedodontics. 2nd ed. India: Paras Medical Publisher; 2009

2.   McDonald RE, Avery DR, Dean JA. Dentistry for the Child and Adolescent. 9th ed. Missouri: Mosby; 2011

Child Abuse

Prof. R. K. Pandey, Dr. Garima Jindal, Department
of Paediatric and Preventive Dentistry

A 5 year old boy reported to the department for his appointment for restoration in his teeth. He had periorbital ecchymosis around his both eyes. He had problem in sitting because of pain in buttocks and had a defected gait. On enquiring from his mother, she said "He fell down while playing."

1. What could be suspected in the above case-

    (A) Buccal space infection.

    (B) Sinusitis

    (C) Physical child abuse

    (D) None of these.

2. What is the duty of dentist in such a case:

    (A) Ignore the injuries.

    (B) Report of a suspicion to appropriate child protective agency.

    (C) Do further investigation.

    (D) Do not perform any dental treatment.

3. A case in which caretaker induces or reports factitious symptoms in a child is called as-

    (A) Physical neglect

    (B) Battered child syndrome

    (C) Shaken baby syndrome

    (D) Munchausen syndrome by proxy.

4. Which of the following is not an indicator of emotional abuse?-

    (A) Destructive behavior

    (B) Poor self esteem.

    (C) Multiple injuries in different stages of healing.

    (D) Alcohol or drug abuse.

5. The term battered child syndrome was coined by-

    (A) E.Jordan

    (B) Kempe

    (C) Humphrey

    (D) Croll

6. Which of the following is not a form of child neglect-?

   (A) Educational neglect
   (B) Recreational neglect
   (C) Dental neglect
   (D) Failure to thrive.

Answers:

1. C

   poorly explained multiple injuries indicate physical child abuse. Falling in the playground does not explain both injury to forehead causing periorbital ecchymosis and pain in buttocks [1,2].

2. B

   the duty of the dentist in such a case is to perform required dental treatment and reporting of suspicion of child abuse to appropriate child protective agency [1,2].

3. D

   Munchausen syndrome by proxy is in which caretaker induces or reports factitious symptoms in a child [1,2].

4. C

   Multiple injuries in different stages of healing is seen in physical abuse and all others quoted, in emotional abuse [1,2].

5. B

   Kempe coined the term battered child syndrome [1,2].

6. B

   Recreational neglect is not a form of neglect whereas Educational neglect. Dental neglect and failure to thrive are all forms of child neglect [1,2].

References:

1. Tandon S. Text book of Pedodontics. 2nd ed. India: Paras Medical Publisher; 2009

2. McDonald RE, Avery DR, Dean JA. Dentistry for the Child and Adolescent. 9th ed. Missouri: Mosby; 2011

Chapter - 8

Prosthodontics and Crown and Bridge

Tori

Dr. Pooran Chand, Professor; Dr. Niraj Mishra,
Associate Professor; Dr. Shahid Ahmed Shah, Junior Resident,
Department of Prosthodontics and Crown and Bridge

A healthy 66 years old female patient came to a dental clinic for fabrication of complete dentures. On examination of the mandibular arch two large bony protuberances were observed on either side of the lingual aspect of the mandible in the premolar region. The protuberances were smooth, rounded, fixed and the covering mucosa was slightly blanched and sensitive to pressure.

1. The provisional diagnosis of the bony protuberances can be

    (A) Peripheral Ossifying Fibroma
    (B) Tori
    (C) Denture Granuloma
    (D) Osteoma

2. Management of large mandibular tori is best done by

    (A) Surgical removal
    (B) Providing relief in the denture
    (C) Covering the tori with soft liner
    (D) None of the above

3. Mandibular tori are most commonly present in which region

    (A) Incisor region on the labial side
    (B) Incisor region on the lingual side
    (C) Premolar region on the lingual side
    (D) Premolar region on the buccal side

4. Which of the following is *false* in relation to mandibular tori?

    (A) Adequate denture relief can be provided without breaking the denture seal
    (B) They are covered by thin mucoperiosteum
    (C) May occur singly or in rows
    (D) Large mandibular tori prevent complete seating of impression trays and denture.

5. Mandibular tori occurs in approximately what percentage of population

    (A) 7-10%
    (B) 20-25%
    (C) 30-35%
    (D) 40-45%

Answers:

1. B

   Tori are smooth rounded anatomical protuberances sometimes seen on the lingual surface of the mandible and the midline of the hard palate. Tori are covered with a thin mucoperiosteum; consequently, they are very hard and sensitive to pressure.[1]

2. A

   It often is difficult to provide adequate denture relief for large mandibular tori because it would break the border seal of the denture. If adequate accommodation through relief cannot be anticipated, surgical removal is indicated.[1]

3. C

   Mandibular tori occur singly or in rows just above the floor of the mouth and are most commonly found on the lingual side in the premolar region.[1]

4. C

   Adequate denture relief cannot be provided without breaking the denture seal, therefore, large mandibular tori should be surgically removed.[1]

5. A

   Mandibular tori are present in approximately 7-10% of the population.[1]

Reference:

1. Zarb, George A., Fenton, Aaron H. Prosthodontic treatment for edentulous patients: complete dentures and implant-supported prostheses. St. Louis, MI: Mosby; 2013:88

Combination Syndrome

Dr. Pooran Chand, Professor; Dr. Niraj Mishra, Associate Professor; Dr. Shahid Ahmed Shah, Junior Resident, Department of Prosthodontics and Crown and Bridge

A 45 year old male patient came to a dental clinic for replacement of missing teeth. The patient was wearing a maxillary complete denture and a mandibular distal extension partial denture since the past 4 years. The patient complained of a poorly fitting maxillary denture. On examination the maxillary ridge in the anterior region was hyperplastic and the natural mandibular anterior teeth were extruded.

1. The term used to collectively describe the present situation is

    (A) Combination Syndrome
    (B) Costen Syndrome
    (C) Christenson Syndrome
    (D) Gardner Syndrome

2. Which of the following is *not* a feature of combination syndrome

    (A) Hyperplasia of anterior maxillary ridge
    (B) Enlargement of the tuberosities
    (C) Intrusion of mandibular anterior teeth
    (D) Loss of vertical dimension of occlusion

3. Which impression technique is used for making impressions of hyperplastic ridges

    (A) Window technique
    (B) Mucocompressive technique
    (C) Selective pressure technique
    (D) None of the above

4. The term combination syndrome was coined by

    (A) Kelly
    (B) Jensen
    (C) McFadden
    (D) Carlson

5. Combination syndrome may be accompanied by which of the following features

    (A) Epulis fissuratum
    (B) Occlusal plane discrepancy
    (C) Anterior spatial repositioning of the mandible
    (D) All of the above

Answers:

1. A

Combination syndrome is a dental condition that is commonly seen in patients with a completely edentulous maxilla and partially edentulous mandible with preserved anterior teeth. This syndrome consists of severe anterior maxillary resorption combined with hypertrophic and atrophic changes in different quadrant of maxilla and mandible.[1]

2. C

Extrusion of mandibular anterior teeth occurs in combination syndrome[1]

3. A

Window technique as described by Zaffarulla Khan is used for making impressions of hyperplastic ridges.[1]

4. A

Ellsworth Kelly coined the term combination syndrome. He described 3 key features of combination syndrome: reduction of anterior maxillary bone, enlargement of maxillary tuberosities, and bone resorption under the mandibular RPD bases.[1]

5. D

Saunders added to the description of the combination syndrome byincluding destructive changes such as loss of occlusal vertical dimension, occlusal plane discrepancy, anterior spatial repositioning of the mandible, poor adaptation of the prostheses, epulis fissuratum and periodontal changes.[1]

Reference:

1. Tolstunov Len. Combinationsyndrome: Classification and case report. J Oral Implantol .2000;33:139-51.

Severely Resorbed Mandibular Ridge with Hyperactive Muscles

Dr. Pooran Chand, Professor; Dr. Niraj Mishra, Associate Professor; Dr. Shahid Ahmed Shah, Junior Resident, Department of Prosthodontics and Crown and Bridge

A 59 year old female patient came to a dental clinic with a complaint of a loose mandibular denture made one year back. On examination the mandibular ridge was severely resorbed both in the anterior and posterior regions and muscle attachments present very close the crest of the ridge. The mandibular denture had poor extensions and lacked any stability and there was minimal retention.

1. In the present case what should be expected cause for compromised stability of mandibular denture

   (A) Residual ridge resorption
   (B) Hyperactive muscles
   (C) Poor extensions of the existing denture
   (D) All of the above

2. Neutral zone technique is used for the management of

   (A) Hyperplastic ridges
   (B) Well formed ridges
   (C) Ridges with severe undercuts
   (D) Highly resorbed ridges

3. The potential space between the cheeks and lips on one side and the tongue on the other, that area or position where the forces between the tongue and cheeks or lips are equal is known as the

   (A) Neutral zone
   (B) Donder's space
   (C) Silverman's space
   (D) None of the above

4. The closed mouth impression technique using tissue conditioners for making final impression of highly resorbed mandibular ridge was given by

   (A) Winkler
   (B) Klein
   (C) Shanahan
   (D) Levine

5. Factors enhancing the stability of mandibular denture are
   (A) Proper contours of the denture flanges
   (B) Overextension of the dentures flanges
   (C) Increasing thickness of the denture flanges
   (D) Underextension of the dentures flanges

Answers:

1. D

   Residual ridge resorption, hyperactive muscles lying close to the crest of the ridge and poor extensions of the denture base result in lack of stability of mandibular denture.[1]

2. D

   The neutral zone philosophy for management of highly resorbed ridges is based on the concept that for each individual patient, there exists within the denture space a specific area where the function of the musculature will not unseat the denture and at the same time, where the forces generated by the tongue are neutralized by the forces generated by the lips and cheeks.[1]

3. A

   The potential space between the cheeks and lips on one side and the tongue on the other, that area or position where the forces between the tongue and cheeks or lips are equal is known as the neutral zone. Several other terms have also been coined for describing this space like zone of equilibrium, zone of minimal conflict, biometric denture space, zone of least interference.[1]

4. A

   Winkler described the closed mouth technique for making impressions of resorbed ridges using tissue conditioners and a final impression is made using light body elastomeric material[1]

5. A

   Proper contours of the polished surface of the denture, ideal tongue position to gain an effective lingual border seal and maximum physiologic tissue coverage of the denture bearing area by applying minimum pressure help in improving the stability of the mandibular denture.[1]

Reference:

1. Beresin VE, Schiesser FJ. The neutral zone in complete dentures. J Prosthet Dent. 2006;95:93–100.

<u>Costen's Syndrome</u>

Dr. Niraj Mishra, Associate Professor; Dr.Sunit Kumar Jurel, Associate Professor; Dr. Shahid Ahmed Shah, Junior Resident, Department of Prosthodontics and Crown and Bridge

A 60 year old male patient reports to the dental clinic with complaints of difficulty in chewing food, a dull aching pain in the face, ear ache particularly in the morning and reduced ability to open or close the mouth. The patient is wearing a complete denture since the past six years. Examination reveals over closure of the vertical dimension. Angular cheilitis is also present.

1. The provisional diagnosis of the present case scenario can be

    (A) Costen's Syndrome
    (B) Migraine
    (C) Myofacial pain dysfunction syndrome
    (D) None of the above

2. Pain in Costen's syndrome can be due to

    (A) Overclosure of the vertical dimension
    (B) Pressure on the glossopharyngeal nerve
    (C) Pressure on the sphenopalatine nerve
    (D) Raised vertical dimension

3. Symptoms of Costen's syndrome include

    (A) Pain in the ear, head, sinus and tongue
    (B) Clicking of the TMJ
    (C) Bruxism
    (D) All of the above

4. Angular cheilitis in the present case is due to

    (A) Increased vertical dimension of occlusion
    (B) Decreased vertical dimension of occlusion
    (C) Poor oral hygiene
    (D) Both a and c

5. Management of Costen's syndrome includes

    (A) Restoring the lost vertical dimension of occlusion
    (B) Using monoplane occlusion
    (C) Using surgery as the first option.
    (D) Reducing the vertical dimension

Answers:

1. A

   Poorly made complete dentures with loss of vertical dimension of occlusion, dull aching pain in the face, tenderness of the jaws and angular chelitis are all presenting features of Costen's syndrome.[1]

2. A

   In overclosure of the vertical dimension there is erosion of the roof of the glenoid fossa leaving either a perforation or very thin bone between the condyle and the dura mater. On closure there is pain from the rich nerve supply of the dura and this causes a dull vertex pain. Pain may also occur due to pressure on the auriculotemporal nerve and chorda tympani nerve.[1]

3. D

   Symptoms of Costen's syndrome include pain in the ear, head, sinus and tongue, clicking and snapping sounds in the TMJ, bruxism, difficulty in chewing food, tinnitus and hearing loss.[1]

4. B

   Angular cheilitis is seen in patients with excessive overclosure of the vertical dimension due to drooling of saliva and fungal infections [1]

5. A

   Management of Costen's syndrome includes restoring the lost vertical dimension of occlusion, pain relief with analgesics, gentle stretching and relaxation jaw exercises, occlusal splint therapy, and surgery is the last resort.[1]

References:

1. Wing G. The status of costen's syndrome. Aus Dent Jrnl. 1959;98-103.

Closest Speaking Space

Dr. Niraj Mishra, Associate Professor; Dr.Sunit Kumar Jurel,
Associate Professor; Dr. Shahid Ahmed Shah, Junior Resident,
Department of Prosthodontics and Crown and Bridge

A 72 year old complete denture wearer reports to the dental clinic with complaints of difficulty in chewing food and inability to speak properly. Complete dentures were made two months back. Examination reveals increased vertical dimension of occlusion and lack of freeway space to perform functions normally.

1. The term 'closest speaking space' was coined by

    (A) Silverman
    (B) Niswonger
    (C) Thompson
    (D) Sharry

2. Closest speaking space is measured in which area

    (A) Incisor region.
    (B) Canine region
    (C) Premolar region
    (D) Molar region

3. In class I situation, Ideal freeway space for performing normal functions should be

    (A) Less than 2 mm
    (B) 2-4 mm
    (C) More than 4 mm
    (D) 6-8 mm

4. While measuring the closest speaking space, the patient should be seated in which position

    (A) Supine position
    (B) Semisupine position
    (C) Upright position without the use of headrest
    (D) Upright position with the use of headrest

5. The closest speaking space occurs when the patient pronounces

    (A) S sound
    (B) F sound
    (C) V sound
    (D) M sound

Answers:

1. A

The term closest speaking space was coined by Meyer M Silverman.[1]

2. C

Closest speaking space is measured in the premolar region.[1]

3. B

Ideal freeway space for performing normal functions should be 2-4 mm.[1]

4. C

While measuring the closest speaking space the patient is seated in an upright position without the use of the headrest, with the eyes forward, and the occlusal surfaces of the upper posterior teeth parallel to the floor.[1]

5. A

The closest speaking space occurs when the patient pronounces the S sound.[1]

Reference:

1. Silverman M. The speaking method in measuring vertical dimension.J Prosth. Dent. 1953 March 3;2:193-99

Dentogenics Concept

Dr. Niraj Mishra, Associate Professor; Dr.Sunit Kumar Jurel,
Associate Professor; Dr. Shahid Ahmed Shah, Junior Resident,
Department of Prosthodontics and Crown and Bridge

A 54 year old female complete denture wearer reports to the dental clinic with complaints of poor appearance of her dentures. Complete dentures were made two months back. Examination reveals improper tooth selection and arrangement not consistent with the patient's personality. The teeth appear to be too large in size and the shade does not match the patient's facial complexion.

1. The art, practice and technique of creating the illusion of natural teeth in artificial dentures based on the elementary factors of sex, personality and age is known as

    (A) Golden proportion
    (B) Dentogenics
    (C) Divine proportion
    (D) None of the above

2. The concept of dentogenics for selection of artificial teeth was given by

    (A) Frush and Fisher
    (B) Niswonger
    (C) Jameson
    (D) Levine

3. The three basic components of colour while selecting artificial teeth include all of the following *except*

    (A) Hue
    (B) Chroma
    (C) Value
    (D) Translucency

4. According to dentogenic concept, age factor can be incorporated in denture teeth by

    (A) Grinding incisal edges of upper anterior teeth
    (B) Rotating canines
    (C) Using squarish teeth
    (D) Using angular teeth

5. While arrangement of artificial teeth, all of the following factors result in feminine appearance *except*,

    (A) Slight overlapping of maxillary lateral incisor over maxillary central incisor
    (B) Raising maxillary canine slightly above occlusal plane
    (C) Using narrow lateral incisors
    (D) Using square arch form

Answers:

1. B

    Dentogenics is the art, practice and technique of creating the illusion of natural teeth in artificial dentures and is based on the elementary factors of sex, personality and age.[1]

2. A

    The concept of dentogenics for selection of artificial teeth was given by James Frush and Roland Fisher.[1]

3. D

    The three basic components of colour while selecting artificial teeth include hue, chroma and value.[1]

4. A

    Age factor can be incorporated in denture teeth by grinding incisal edges of upper anterior teeth, by shortening the papillae and by raising gingival gum line, selecting long teeth, contouring the wax and positioning the tooth properly to suggest recession.[2]

5. D

    Feminine appearance can be incorporated in artificial teeth by slight overlapping of maxillary lateral incisor over maxillary central incisor, raising maxillary canine slightly above occlusal plane, using narrow lateral incisors and using ovoid arch form.[3]

References:

1. Frush JP, Fisher RD. Introduction to dentogenic restorations. J Prosthet Dent 1955; 5:586-95

2. Frush JP, Fisher RD. The age factor in dentogenics. J Prosthet Dent 1957; 7;5-13

3. Frush JP, Fisher RD. How dentogenic restorations interpret the sex factor. J Prosthet Dent 1956; 6:160-172

Neuromuscular Disorder

Dr. Sunit Kumar Jurel, Associate Professor; Dr. Kaushal Kishor Agrawal, Assistant Professor; Dr. Rohan Grover, Junior Resident, Department of Prosthodontics and Crown and Bridge

A 58 year old completely edentulous male patient reported to OPD of the Department of Prosthodontics, with facial paralysis of right half and inability to chew food since three years. Extra-oral clinical examination revealed facial asymmetry with reproducible left side mandibular deviation during mouth opening. Patient was unable to close his right eye completely, unable to blow air from mouth, unable to lift his right eyebrows.

1. A patient with poor neuromuscular control present with occlusal prematurities. Occlusion can be corrected by

    (A) Direct method
    (B) No need to establish correct occlusion
    (C) Patient is asked to bite carborundom paste
    (D) Take interocclusal record and correct on articulator

2. Difficulty may occur in following step during fabrication of complete denture in a Bell's palsy patient

    (A) Impression taking
    (B) Border moulding
    (C) Teeth setting
    (D) Jaw relation

3. In the patient of Bell's palsy, excessive horizontal overlap in posteriors teeth is given

    (A) To avoid cheek biting
    (B) It helps in speech
    (C) It helps in retention
    (D) Provide balanced occlusion

4. Which of the following duct is affected in Bell's palsy

    (A) Stenson's
    (B) wharton's
    (C) nasolacrimal
    (D) lacrimal

5. Following type of teeth are indicated in patient of Bell's palsy

(A) Anatomic

(B) Semianatomic

(C) Non anatomic

(D) any type

Answers:

1. D

Due to neuromuscular disability in such patients, the correct centric relation can not be recorded. Due to it eccentric relations are recorded which leads to occlusalprematurities. To correct these occlusalprematurities best method is to rearticulate on articulator with new centric relation and correcting the occlusion.[1]

2. D

Refer to question no. 1 explaination.

3. A

In the patient of bell's palsy excessive horizontal overlap in posteriors teeth is given to avoid cheek biting since muscles are paralysed and have no control of these muscle on movement.[1]

4. A

Duct of parotid gland pierces the buccinator muscle and open in the region of 2nd molar. Since the buccinator is paralysed the opening of the parotid gland is also affected.[1]

5. C

In patient of bell's palsy is non anatomic teeth are indicate to minimize lateral forces.[1]

Reference:

1. Herbert Sherman denture insertion, In:Essentials of complete denture prosthodontics: Sheldon winkler:AITBS Indian edition 2000

Immediate Denture

Dr. Sunit Kumar Jurel, Associate Professor; Dr. Kaushal Kishor Agrawal, Assistant Professor; Dr. Rohan Grover, Junior Resident, Department of Prosthodontics and Crown and Bridge

A musician of 55 year-old, visited to OPD, with no significant medical history. She presented complete edentulous mandibular arch and a Kennedy class I maxillary arch with an anterior fixed partial denture (#13- 22) that had been placed several years back. The three remaining abutments presented advanced periodontal disease. The patient was adamant that she could not be edentulous for any length of time.

1. Most appropriate treatment option for this patient is

    (A) Immediate denture
    (B) Complete denture
    (C) Partial denture
    (D) Overdenture

2. Which of the following is NOT an advantage of immediate dentures

    (A) Reduced post operative pain
    (B) Easy adaptation
    (C) Less chairside time
    (D) None

3. In the construction of complete arch immediate denture, anterior teeth are extracted

    (A) in first appointment
    (B) before construction of denture
    (C) after denture construction
    (D) after posterior teeth extaction

4. One of the major disadvantage of immediate denture is

    (A) pain associated with treatment
    (B) difficulty in managing occlusion
    (C) need for reline
    (D) no control over tooth placement and shape

5. When both maxillary and mandibular complete dentures are proposed then it is advisable to construct

   (A) maxillary followed by mandibular
   (B) mandibular followed by maxillary
   (C) both simultaneously
   (D) none

Answers:

1. A

   Indication of immediate denture
   a. public dealing
   b. social appearance
   c. patient does not want any edentulous periods[1]

2. Greater chairside time is one the major disadvantage of immediate denture[1]

3. Treatmment procedure of immediate denture
   a. The posterior teeth are extracted and socket are allowed to heal
   b. Impression are made
   c. Anterior teeth in master cast are broken and trimmed upto the cervical margin
   d. Denture is fabricated
   e. During the insertion appointment the remaining anterior teeth are extracted
   f. The denture is inserted1

4. Disadvantages of immediate denture
   a. The fit, appearance or comfort is very difficult to predict
   b. There is no try in
   c. Often require tissue conditons during healing phase
   d. Need a definitive reline1

5. Both denture are inserted simultaneously to any irregularity in centric occlusion[1]

Reference:

1. Nancy S. Arbree: Immediate dentures:In:Prosthodontic treatment for edentulous patients: Zarb Bolender:Mosby(Elsevier), New Delhi India:123-159

Midline Fracture of Complete Denture

Dr. Sunit Kumar Jurel, Associate Professor; Dr. Kaushal Kishor Agrawal, Assistant Professor; Dr. Rohan Grover, Junior Resident, Department of Prosthodontics and Crown and Bridge

A 62 years male patient comes to OPD Department of prosthodontics with chief complaints of missing all upper jaw teeth and several lower jaw teeth. Intra oral examination revealed high frenum attachment in maxilla. The opposing complement of natural dentition was present. Maxillary denture was got fractured from midline and repaired two times in a private clinic.

1. The possible reason of midline fracture of maxillary complete denture is

    (A) Excessive forceful bite by mandibular natural teeth
    (B) Excessive resorption of alveolar ridges
    (C) Very thin acrylic resin
    (D) None

2. Midline fracture of maxillary denture is usually a result of

    (A) impact fracture
    (B) fatigue fracture
    (C) accidental dropping
    (D) None

3. For repair of maxillary midline fractured denture, a long rounded bevel is made on each side of opening about _____mm wide along the entire midline and onto the labial surface.

    (A) 1
    (B) 2
    (C) 5
    (D) 10

4. The load required to fracture denture range from

    (A) 180-800 Ib
    (B) 1000-1200 Ib
    (C) 1200-1400 Ib
    (D) None

Answers:

1. A

   Patient are able to exert extreme pressure on maxillary denture when they occlude against natural mandibular teeth which leads to fracture of maxillary complete denture.[1]

2. B

   Midline fracture of maxillary denture is usually a result of fatigue fracture.[1]

3. C

   For repair of maxillary midline fractured denture, a long rounded bevel is made on each side of opening about 5 mm wide along the entire midline and onto the labial surface.[1]

4. A

   Most common denture fracture of maxilla and mandible are midline fracture.[1]

Reference:

1. L Rush bailey: Denture repairs, IN: Essentials of complete denture prosthodontics: Sheldonwinkler: AITBS publishers India 2012:352-60

Overdenture

Dr. Kaushal Kishor Agrawal, Assistant Professor; Dr. Pooran
Chand, Professor; Dr. Rohan Grover, Junior Resident,
Department of Prosthodontics and Crown and Bridge

A Patient reported to the Department of Prosthodontics with the chief complaint of missing teeth in upper jaw. On examination maxillary arch showed only maxillary canines (13 and 23) and second molar (17) were present. All teeth were periodontally sound. The situation can be classified as a Kennedy's class II modification Patient had given a history of multiple temporary partial dentures that she was not satisfied. The chief reason for dissatisfaction was poor retention. Sufficient inter arch space was present.

1. The suitable treatment option for this case is

   (A) Overdenture
   (B) Partial denture
   (C) Complete denture
   (D) None of the above

2. All are the advantage of overdenture EXCEPT

   (A) Preservation of alveolar bone
   (B) Aesthetic
   (C) Support
   (D) Retention

3. Which of the following is not an advantage of overdenture

   (A) Prevention of alveolar bone
   (B) Retention
   (C) Support
   (D) Caries prevention

4. Which of the following teeth provide better support for overdenture

   (A) Bilateral Central incisor
   (B) Bilateral Lateral incisor
   (C) Bilateral Canine
   (D) Bilateral molar

5. True about overdenture is

   (A) Anterior abutments are preferred over posterior abutment
   (B) Maintenance of vertical height of occlusion
   (C) Improve stability
   (D) All

Answers:

1. A

   The treatment option in this case is overdenture, since it provide preservation of alveolar bone, support, retention, periodontal maintenance.[1]

2. B

   Advantages of overdenture
   i.   Preservation of alveolar bone
   ii. Support
   iii. Retention
   iv. Periodontal maintenance[1]

3. D

   Caries susceptibility is disadvantage of an overdenture.[1]

4. C

   For an overdenture strategic tooth position ang root length is very important factor. The canines and premolars are considered best tooth for an overdenture.[1]

5. D

   Advantages of overdenture
   i.   Preservation of alveolar bone
   ii. Support
   iii. Retention
   iv. Periodontal maintenance
   v.   Harmony of arch form1

Reference:

1.   Robert defranco: Overdentures, In:Essentials of complete denture prosthodontics: Sheldon Winkler: AITBS Indian edition 2012 384-402

Radiotherapy

Dr. Kaushal Kishor Agrawal, Assistant Professor; Dr. Pooran Chand, Professor; Dr. Rohan Grover, Junior Resident, Department of Prosthodontics and Crown and Bridge

A patient aged 65 years reported to OPD, with the chief complaint of difficulty in mastication and a dry mouth. He presented with the history of radiotherapy since last 2 years and extraction of all his teeth 8 months prior to radiotherapy. Intra-orally, irregular maxillary and mandibular ridges with very scanty saliva were found.

1. Reduced salivary flow following irradiation is dose dependent, at what dose the flow reach essentially zero

   (A) 4000 rads
   (B) 5000 rads
   (C) 6000 rads
   (D) 7000 rads

2. Most sensitive phase in cell division to radiation is

   (A) G1 phase
   (B) G2 phase
   (C) S phase
   (D) None

3. A patient requires extraction from an area that has been subjected to radiation therapy. Which of the following condition represent the greatest danger to this patient?

   (A) Alveolar osteitis
   (B) Osteoradionecrosis
   (C) Prolonged healing
   (D) Fracture of mandible

4. First complication after radiotherapy is

   (A) Mucositis
   (B) Candidiasis
   (C) Alopecia
   (D) Xerostomia

5. Radiation causes changes in blood flow by

   (A) Anemia
   (B) Endarteritis of small blood vessels
   (C) Infection
   (D) All of the above

Answers:

1. C

The extent of reduced flow is dose dependentandand reaches to zero at 60 GY[1]

2. B

G2 phase is more radiosenstive and S phase is radioresistant[1]

3. B

Wwhen bone is irradiated the marrow become hypoxic, hypocellular and hypovascular. If tooth extraction is done the mucous membrane breaks and infection gains entry in to the bone leaving a non healing wound resulting in osteoradionecrosis[1]

4. A

Mucositisone of the earliest complication it appears at the end of 2nd week[1]

5. B

The long term deterministic effect of radiation on tissue and organs depends primarily on the extent of damage to the fine vasculature irradiation of of capillaries causes swelling, degeneration, and necrosis, which increases capillary permeability and initiate progressive fibrosis around the vessels, leading to deposition of scar tissue.[1]

Reference:

1. Stuart C. White, Michael J. Pharaoh:Radiobiology. In, Oral Radiology:Elsevier, Noida India 2009:18-30

Rebasing of Complete Denture

Dr. Kaushal Kishor Agrawal, Assistant Professor; Dr. Pooran
Chand, Professor; Dr. Rohan Grover, Junior Resident,
Department of Prosthodontics and Crown and Bridge

A 50 year male patient reported to the OPD, Department of Prosthodontics, with a chief complaint of loose mandibular complete denture. There was no any relevant medical history. Patient was completely edentulous since 5 months. On examination, the patient had partially edentulous maxillary arch and completely edentulous mandibular arch.

1. In which of the following condition relining and rebasing can be done for a loose complete denture

   (A) Excessive alveolar bone loss
   (B) When CO and CR does not coincide
   (C) The patient is poor and cannot afford the new denture
   (D) More than 2 mm loss of alveolar bone height

2. Functional techniques of relining and rebasing utilise

   (A) Wax
   (B) Tissue conditioner
   (C) ZOE
   (D) Alginate

3. During relining/rebasing fear lies in alteration of

   (A) balanced occlusion
   (B) centric occlusion
   (C) vertical dimension
   (D) condylar guidance

4. As compared to relining, in rebasing of a denture a change can occur in

   (A) centric occlusion
   (B) centric relation
   (C) entire denture base
   (D) tissue surface

5. Relining and rebasing of complete denture is required because

   (A) denture base material abrades
   (B) ridge resorption is a continous process
   (C) it prolongs the longevity of the denture
   (D) all the above

Answers:

1. C

   "Relining is the process of adding some material to the tissue side of a denture to fill the space between the tissue and the denture base"

   "Rebasing is the process of replacing all the base material of a denture. The purpose of such a process is to fill the space between the tissue and the denture base without changing the position of teeth and the relation of the denture"

   Indication of relining or rebasing:
   i. Immediate denture at 3-6 months after their original construction
   ii. When residual alveolar ridge is resorbed and adaptation of the denture base to the ridge is poor
   iii. When the patient cannot afford the cost of the treatment[1]

2. B

   In functional technique of relining and rebasing tissue conditioners are used because with these material good functional impression can be made[1]

3. C

   Many dentistbelive that the replacement of the palatal portion of a maxillary denture is necessary to avoid to increase in vertical dimension[1]

4. C

   Rebasing is a process of replacing all the base material of denture[1]

5. D

   Indication of relining and rebasing
   i. immediate denture at 3-6 months after their original construction
   ii. to adopt to the resorbing ridge
   iii. when the patient cannot afford the cost of the treatment[1]

Reference:

1. Nikzad S. Javid and John F. Bowman; Relining and rebasing techniques. In Essentials of complete denture prosthodontics. Sheldon Winkler;AITBS publisher India 2012:341-351

Classifications of RPD

Dr. Mayank Singh, Assistant Professor; Dr. H.A. Alvi, Professor; Dr. Ronak Bhatt, Junior Resident, Department of Prosthodontics and Crown and Bridge

A 55 year old patient reported to the Department of Prosthodontics with the chief complaint of inability to chew food due to loss of teeth. On examination the patient had bilaterally missing teeth in the mandibular posterior region and edentulous span in maxillary left posterior region. Patient is partially edentulous since 8 months. The patient wanted replacement for the same.

1. To which Kennedy's class does the maxillary partially edentulous state of above patient belong?

   (A) Class I
   (B) Class II
   (C) Class III
   (D) Class IV

2. The distal extension RDP in mandibular posterior region is?

   (A) Tooth borne
   (B) Tissue borne
   (C) Mostly Tissue and partially tooth borne
   (D) Mostly tooth and partially tissue borne

3. Which class of RDP best resists the forces to which it is subjected?

   (A) Class I
   (B) Class II
   (C) Short span Class III
   (D) Class IV

4. The edentulous areas other than those determining the main type of classification are called as?

   (A) Class
   (B) Modification
   (C) Edentulous area
   (D) Missing area

5. To which Kennedy's class does the Mandibular partially edentulous state of above patient belong?
   (A) Class I
   (B) Class II
   (C) Class III
   (D) Class IV

Answers:

1. C

   Kennedy's classification

   Class I- bilateral edentulous areas located posterior to remaining teeth.

   Class II- unilateral edentulous area located posterior to remaining teeth.

   Class III- unilateral edentulous area with natural teeth remaining both anterior and posterior to it.

   Class IV- a single but bilateral edentulous area located anterior to remaining natural teeth.[1]

2. C

   Class I and II are tooth and tissue borne for RDP design; class III is mainly tooth borne due to tooth support at both ends; and class IV depends on the edentulous ridge span (short span – tooth supported, long span – tooth and tissue supported).[1]

3. C

   The class III (tooth borne) being supported at both the ends of edentulous spaces best resists the forces. It also normally does not tend to rotate or lift. Short span resists the forces better than long span.[2]

4. B

   Edentulous area other than those determining the main types (spaces other than the original classes) are designated as modification spaces.[2]

5. A

   refer to explanation of question number 1.

References:

1. Alan B, David T. McCracken's Removable Partial Prosthodontics. 12th edition. St.Louis: Elsevier Mosby; 2012.

2. Phoenix, Rodney D, David R, Charles F. Stewart's Clinical Removable Partial Prosthodontics. Fourth edition. Quintessence publishing co, Inc; 2008.

Indirect Retainer

Dr. Mayank Singh, Assistant Professor; Dr. Balendra Pratap
Singh, Associate Professor; Dr. Ronak Bhatt, Junior Resident,
Department of Prosthodontics and Crown and Bridge

A 45 year old patient reported to the Department of Prosthodontics with the chief complaint of inability to chew food due to loss of teeth since 8 months. On examination the patient had bilaterally missing teeth in the mandibular posterior region. The patient wanted replacement for the same.

1. The minor connector in the RDP should cross the gingival margin at?

    (A) Acute angle
    (B) Obtuse angle
    (C) Right angle
    (D) Should not cross gingiva

2. The function of occlusal rests in the above patient will be?

    (A) To resist vertical force of occlusion
    (B) Stabilize the denture
    (C) To increase retention of RPD
    (D) To prevent lateral forces acting on tooth

3. Guiding planes are?

    (A) Located adjacent to edentulous area
    (B) Located far anterior to edentulous area
    (C) Helps in stability of denture
    (D) Provides a different path of insertion and removal

4. The angle between the occlusal rest and the vertical minor connector from which it will originate will be?

    (A) 90 degrees
    (B) 100 degrees
    (C) 120 degrees
    (D) Less than 90 degrees

5. Where should the indirect retainer be located in relation to the fulcrum line?

    (A) As near as possible to the fulcrum line
    (B) As far as possible to the fulcrum line
    (C) In the line of fulcrum line
    (D) Can be located anywhere

Answers:

1. C

the minor connector always crosses the gingiva abruptly making 90 degree angle with gingiva.[1]

2. A

occlusal rest resists vertical forces, retentive arm resists dislodging forces, reciprocating arm resists horizontal forces in the direct retainers.[1]

3. A

All proximal surfaces of teeth adjacent to edentulous areas must be parallel to the previously determined path of insertion.[2]

4. D

the angle formed by the occlusal rest and the vertical minor connector from which it originates should be less than 90 degrees. This helps in directing the occlusal forces along the long axis of abutment tooth.[2]

5. B

the indirect retainer resists the movement of the rdp away from the tissue. It resists the dislodging forces best when it is located as far as possible from the fulcrum line.[2]

References:

1. Alan B, David T. McCracken's Removable Partial Prosthodontics.12th edition. St.Louis: Elsevier Mosby; 2012.

2. Phoenix, Rodney D, David R, Charles F. Stewart's Clinical Removable Partial Prosthodontics. Fourth edition. Quintessence publishing co, Inc; 2008.

Direct Retainers

Dr. Mayank Singh, Assistant Professor; Dr. Kamleshwar
Singh, Associate Professor; Dr. Ronak Bhatt, Junior Resident,
Department of Prosthodontics and Crown and Bridge

A 50 year old patient reported to the Department of Prosthodontics with the chief complaint of inability to chew food due to missing teeth since one year. On examination the patient had edentulous span in maxillary left posterior region. The patient wanted replacement for the same.

1. The means by which one part of RDP opposes the action of the retainer in the function is called?

    (A) Tripoding
    (B) Reciprocation
    (C) Retention
    (D) Stress breaking

2. The terminal end of the retentive arm of direct retainer will be placed at?

    (A) Middle of gingival third
    (B) Middle of middle third
    (C) Middle of occlusal third
    (D) Under gingival sulcus

3. The direct retainers will be placed on which tooth in maxillary arch?

    (A) 23 and 27
    (B) 17 and 27
    (C) 13 and 23
    (D) 13 and 17

4. If RPI clasp is used in above case, what does it stand for?

    (A) Occlusal rest, proximal plate, I bar
    (B) Cingulum rest, proximal plate, I bar
    (C) Rest, proximal guide plane, I bar
    (D) Rest, proximal plate, indirect retainer

5. Which of the following is not the component of a direct retainer?

    (A) Retentive arm
    (B) Reciprocating arm
    (C) Occlusal Rest
    (D) Guide plane

Answers:

1. B

   the rigid reciprocal arm helps in reciprocating stress generated against the tooth by the retentive arm. It also stabilizes the denture against horizontal movement and is always situated above the height of contour.[1]

2. A

   in posterior tooth mainly the maximum bulge of teeth is at middle third, hence undercut is naturally formed in gingival third which is engaged by terminal end of retentive arm for retention of RDP.[1]

3. A

   the directs retainers are those which engage the teeth adjacent to the edentulous areas. Hence the direct retainers in maxillary arch in above case will be on 22 and 27 teeth.[1]

4. A

   R- occlusal rest, P- proximal plate, I- I bar. This system was introduced by Kroll. [2]

5. D

   guide planes are prepared on the proximal surface of the tooth on which direct retainer is placed. The compoents of direct retainers are retentive arm, reciprocal arm, minor connector and an occlusal rest.[2]

References:

1. Alan B, David T. McCracken's Removable Partial Prosthodontics. 12th edition. St.Louis: Elsevier Mosby; 2012.

2. Phoenix, Rodney D, David R, Charles F. Stewart's Clinical Removable Partial Prosthodontics. Fourth edition. Quintessence publishing co, Inc; 2008.

Minor Connectors in RPD

Dr. Kamleshwar Singh, Associate Professor; Dr. HA Alvi, Professor; Dr. Varuni Arora, Senior Resident, Department of Prosthodontics and Crown and Bridge

A 36-year-old woman had been wearing an interim removable partial denture for 4 years to replace missing maxillary anterior teeth and the left second premolar. She was diagnosed with generalized aggressive periodontitis with an average of 40 to 50% bone loss with 3 to 7 mm of attachment loss. Her most recent treatment consisted of the extraction of 2 teeth with a poor prognosis (maxillary right second and third molars), scaling/root planing, and open flap debridement of the maxillary right quadrant. Restorative treatment was initiated with caries control. The maxillary right second premolar was restored with a mesio-occluso-distal amalgam. The maxillary left second molar received endodontic treatment due to pulpal necrosis.

1. While designing RPD for this patient, which minor connector would you chose between left first premolar and left first molar?

   (A) Ladder like
   (B) Meshwork
   (C) Metal base with beads
   (D) Acrylic extension only

2. The junctions of these mandibular minor connectors with the major connectors should be

   (A) 90 degrees
   (B) Less than 90 degrees
   (C) More than 90 degrees
   (D) Angle doesn't matter. They should be strong

3. Minor connectors must cross gingival tissue should do so

   (A) abruptly, joining the major connector at nearly a right angle
   (B) obtusely, joining the major connector
   (C) acutely, joining the major connector
   (D) a and b both correct

4. An open latticework or ladder type of design is conveniently made by using preformed

   (A) 12-gauge half-round and 18-gauge round
   (B) 18-gauge half-round and 12-gauge round
   (C) 12-gauge half-round and 16-gauge round
   (D) 16-gauge half-round and 18-gauge round

5. The minor connector for the mandibular distal extension base should extend posteriorly

    (A) about two thirds the length of the edentulous ridge
    (B) about half the length of the edentulous ridge
    (C) full edentulous ridge
    (D) about three fourths the edentulous ridge

Answers:

1. C

    This region is tooth supported and hence would not require relining. In such cases metal with beads is preferable.[1]

2. A

    Marginal gingiva should be covered by the minor connector in as short a span as possible (90°). [2]

3. A

    Same as Answer [2]

4. A [2]

5. A

    For the maxillary distal extension base, the minor connector should extend upto the maxillary tuberosity. [2]

References:

1. Polly MS, Brudvik JS. Managing the maxillary partially edentulous patient with extensive anterior tooth loss and advanced periodontal disease using a removable partial denture: A clinical report. J Prosthet Dent 2008;100:259-263

2. Carr AB, McGivny GP, Brown DT. Mc Cracken's Removable Partial Prosthodontics. 11th ed Mosby. Elsevier.2012.

Rest and Rest Seats in RPD

Dr. Kamleshwar Singh, Associate Professor; Dr. Mayank
Singh, Assistant Professor, Dr. Varuni Arora, Senior Resident;
Department of Prosthodontics and Crown and Bridge

A 61 year old female was treated in the following manner. The second maxillary right molar, first maxillary left premolar, second left mandibular molar, and second left mandibular premolar were extracted. Endodontic therapy of the right and left maxillary canine and the second and maxillary left premolar was performed. In the mandibular arch, crown was placed on right third molar. The mandibular arch was edentulous posterior to right and left canines. The residual alveolar ridge was firm. A maxillary partial fixed dental prosthesis and a mandibular traditional RDP were fabricated.

1. Which teeth do you think would be bearing rest seats for the conventional RPD given to her?

   (A) Third molar and premolars
   (B) Right third molar and left premolar
   (C) Third molar and incisors
   (D) Both premolars and canine

2. Floor of the rest seat should be at

   (A) 86 °
   (B) 90°
   (C) 100°
   (D) 120°

3. When floor of the occlusal rest seat is inclined more than 90°, then the prosthesis behaves like which simple machine

   (A) Wedge
   (B) Screw
   (C) Inclined plane
   (D) Lever

4. Fluoride gel should be applied to the abutment teeth following enamel recontouring

   (A) Five minutes before impression with an irreversible hydrocolloid
   (B) Half an hour before impression with an irreversible hydrocolloid
   (C) A day before impression with an irreversible hydrocolloid
   (D) After impression with an irreversible hydrocolloid

5. Pear shaped multifluted burs can be used for
    (A) Cingulum rests
    (B) Rounding marginal ridges
    (C) Both of the above
    (D) Height of contour adjustments

Answers:

1. A

    Teeth adjacent to an edentulous span are ideally the primary abutments.. [1]

2. A

    This angle should always be less than 90[0.] to direct forces towards the centre of the tooth. [1]

3. C

    This inclined plane transfers undesirable tipping forces to the tooth.[1]

4. D

    Fluoride gel may be displaced by the irreversible hydrocolloid. [1]

5. C

    Pear shaped burs facilitate proper smoothening and rounding of the preparation. [1]

Reference:

1. Carr AB, McGivny GP, Brown DT. Mc Cracken's Removable Partial Prosthodontics. 11th ed Mosby. Elsevier.2012

Major Connector in RPD

Dr. Kamleshwar Singh, Associate Professor; Dr. Balendra Pratap Singh, Associate Professor, Dr. Varuni Arora, Senior Resident, Department of Prosthodontics and Crown and Bridge

An 88-year-old man had remaining teeth that were periodontally sound, heavily restored, and had extensive marginal and root caries. Maxillary and mandibular wrought wire and acrylic resin interim partial dentures showed evidence of several repairs and addition of missing teeth (Fig. 1). The prognosis for the remaining teeth was deemed poor because of a high caries risk and extensive restorations. Likewise, the prognosis for a complete denture was guarded because of an unfavorable arch form and minimal vestibular depth.

1. Which major connector would be planned in this patient?

   (A) Anteroposterior double palatal bar
   (B) Complete palatal
   (C) Closed horse shoe
   (D) Posterior palatal bar

2. To differentiate between a palatal bar and a palatal strap, palatal bar should have palatal connector component

   (A) Less than 6 mm
   (B) More than 6 mm
   (C) Less than 8 mm
   (D) More than 8 mm
   (E) 10 mm in width

3. Palatal connectors require relief

   (A) Over torus
   (B) Over median palatal suture
   (C) Over the posterior two-thirds of the hard palate
   (D) A and b

4. In which form can a palatal plate not be used?

   (A) as a plate of varying width that covers the area between two or more edentulous areas
   (B) in the form of an anterior palatal connector with a provision for extending an acrylic resin denture base posteriorly
   (C) both a and c
   (D) none

5. When the last remaining abutment tooth on either side of a Class I arch is the canine or first premolar tooth and the residual ridges have undergone excessive vertical resorption, major connector strongly advised is
   (A) Anteroposterior double palatal bar
   (B) Complete palate
   (C) Closed horse shoe
   (D) Posterior palatal bar

Answers:

1. B

   Number of abutments in maxillary arch is less and compromised. This situation requires complete palatal coverage.[1]

2. C[2]

3. D

   Palatine tori and median palatine raphe are areas where the mucosa/ submucosa is thin and friable, thereby needing relief. [2]

4. D

   Complete Palate connector should be used in both the given situations. [2]

5. B

   This situation requires maximum stress distribution and coverage. [2]

References:

1. Waliszewski MP, Brudvik JS. The conversion partial denture: A clinical report. J Prosthet Dent 2004;91:306-9

2. Carr AB, McGivny GP, Brown DT. Mc Cracken's Removable Partial Prosthodontics. 11th ed Mosby. Elsevier.2012

Gypsum Products

Dr. Pooran Chand, Professor; Dr Niraj mishra, Associate Professor, Dr. Pradeep Kumar, Senior Resident, Department of Prosthodontics and Crown and Bridge

A patient reported to the Department of Prosthodontics with the chief complaint of difficulty in eating food due to missing teeth. On clinical evaluation, he was found to be completely edentulous with flabby tissue in mandibular anterior region. So, it was planned to fabricate maxillary and mandibular complete denture for this patient.

1. Which of the following type of gypsum product should be used to make diagnostic cast for this patient?

   (A) Type I
   (B) Type II
   (C) Type III
   (D) Type IV

2. Which of the following which of the following type of gypsum product should be used to make definitive cast for this patient?

   (A) Type I
   (B) Type II
   (C) Type III
   (D) Type IV

3. Which method is used to disinfect gypsum casts?

   (A) Microwave irradiation
   (B) Infrared irradiation
   (C) Ultraviolet disinfection
   (D) Autoclave

4. Which of the following type of gypsum product can be used to impress flabby tissue?

   (A) Type I
   (B) Type II
   (C) Type III
   (D) Type IV

Answers:

1. B

    ADA Specification No.25 classifies gypsum products into following five types:

    Type I- Plaster, impression-Used to impress flabby tissues.

    Type II- Plaster, model- Used for making diagnostic casts and to fill flask during denture construction.

    Type III- Dental stone- Used for making master cast.

    Type IV- Dental stone, high strength- It is also known as die stone and is used for making dies.

    Type V- Dental stone, high stone, high expansion- Used as investment material. (1)

2. C

    Dental stone as it has higher strength than model plaster. (1)

3. A

    If an impression has not been disinfected, then it is necessary to disinfect the stone casts. Disinfection solutions that do not adversely affect the quality of gypsum cast can be used. Alternatively, disinfectants can be incorporated either in the powder or dissolved in mixing water. Microwave irradiation for 5-min at 900W can be used to disinfect stone casts. (1)

4. A.

    As it is free flowing and results in mucostatic impression. (1)

Reference:

1. Anusavice KJ, Shen C, Rawls HR, eds. Phillips' Science of Dental Materials. 12th ed. St Louis, Mo: Saunders; 2013:182-93.

Impression Materials Used in Complete Dentures

Dr. Pooran Chand, Professor; Dr Sunit Kr Jurel, Associate Professor, Dr. Himanshi Aggarwal, Senior Resident; Department of Prosthodontics and Crown and Bridge

A patient reported to the Department of Prosthodontics with the chief complaint of difficulty in eating food due to missing teeth. On clinical evaluation, he was found to be completely edentulous so it was planned to fabricate maxillary and mandibular complete denture for this patient.

1. Which of the following is the most commonly used reversible primary impression material?
    (A) Alginate
    (B) Impression compound
    (C) Impression waxes
    (D) Elastomers

2. Which of the following material results in a muco-compressive impression?
    (A) Alginate
    (B) Impression compound
    (C) Impression waxes
    (D) Impression plaster

3. Which of the following material is most commonly used for making definitive impression for edentulous arches?
    (A) Alginate
    (B) Impression compound
    (C) Impression waxes
    (D) Zinc Oxide eugenol impression paste

4. Which of the following impression material cannot be used for making impression of the flabby ridges?
    (A) Alginate
    (B) Impression compound
    (C) Impression waxes
    (D) Impression plaster

Answers:

1. A.

   As it is cheap, easily available and thermoplastic material. Both alginate and elastomers are irreversible impression materials. (1)

2. B.

   As it is a highly viscous material and flows only under pressure. (1)

3. D.

   As it is dimensionally more stable, produces accurate details and is easy to manipulate. (1)

4. B

   As it results in a mucocompressive impression owing to its high viscosity. All other given materials are free flowing and do not compress the tissues, resulting in a mucostatic impression. (1)

Reference:

1. Anusavice KJ, Shen C, Rawls HR, eds. Phillips' Science of Dental Materials. 12th ed. St Louis, Mo: Saunders; 2013:151-81.

Impression Procedures for Removable Partial Dentures

Dr. H.A.Alvi, Professor, Dr Balendra Pratap Singh, Associate
Professor, Dr.Himanshi Aggarwal, Senior Resident;
Department of Prosthodontics and Crown and Bridge

A 48 year old patient reported to Prosthodontics department with complaint of difficulty in eating due to missing teeth. On clinical examination, it was found that maxillary posterior teeth on both sides and mandibular premolars and first molar on one side were missing. Following diagnosis and through evaluation, it was planned to fabricate maxillary and mandibular cast removable partial dentures for the patient as he was not willing for any fixed treatment due to financial constraints.

1. Which of the following technique should be used to make maxillary impression?

    (A) Mucocompressive impression technique
    (B) Mucostatic impression technique
    (C) Anatomic impression technique
    (D) Dual impression technique

2. Which of the following technique should be used to make mandibular impression?

    (A) McLean's and Hindels' method
    (B) Functional Relining technique
    (C) Mucostatic impression technique
    (D) Dual impression technique

3. Which one of the following is a fluid wax?

    (A) Utility wax
    (B) Korrecta wax no.4
    (C) Modelling wax
    (D) Beading wax

4. In which of the following condition, dual impression technique is not indicated?

    (A) Kennedy's Class I
    (B) Kennedy's Class II
    (C) Kennedy's Class III
    (D) Short span Kennedy's Class IV

Answers:

1. D

    According to Kennedy's classification, maxilla is Class I and mandible is Class III partially edentulous arch. For Class I, II and long span Class IV (tooth tissue supported conditions), dual impression technique is recommended. This includes following techniques:

    -Physiologic or functional impression technique: McLean's and Hindels' method, Functional Relining technique and fluid wax technique.

    -Selected pressure impression technique. (1)

2. C

    As Kennedy's Class III is a tooth supported condition, anatomic or mucostatic impression technique should be used. (1)

3. B

    Fluid waxes are those waxes that are firm at room temperature and have the ability to flow at room temperature. The most commonly used fluid waxes are Iowa wax and Korrecta wax no.(1, 2)

4. C.

    Refer to Q1.

References:

1. Stewart KL, Rudd KD, Kuebker WA, eds. Clinical Removable Partial Dentures. 2nd ed. Medico Dental Media International Inc, USA; 2005: 373-92.

2. Carr AB, McGivney GP, Brown DT, eds. McCracken's Removable Partial Prosthodontics, 11th ed. St Louis, Mo: Mosby; 2005:271-85.

Jaw Relations for Removable Partial Dentures

Dr. H.A.Alvi, Professor, Dr Kamleshwar Singh, Associate Professor, Dr. Pradeep Kumar, Senior Resident; Department of Prosthodontics and Crown and Bridge

A 48 year old patient reported to Prosthodontics department with complaint of difficulty in eating due to missing teeth. After clinical examination, it was diagnosed as a case of Kennedy's Class I maxillary arch and Kennedy's Class III mandibular arch. So, it was planned to fabricate maxillary and mandibular cast removable partial dentures for this patient

1. Which of the following material cannot be used for recording centric relation in this patient?

   (A) Wax
   (B) Irreversible hydrocolloid
   (C) Metallic oxide bite registration paste
   (D) Elastomeric material

2. Which material is most likely to be least satisfactory for recording centric relation?

   (A) Wax
   (B) Polyether bite registration material
   (C) Metallic oxide bite registration paste
   (D) Elastomeric material

3. Which method can't be used for establishing interocclusal relations for Kennedy's Class I situation?

   (A) Direct apposition of casts
   (B) Functionally generated path technique
   (C) Using occlusal rims on record bases
   (D) Using metal framework

4. Which of the following is not essential for establishing a satisfactory occlusion in this case?

   (A) Analysis of existing occlusion
   (B) Correction of existing occlusal disharmony
   (C) Establishing a new plane of occlusion
   (D) Recording centric and eccentric jaw relations

Answers:

1. B

   As alginate is dimensionally unstable. (1)

2. A

   As distortion of wax during or after removal from the mouth may interfere with accurate seating. Excess wax that contacts mucosal surfaces may distort soft tissue, thereby preventing accurate seating of wax record onto the stone casts. (1, 2)

3. A

   As the opposing casts cannot be articulated accurately by hand because of lack of posterior occlusion, especially in Kennedy's Class I and II partially edentulous arches. (1, 3)

4. C

   As establishing a new plane of occlusion is not always required. (1)

References:

1. Carr AB, McGivney GP, Brown DT, eds. McCracken's Removable Partial Prosthodontics, 11th ed. St Louis, Mo: Mosby; 2005:301-18.

2. Carr AB, McGivney GP, Brown DT, eds. McCracken's Removable Partial Prosthodontics, 11th ed. St Louis, Mo: Mosby; 2005:189-229.

3. Stewart KL, Rudd KD, Kuebker WA, eds. Clinical Removable Partial Dentures. 2nd ed. Medico Dental Media International Inc, USA; 2005: 393-437.

Diagnosis and Treatment Planning in Removable Partial Dentures

Dr. H.A.Alvi, Professor, Dr Mayank Singh, Assistant Professor, Dr Kamleshwar Singh, Associate Professor, Department of Prosthodontics and Crown and Bridge

A 50 year old patient reported to the Prosthodontics Department with the complaint of inability to chew food due to pain in lower right first premolar and loss of remaining upper and lower posterior teeth.

1. Sequence of oral examination should begin with

   (A) Thorough and complete oral prophylaxis
   (B) Relief of pain and placement of temporary restoration
   (C) Preliminary impression making
   (D) Thorough IOPA survey

2. Which of the following is not an indication for fabrication of removable partial denture?

   (A) Distal extension situation
   (B) Need for bilateral stabilization
   (C) Single missing tooth
   (D) Long span edentulous condition

3. Which of the following is not a purpose served by diagnostic casts?

   (A) Analysis of existing occlusion from both lingual and buccal aspects
   (B) Fabrication of metallic framework
   (C) Fabrication of individual impression trays
   (D) Permit comprehensive presentation of present and future restorative needs to the patient

Answers:

1. B

   As acute needs of the patient should be addressed first followed by prophylaxis. It is advisable not only to relieve pain and discomfort arising from tooth defects but also to determine the extent of caries and arrest further caries activity until definitive treatment can be instituted. By restoring tooth contours with temporary restorations, impression will not be torn on removal from mouth and a more accurate diagnostic cast may be obtained. (1)

2. C

   As best option for replacing a single missing tooth is an implant retained crown. (1)

3. B

   As fabrication of metallic framework is always done on a master/definitive cast. (1)

Reference:

1. Carr AB, McGivney GP, Brown DT, eds. McCracken's Removable Partial Prosthodontics, 11th ed. St Louis, Mo: Mosby; 2005:189-229.

Biocompatibilty of Dental Materials

Dr. Pooran Chand, Professor; Dr.Himanshi Aggarwal, Senior Resident, Dr. Rani Ranabhatt, Junior Resident; Department of Prosthodontics and Crown and Bridge

Biocompatibility is defined as the ability of the biomaterial to perform its desired function with respect to a medical (or dental) therapy, without eliciting any undesirable local or systemic effects in the recipient or beneficiary of that therapy but generating the most appropriate beneficial cellular or tissue response in that specific situation, and optimizing the clinically relevant performance of that therapy.

1. The biocompatibility of a material does not depend on

    (A) Chemical nature of its components
    (B) Physical nature of its components
    (C) Mechanical nature of its components
    (D) Surface characteristics of the material

2. Estrogenicity which is defined as the potential of a chemical to act in the body in a manner similar to that of estrogen, is shown by

    (A) Gold
    (B) Mercury
    (C) Bisphenol A
    (D) Methacrylates

3. Metal ions produce which type of hypersensitivity reaction?

    (A) Type l
    (B) Type ll
    (C) Type lll
    (D) Type lV

4. Patch test is used for

    (A) Allergic contact dermatitis
    (B) Hypersensitivity
    (C) Mutagenicity
    (D) Estrogenicity

Answers:

1. C

The biocompatibility of a material depends on several factors
   1. Chemical nature of its components
   2. Physical nature of its components
   3. Types and locations of the patient tissues that will be exposed to the device
   4. Duration of the exposure
   5. Surface characteristics of the metal
   6. Amount and nature of substances eluted from the material. (1)

2. C

Bisphenol A (BPA) is a synthetic starting point for bis-GMA composites in dentistry as well as many other plastics. The concern about estrogen in dentistry centers around this chemical. (1)

3. D

Metal ions first interact with a host molecule to produce a Delayed Type IV hypersensitivity reaction which is modulated by monocytes and T cells. (1)

4. A

Most definitive diagnostic test for allergic contact dermatitis. When the suspected allergen is applied to skin, hyperemia, edema, vesicle formation & itching can be seen after 48 to 96 hours to produce small area of allergic contact dermatitis, which is considered as a positive patch test reaction. (1)

Reference:

1. Anusavice KJ, Shen C, Rawls HR, eds. Phillips' Science of Dental Materials. 12th ed. St Louis, Mo: Saunders; 2013:111-47.

Obstructive Sleep Apnea (Osa) and its Treatment Modalities

Dr. Deeksha Arya, Associate Professor; Dr. Raghuwar D Singh, Professor; Dr. Lakshya Kumar, Assistant Professor, Department of Prosthodontics and Crown and Bridge

A 45 year old patient was referred to the Department with complain of snoring and frequent sleep arousal. On Polysomnography it was found that patient having problem of Moderate sleep apnea.

Clinical treatment:

Oral appliances are the effective treatment modality for the Obstructive sleep apnea patients. The patient was given Mandibular advancement device (MAD) as it is most successful treatment. Basic mode of function of these oral appliances is to prevent the tongue from approaching the posterior wall of pharynx and causing an obstruction.

1. What is the gold standard treatment modality of OSA?
    (A) CPAP(Continuous Positive Airway Pressure)
    (B) MAD
    (C) Surgical Treatment
    (D) None

2. MAD is contraindicated in which condition?
    (A) If the patient having nasal obstruction
    (B) Patient having more than 2 missing teeth /quadrant
    (C) Patient having TMJ problem
    (D) All of the above

3. What is the clinical predictor to diagnose OSA?
    (A) Split Night study
    (B) Epworth sleepiness scale (ESS)
    (C) Polysomnography
    (D) None

4. Snoring and Mild OSA can also be corrected by-
    (A) Behavioral Modification
    (B) CPAP
    (C) Surgical Treatment
    (D) None

Answers:

1. A

   Cpap is the standard for treating the symptoms of OSA and it acts by continuously pumping room air under pressure through sealed face mask through the upper airway to the lung.(1)

2. D

   MAD gets its retention from teeth. (1)

3. B

   ESS is the questionnaire, optimally measure a patients likelihood of falling asleep in various situations.(2)

4. A

   Mild OSA can be corrected by modifications in certain area of behavior such as sleep position, alcohol use, sedative use, smoking and patient weight.(2)

References:

1. Meyer JB Jr, Knudson RC. The sleep apnea syndrome. Part I: Diagnosis. J Prosthet Dent 1989;62:675-9.

2. Meyer JB, Knudson RC. The sleep apnea syndrome. Part II: Treatment. J Prosthet Dent 1990; 63:320-4.

Fabrication of Nasal Prosthesis

Dr. Deeksha Arya, Associate Professor; Dr. Raghuwar D
Singh, Professor; Dr. Ramashanker, Associate Professor,
Department of Prosthodontics and Crown and Bridge

A 40-year old male patient reported in the department of Prosthodontics with the chief complaint of unaesthetic appearance due to depressed mid-face. The nasal area of the patient had bands of soft tissue with very little or no bony support.

Clinical Treatment:

It was planned to incorporate the soft tissue band within the prosthesis. For nasal prosthesis, facial mask impression (facial moulage) of the patient was made using alginate impression material. This moulage was used to plan the nasal prosthesis. Nasal prosthesis was fabricated by using silicone material.

1. What is the best material used to fabricate nasal prosthesis?
   (A) Self cure Acrylic resin
   (B) Silicon
   (C) Heat cure Acrylic resin
   (D) None

2. What is the advantage of Moulage impression technique?
   (A) Eliminates the need of Impression tray
   (B) Can be use for any facial defect
   (C) Accurately capture the details of defect
   (D) None

3. Most commonly used impression material for Facial defect:
   (A) Impression compound
   (B) Reversible hydrocolloid
   (C) Irreversible hydrocolloid
   (D) Impression waxes

4. What are the other methods for producing Model of the Facial defect?
   (A) Rapid Prototyping
   (B) Laser Sintering
   (C) Stereo lithography
   (D) All of the Above

Answers:

1. B

   Silicones remain the more widely used materials for facial restorations because of their good surface texture and hardness.(1)

2. A

   This technique for the fabrication of a facial moulage eliminates the need for a custom tray and thus an additional impression of the patient, which reduces laboratory and clinical time.(1)

3. C

   Alginate is the most commonly used impression material for facial defect.(1)

4. D

   CAD/CAM (computer aided design and computer aided manufacturing) system for fabrication of oral and maxillofacial prosthesis is being used. However, its use is limited due to its complexity, cost and nonavailability at many centres.(1)

Reference:

1.   Toljanic JA, Lee J, Bedard JF. Temporary nasal prosthesis rehabilitation: a clinical report. J Prosthet Dent. 1999 Oct;82(4):384-6.

Fabrication of Nasal Stent

Dr. Deeksha Arya, Associate Professor; Dr. Shuchi Tripathi,
Associate Professor; Dr Raghuwar D Singh, Professor, Department
of Prosthodontics and Crown and Bridge

A 57 year old male patient reported in the department with the surgical correction of nasal obstruction done approximately 1 week before. On examination healing wound was seen with no active site of inflammation.

Clinical treatment

A nasal stent has been given to patient for maintaining the patency of the nostril. This stent accurately fits into the place, allows nasal passage and esthetic.

1. What is the use of nasal stent?

    (A) To prevent nasal scar contracture
    (B) To prevent postoperative narrowing
    (C) To reshape the outer nasal passage
    (D) All of the above

2. What is the most commonly used material for final impression?

    (A) Alginate
    (B) Zinc oxide eugenol paste
    (C) Impression plaster
    (D) Impression compound

3. What is the length of time of stenting?

    (A) 2-7 days
    (B) 2 weeks to 6 months
    (C) 6 months to 1 Year
    (D) None

4. What is the main cause of nasal obstruction?

    (A) Trauma
    (B) Deviated nasal septum
    (C) Tumour
    (D) All of the above

Answers:

1. D

    Nasal stents are routinely use to maintain nasal cavity space during initial healing period and also prevent postoperative contracture and shape the nasal passage.(1)

2. A

    Alginate is most commonly used for impression.(1)

3. B

    Stent can be place for 2 weeks to 6 months.(2)

4. D

    Nasal obstruction can be caused by trauma, neoplasm or deviated nasal septum.(2)

References:

1. Egan KK, Kim DW.A novel intranasal stent for functional rhinoplasty and nostril stenosis. Laryngoscope 2005;115:903-909.

2. Weber R,Hochapfel F, Draf W. Packing and stenting in endonasal surgry. Rhinology 2000;38:49-62.

Obturator with Metal Ceramic Crown

Dr. Lakshya Kumar, Assistant Professor; Dr.Raghuwar
D Singh, Professor; Dr. Nehal Solanki, Senior Resident,
Department of Prosthodontics and Crown and Bridge

A 19 year old female reported to the Department of Prosthodontics with a history of ameloblastic fibroma and maxillectomy of the right side performed before 6 months. Defect was not closed surgically. The patient complains of inability to chew and regurgitation into the nasal cavity. The patient has esthetic concerns and belongs to lower middle class. Maxillectomy involves the right palatine process of the maxilla, the right palatine bone and the alveolar process from central incisor to the hamular notch. The remaining dentition is periodontally sound.

Treatment:

After oral prophylaxis, a cast obturator was planned with a vertical semi precision attachment on a porcelain fused to metal crown on the left central incisor, Embrasure clasps was planned on the left molars and circumferential clasps on left premolars.

1. According to Aramany's classification, this defect can be classified as:
    (A) Class 1
    (B) Class 2
    (C) Class 3
    (D) Class 4

2. Which of the following is/are advantage/s of an obturator prosthesis over surgical closure of the defect:
    (A) Better hygiene maintenance in the defect area
    (B) Ability to drain mucus secretions from the defect
    (C) Ability to detect recurrences at an early stage
    (D) All of the above

3. If a precision attachment was contraindicated in this case, which direct retainer would have been the most appropriate?
    (A) Cast circumferential clasp
    (B) I bar clasp
    (C) Ring clasp
    (D) Wrought circumferential clasps

4, The advantages of using a semi precision attachment over conventional direct retainer are all except?

(A) Superior retention
(B) Superior esthetics
(C) Easier to fabricate
(D) Both a and b

5. Which of the following factors favors the use of a clasp in such a case as described?

(A) High smile line
(B) Low smile line
(C) Bony undercut below the facial gingival margin
(D) Shallow vestibule

Answers:

1. A (1)

2. D

Sharma AB, Beumer J. Reconstruction of maxillary defects: the case for prosthetic rehabilitation. J Oral Maxil-lofac Surg 2005;63:1770-177(1)

3. B

Direct retainers. In: Carr A, Brown D. editors. McCracken's removable partial prosthodontics. 12th ed. St. Louis, Missouri: Elsevier; 201(1)

4. C

Grossman Y, Madjar D. Resin-bonded attachments for maxillary obturator retention: A clinical report. J Prosthet Dent 2004;92:229-3(1)

5. B

References:

1. Direct retainers. In: Carr A, Brown D. editors. McCracken's removable partial prosthodontics. 12th ed. St. Louis, Missouri: Elsevier; 2011.

Fabrication of Maxillary Obturator

Dr. Lakshya Kumar, Assistant Professor; Dr. Ramashanker, Associate Professor; Dr. Harit Talwar, Resident, Department of Prosthodontics and Crown and Bridge

A year old male patient reported to the department of prosthodontics with the chief complaint of unesthetic appearance of his face due to the missing portion of his lip. Patient was diagnosed with some chronic granulomatous inflammation but definite diagnose was not being made. Patient also complains of inability to chew and regurgitation into the nasal cavity. On clinical examination oronasal communication in the centre of the palate was found. was also found. Periodontal condition of maxillary teeth was found to be unsatisfactory with grade 2 mobility in 11.

1. According to Aramany classification the defect in palate can be classified into

   (A) Class I
   (B) Class II
   (C) Class III
   (D) Class IV

2. What will be ideal treatment plan?

   (A) Lip prosthesis only
   (B) Maxillary obturator removable prosthesis only
   (C) Both A & B but separate
   (D) Both A & B but conjoint(attached to each other with some mechanical device)

3. Which of the most common material used for fabrication of lip prosthesis

   (A) Acrylic
   (B) PEMA
   (C) Silicon
   (D) PEEK

4. While fabricating maxillary prosthesis which type of retention will be preferred?

   (A) Extra coronal
   (B) Intra coronal
   (C) Intra radicular
   (D) Circumferential clasp/ I bar

5. Which of the following mechanical retention aid can be used in jointing the maxillarycomponentand lip component of the prosthesis?
    (A) Magnets
    (B) clasps
    (C) wire
    (D) All of the above

Answers:

1. C 1

2. D 1

3. C 1

4. C 1

5. A 1

References:

1. Oki M1, Ozawa S, Taniguchi H.A maxillary lip prosthesis retained by an obturator with attachments: A clinical report.J Prosthet Dent. 2002 Aug;88(2):135-8.

Fabrication of Finger Prosthesis

Dr. Lakshya Kumar, Assistant Professor; Dr. Deeksha Arya,
Associate Professor; Dr. Rohan Grover, Junior Resident,
Department of Prosthodontics and Crown and Bridge

A 24 year old female patient reports to the maxillofacial clinic with a chief complaint of 3 missing fingers of her left hand. The index, middle and ring fingers were lost when she was 4 years old when she accidently put her hand in a chaff cutter machine. The fingers were amputated at the junction of the proximal and middle phalanx. The patient wants replacement of her lost fingers with a life like prosthesis.

1. Amputated fingers can be replaced by which of the following methods

   (A) Glove type finger prosthesis

   (B) Implant retained finger prosthesis

   (C) Reconstruction

   (D) All of the above

2. The most common material used in maxillofacial prosthetics for replacement of extraoral missing structures is

   (A) Silicone

   (B) Acrylic resin

   (C) Titanium

   (D) Waxes

3. Which type of silicone material is preferred in maxillofacial practice?

   (A) HTV (High temperature vulcanization)

   (B) RTV (Room temperature vulcanization)

   (C) Combination of RTV and HTV

   (D) None of the above

4. Which of the following materials may be used for characterization of extraoral prosthesis

   (A) Pigments

   (B) Stains

   (C) Flock

   (D) All of the above

1. Which of the following is not an advantage of high temperature vulcanization silicone
   (A) Improved life like feel of prosthesis
   (B) Low tear resistance
   (C) High resistance to chemicals and solvents
   (D) Improved staining properties

Answers:

1. D

   All the above treatment modalities may be used to restore amputated digits. (1)

2. A

   Silicone provides the best esthetic, physical and mechanical properties in the currently available maxillofacial prosthetic materials. (2)

3. A

   HTV silicones have higher strength and durability. (1)

4. D

   All of the above can be used for color characterization of maxillofacial prosthesis.(1)

5. B

   Thin margins of silicone have low tear strength. (2)

References:

1. M Suresh Babu, A Gopinadh, C Sandeep, B Sreedevi, K Krishna Kishore, M Sanjay Dutt. An innovative technique for fabrication of finger prosthesis – A case report. J Orofacial Sci. 2011;3(1):14–16.

2. Pillet Jean, O Evelyn J Mackin, library P. Aesthetic Restoration. Atlas of Limb Prosthetics: Surgical, Prosthetic, and Rehabilitation Principles: Partial-Hand Amputations.

Fabrication of Ocular Prosthesis

Dr.Raghuwar D Singh, Professor; Dr. Deeksha Arya, Associate
Professor and Dr. Himanshi Aggarwal, Senior Resident,
Department of Prosthodontics and Crown and Bridge

A 51-year-old male patient reported to the department of Prosthodontics with the complaint of unaesthetic facial appearance due to sunken appearance of right eye. Patient has a history of trauma 10 years back, net resulted in gradual loss of vision and shrinkage of eye ball. Based on history and clinical examination it was diagnosed a case of 'Phthisis bulbi.'

Clinical treatment:

After careful examination of the area of the defect and treatment planning, it was planned to fabricate a custom ocular prosthesis for the patient. Impression techniques for custom ocular prosthesis vary depending upon operator preference and defect morphology. Alginate impression material was used to take the impression of the defect site. A split cast was prepared for making the wax pattern. The shade of sclera was determined according to the patient's natural eye sclera colour. Heat cured acrylic resin was used to make the ocular prosthesis.

1. The most common impression technique for custom ocular prosthesis is:

    (A) Stock ocular tray technique
    (B) External tray technique
    (C) Syringe technique
    (D) Custom tray technique

2. Most commonly used impression material for ocular defect:

    (A) Impression compound
    (B) Reversible hydrocolloid
    (C) Irreversible hydrocolloid
    (D) Impression waxes

3. The material used in fabrication of ocular prosthesis is:

    (A) Self cure acrylic resin
    (B) Heat cure acrylic resin
    (C) Either of the above
    (D) Light cure resin

4. A properly fitted ocular prosthesis has following feature:
    (A) Retains the shape of the defect socket,
    (B) Prevent collapse or loss of shape of the lids.
    (C) Prevent accumulation of fluid in the cavity.
    (D) All of the above

Answers:

1. A

    the external tray technique is particularly useful for patients with less desirable morphology of the defect. [1]

2. C

    Alginate is the most commonly used impression material for ocular defect. Elastomers are the other material which can be used for the same purpose. [1]

3. C

    clear acrylic resin is used for fabrication of ocular prosthesis. [2]

4. D

    Properly fitted ocular prosthesis should maintain the shape of the defect socket. [1]

References:

1. Thomas D Taylor. Clinical maxillofacial Prosthodontics. Quintessence: Chicago, 2000; 265-7.

2. Aggarwal H, Singh RD, Kumar P, Gupta SK, Alvi HA. Prosthetic guidelines for ocular rehabilitation in patients with phthisis bulbi: a treatment-based classification system. J Prosthet Dent. 2014;111(6):525-8.

Fabrication of Guide Flange Prosthesis in Hemi-Mandibulectomy Patient

Dr. Raghuwar D Singh, Professor; Dr. Ramashanker,
Associate Professor; Dr. Deeksha Arya, Associate Professor,
Department of Prosthodontics and Crown and Bridge

A 45-year-old female patient reported to the department of Prosthodontics for prosthetic rehabilitation following a hemi-mandibulectomy from left condyle to left parasymphyseal region. The deviation of mandible was observed towards the reconstructed (left) side on opening due to the effect of the normal right mandibular depressor muscles action.

Clinical treatment:

During the initial healing period following hemi-mandibulectomy, prosthodontic intervention is required for preventing the mandibular deviation. Guide flange prosthesis helps patient moving the mandible normally without deviation during functions like speech and mastication.

1. What is the appropriate treatment for an edentulous patient having squamous cell carcinoma of lip with invasion into the alveolus:
    (A) Segmental mandibulectomy
    (B) Resection mandibulectomy
    (C) Hemi-mandibulectomy
    (D) Commando operation

2. What is the main function of Guide flange prosthesis?
    (A) Prevent deviation of the mandible
    (B) Help in mastication
    (C) Protect the underlying tissue to injury
    (D) Act as a post surgical template

3. After hemi-mandibulectomy, deviation of mandible occurs on:
    (A) Mediolateral
    (B) Unresected side
    (C) Resected side
    (D) Forward

4. Deviation of the mandible occurs due to the action of following muscle:
    (A) Mandibular depressor muscle of resected side
    (B) Mandibular depressor muscle of unresected side
    (C) Simultaneous action of resected and unresected side depressor muscle
    (D) Masseter muscle

Answers:

1. D

   Commando operation attributed for the en bloc removal of an advanced 1° malignancy of the oral cavity, usually squamous cell carcinoma. In a segmental resection, the condyle-to-condyle continuity is disrupted by removing all or a portion of the ramus, angle, body and parasymphysis, which is usually performed for tumours. (1)

2. A

   Guide flange prosthesis prevent deviation of mandible during speech and mastication. (1)

3. C (1)

4. B

   Muscle evolved in deviation of mandible are those which are on unresected side. (1)

Reference:

1. Taylor TD. Diagnostic considerations for prosthodontic rehabilitation of the mandibulectomy patient. In: Taylor TD, editor. Clinical maxillofacial prosthetics. Chicago: Quintessence Publishing; 2000. pp. 155–170.

Clinical Significance of Noneugenol Impression Paste

Dr. Raghuwar D Singh, Professor; Dr. Lakshya Kumar, Assistant Professor;
Dr. Ramashanker, Associate Professor, Department
of Prosthodontics and Crown and Bridge

A 55-year-old patient reported to Prosthodontic department with complaint of difficulty in mastication and unaesthetic appearance due to complete loss of maxillo-mandibular teeth for one year.

Clinical treatment:

Through oral examination, complete denture was planned for the patient. Patient was uncomfortable and complained for burning sensation in the mouth during making the final impression with zinc oxide eugenol paste. One of the chief disadvantages of the zinc oxide eugenol pastes is the possible stinging or burning sensation caused by the eugenol that leaches out and contacts soft tissues. Hence, noneugenol paste containing Orthoethoxybenzoic acid is recommended in this type of cases.

1. What is the most commonly used material for final impression?
    (A) Alginate
    (B) Zinc oxide eugenol paste
    (C) Impression plaster
    (D) Elastomeric impression material with putty consistency

2. Which following component in ZnO eugenol paste causes burning sensation in the mouth?
    (A) Zinc oxide
    (B) Lanolin
    (C) Eugenol
    (D) Resinous balsam

3. In noneugenol paste, eugenol is replaced by which material?
    (A) Benzoic acid
    (B) Lanolin
    (C) Orthoethoxybenzoic acid
    (D) Ethyline dioxide

4. Setting time of ZnO eugenol impression paste can be shortened by using:
    (A) Accelerator
    (B) Retarder
    (C) Plastisizer
    (D) Cooling the spatula & mixing slab

Answers:

1. B

ZnO Eugenol is also known as 'wash impression' material and record more accurate impression compare to other impression materials.(1)

2. C

The chief disadvantages of ZnO Eugenol paste is burning sensation, caused by Eugenol that leaches out and contacts the soft tissues.(1)

3. C

Orthoethoxybenzoic acid is a valuable substitute for eugenol.(1)

4. A

Setting time can be shortened by adding a small amount of accelerator, a drop of water or extending the mixing time.(1)

Reference:

1. Kenneth J Anusavice. Impression materials. Phillips Science of Dental materials. Elsevier Health Sciences pub. 11th edition. pp. 251-54.

Fabrication of Maxillary Obturator

Dr. Ramashanker, Associate Professor; Dr. Raghuwar D Singh, Professor; Dr. Harit Talwar, Resident, Department of Prosthodontics and Crown and Bridge

A 60 year old male patient reported to the department of prosthodontics with the history of maxillectomy due to Squamous Cell Carcinoma of maxilla. Patient complains of inability to chew and regurgitation into the nasal cavity. On clinical examination it was observed that teeth and alveolar process on one side not crossing the midline was excised. There were few missing teeth and periodontal condition of rest of the remaining teeth was found to be satisfactory.

1. According to Aramany classification this defect can be classified into

   (A) Class I
   (B) Class II
   (C) Class III
   (D) Class IV

2. Design of metal framework in maxillary obturator will be

   (A) Linear design
   (B) Tripodal design
   (C) Quadrilateral design
   (D) Bilateral design

3. Which of the following types of bulb design complicates hygiene

   (A) Open bulb
   (B) Closed bulb
   (C) Closed hollow bulb
   (D) Hygiene is not dependent on bulb type

4. During the follow up recurrence was detected and alveolar process was also excised up to the contralateral canine. The defect is reclassified into

   (A) Class I
   (B) Class II
   (C) Class III
   (D) Class IV

5. Implants can aid in an obturator prosthetics as

   (A) Direct retention
   (B) Rest
   (C) In eliminating cantilever
   (D) All of the above

Answers:

1. B

   As the defect does not cross the midline, this is an Aramany Class II condition.–(1)

2. B

   Tripodal design facilitates stabilization. – (2)

3. A

   Open bulb leads to accumulation of secretions which complicates hygiene.– (2)

4. D

   As the defect has now crossed the midline, it becomes an Aramany Class IV condition. (1)

5. D

   Implant placement greatly improves obturator prognosis from all aspects.2

References:

1. Aramany, M. A. Basic principles of obturator design for partially edentulous patients. Part I : Classification, J Prosthet Dent. 2001; 559–561.

2. Aramany, M. A. Basic principles of obturator design for partially edentulous patients. Part II : Design principles. J ProsthetDent. 2001; 86(6):562–568.

Fabrication of Orbital Prosthesis

Dr. Ramashanker, Associate Professor; Dr.Deeksha Arya, Associate Professor; Dr. Vinit Shah, Jumior Resident, Department of Prosthodontics and Crown and Bridge

A 58-year-old male patient reported to the department of Prosthodontics with the complaint of unaesthetic facial appearance due to loss of left eye and surrounding structures. Patient has a history of trauma 7 years back. Clinical treatment:

After careful examination of the area of the defect and treatment planning, it was planned to fabricate a custom orbital prosthesis for the patient. Alginate impression material was used to take the impression of the defect site. A split cast was prepared for making the wax pattern. The shade of sclera was determined according to the patient's natural eye sclera colour. Heat cured acrylic resin was used to make the orbital prosthesis.

1. Which of the following is a NOT a type of adhesive system used in maxillofacial prosthetics?
   (A) Spray-on adhesives
   (B) Pastes form adhesives
   (C) Double sided tapes
   (D) None of the above

2. Which of the following is a type of colour pigment used in maxillofacial prosthetics?
   (A) Oil based
   (B) Dry earth based
   (C) Silicone
   (D) All of the above

3. Which of the following is / are polymer material/s used in fabrication of maxillofacial prosthesis?
   (A) RTV silicone
   (B) Chlorinated polyethylene
   (C) Polyphosphazenes
   (D) All of the above

4. Removal of the globe along with all the soft tissues of the orbit is called:
   (A) Enucleation
   (B) Evisceration
   (C) Exenteration
   (D) None of the above

5. Which of the following can be used for impression of an orbital defect?
   (A) Digital impression using phase measuring profilometry
   (B) Irreversible hydrocolloid
   (C) Light bodied polysulfide
   (D) All of the above.

Answers:

1. D (1)

2. D

   All of the three can be used as a colour pigment in maxillofacial prosthesis. (1)

3. D (1)

4. B

   Evisceration is the removal of the contents of the globe while leaving the sclera and extraocular muscles intact. Enucleation is the removal of the eye from the orbit while preserving all other orbital structures. Exenteration is the most radical of the three procedures and involves removal of the eye, adnexa, and part of the bony orbit. (1)

5. D (1)

Reference:

1. Gettleman LM: Chlorinated polyethylene and polyphosphozenes. In Materials research in maxillofacial prosthesis. L. Gettleman and Z. Khan, Cochairs. J. Setcos, Editor. Trans Acad of Dental Mater. 1992; 5(1):156-172.

Metallic Denture Base

Dr. Ramashanker, Associate Professor; Dr. Lakshya Kumar, Assistant Professor; Dr. Vinit Shah, Jumior Resident, Department of Prosthodontics and Crown and Bridge

Although allergy to acrylic or its components is a relatively uncommon occurrence but it has still been reported and can be a real challenge to manage. One of the options in such a case is using a metal denture base.

1. Epithelium that lines oral cavity is:

    (A) Keratinized
    (B) Non-keratinized
    (C) Para-keratinized
    (D) Stratified squamous type

2. Mucosa on hard palate is:

    (A) Non-keratinized
    (B) Para-keratinized
    (C) Keratinized
    (D) specialized

3. Following is true for sublingual flange area, during construction of complete denture:

    (A) If used correctly can aid in retention of lower denture
    (B) It extends from canine to canine
    (C) Flange in this area should be extended vertically
    (D) It cannot form a valve seal

4. The residual monomer level in denture bases:

    (A) Is about 3% in correctly polymerized heat cured resin
    (B) Is about 30% in correctly polymerized heat cured resin
    (C) Is likely to be high if a short curing cycle is employed
    (D) Both 'A' and 'C' are correct

5. Denture stomatitis:

    (A) Is usually associated with a sore mouth
    (B) Is usually associated with wearing denture at night
    (C) Is more common in men than women
    (D) Both A and B are correct

Answers:

1. D

Stratified squamous epithelium lining of the oral cavity may be keratinized, non keratinized, para keratinized or specialized.(1)

2. C (2)

3. A

The sublingual flange area is a crucial area to gain retention and support in patients having resorbed residual ridges.(3)

4. D

Shorter curing cycles lead to less polymerization of residual monomer.(4)

5. D

Denture stomatitis is more common in females. (5)

References:

1. Sim J. Allergic reaction to Denture Base Material. *J. Can. Dent. Assoc.* 1958: 24; 292–294.

2. Strain J C. Reactions associated with acrylic denture base resins. *J. Prosthet. Dent.* 1967: 18; 465–468.

3. Stungis T E, Fink J N. Hypersensitivity to acrylic resin. *J. Prosthet. Dent.* 1969;22: 425–428.

4. Guinta J L, Grauer I, Zablotsky N. Allergic contact stomatitis caused by acrylic resin. *J. Prosthet. Dent.* 1979: 42; 188–190.

5. Devlin H, Watts D C. Acrylic 'Allergy'. *Br. Dent. J.* 1984: 157; 272–75.

Removable Dental Prostheses:Treatment Planning

Dr. Balendra Pratap Singh, Associate Professor; Dr. Kamleshwar Singh, Associate Professor, Dr. Niharika Yadav, Junior Resident; Department of Prosthodontics and Crown and Bridge

A 45 years old male patient reported to the department with complaint of poor esthetics due to several missing anterior maxillary teeth. Patient is teacher by profession and lost the teeth in an accident. On clinical examination, remaining teeth do not reveal any pathology. In the treatment planning it is decided to fabricate removable dental prosthesis to replace the missing teeth.

1. Best possible support for removable prosthesis will be provided by:
    (A) Anterior splint bar (10 gauge)
    (B) Occlusal or lingual rests
    (C) Anterior splint bar (13 gauge)
    (D) Gold alloy bars

2. If both the canines are used as abutment then their support depends on:
    (A) Alveolar bone morphology
    (B) Crown and root morphology
    (C) Design of minor connector
    (D) Design of major connector

3. Removable dental prosthesis is preferred over fixed dental prosthesis in this case, reason for this treatment planning can be:
    (A) Short length of edentulous span
    (B) Less amount of residual ridge resorption
    (C) Esthetic will be good by adding teeth to denture
    (D) Too less vertical space for fixed prosthesis

4. Guiding planes will be prepared on the abutment teeth to direct prosthesis during insertion and removal. Which of the following is untrue about guiding plane:
    (A) It eliminate gross food trap between abutment and denture
    (B) It can be prepared on more than one axial surface of abutment
    (C) Proximal guiding flange include about two third of buccal lingual width of teeth
    (D) Minor connector have same curvature as that of guiding plane

Answers:

1. A (1)

2. B

   Root morphology decides how much support a tooth can provide. (1)

3. C

   When the residual ridge is resorbed, RDP's can restore esthetics better than FDP's.(1)

4. C

   Guiding flanges should be half the bucco-lingual width of teeth.(1)

Reference:

1. Alan B, David T. McCracken's Removable Partial Prosthodontics.12th edition. St.Louis: Elsevier Mosby; 2012.

Treatment Planning for Removable Dental Prostheses

Dr. Balendra Pratap Singh, Associate Professor;
Dr. Mayank Singh, Assistant Professor, Dr. Niharika Yadav, Junior
Resident; Department of Prosthodontics and Crown and Bridge

A 43 years old male reported to department with grossly carious right first and second molar in maxillary arch. Due to poor prognosis molars were extracted. Now healing is complete and missing teeth are to be replaced. Dentition on other side of arch is complete and healthy.

1. In above mentioned case, cantilever fixed prosthesis can be most successful if:

   (A) If cantilever pontic is wider buccolingually
   (B) Cantilever prosthesis can not be given
   (C) If second molar is to be ignored
   (D) If cantilever pontic do not occlude with less than one half to two thirds of opposing tooth

2. In designing unilateral distal extension RPD major and minor connectors we may not consider:

   (A) Opposing teeth
   (B) Effect of maxillary tuberosity
   (C) Circumferential clasp on abutment
   (D) Rigidity of major connector

3. To fabricate removable dental prosthesis in this case, chromium cobalt alloy will be preferred. Popularity of this alloy over gold alloy is because of:

   (A) More weight than gold alloys
   (B) Greater Stiffness than gold alloys
   (C) Higher proportional limit than gold alloys
   (D) More yield strength than gold

4. In above mentioned case, it was preferred to remove the molars. Extraction will not be indicated in the following case:

   (A) If it will permit less complicated prosthesis design
   (B) Unesthetically positioned teeth
   (C) Sound Abutment with multiple roots and good alveolar bone support
   (D) Inadequate bone support

Answer:

1. C

   If a cantilever prosthesis has to be given in this situation, it would need to have both premolars as abutments and only 1ˢᵗ molar as pontic, respecting Ante's law. (1)

2. B

   The major or minor connector should not cover the maxillary tuberosity.(1)

3. B

   Greater stiffness of cobalt chrome alloy leads to higher rigidity of major connectors. (1)

4. C

   Unesthetically positioned teeth, inadequate bone support and complication in prosthesis design are all indications of extraction of teeth. (1)

Reference:

1. Alan B, David T. McCracken's Removable Partial Prosthodontics.12ᵗʰ edition. St.Louis: Elsevier Mosby; 2012.

Surveying

Dr. Balendra Pratap Singh, Associate Professor;
Dr. H.A. Alvi, Professor, Dr. Niharika Yadav, Junior Resident;
Department of Prosthodontics and Crown and Bridge

A 47 years old female lost her teeth in lower arch due to caries, with missing 35, 36 and 46. Now she wants fabrication of RPD to replace missing tooth. Surveying of the master cast is done.

1. During surveying, undercut must be eliminated by blockout in the diagram. Blocking out do not include-

   (A) Areas not involved should be blocked out
   (B) Ledges on which clasp patterns are not placed
   (C) Relief beneath connectors
   (D) Relief where denture will attach to framework

2. Which of the following factors do not determine path of placement during surveying:

   (A) Guiding planes
   (B) Interference
   (C) Esthetics
   (D) Location of abutment tooth

3. While surveying areas to be modified and location of rests are respectively colored in

   (A) Blue and red
   (B) Red and blue
   (C) Both in blue
   (D) Both in red

4. In surveying worn carbon marker should be discarded because worn out carbon marker

   (A) Single marker is indicated for every five teeth
   (B) They can now only be used for soft tissues
   (C) They give wrong height of contour
   (D) They give correct height of contour but mark is very dull

Answer:

1. B

   This portion is not to be included in connector design and hence needs not to be blocked out. (1)

2. D

   Guiding planes, Interference and Esthetics are important factors determining path of placement.(1)

3. D

   Areas needing preparation or modification are colored in red.(1)

4. C

   Worn out carbon marker does not contact the abutment at a single point.(1)

Reference:

1. Alan B, David T. McCracken's Removable Partial Prosthodontics.12th edition. St.Louis: Elsevier Mosby; 2012.

Failures in Fixed Partial Dentures

Dr. Jitendra Rao, Professor; Dr. Saumyendra V. Singh, Professor; Dr. Shuchi Tripathi, Associate Professor, Department of Prosthodontics and Crown and Bridge

A 35-yr old patient came with a complaint of sensitivity and inability to chew and masticate. History revealed that the area of problem was a fixed-fixed bridge which was fabricated 8 years back. It was concluded that this was a failed case. Types of failure can be: Failures due to clinical procedure, Failures due to laboratory procedures, Failures due to material's limitation, Biologic failures (e.g. Dental caries, Pulp degeneration, periodontal breakdown, Occlusal problems, Tooth perforation) and Mechanical failures (e.g. Loss of retention, Connector failure, Occlusal wear, Tooth fracture, Porcelain fracture)

1. One of the most common biologic failures is

    (A) Periodontal breakdown
    (B) Pulp degeneration
    (C) Dental caries
    (D) Tooth perforation

2. Most common cause of Clinical fracture of Fixed Partial Denture is

    (A) Excessive firing
    (B) Improper condensation
    (C) Improper moisture control
    (D) Poor framework design

3. Suck- back porosity in casting of FPD is caused by

    (A) Improper W/P ratio
    (B) Improper pattern position
    (C) Too rapid solidification
    (D) Inadequate mold & casting temperature

4. Most retentive cement for cementation of FPD is

    (A) Adhesive resin cements
    (B) Glass ionomer
    (C) Polycarboxylate cement
    (D) Zinc phosphate

5. Super floss are used for the regular maintenance of which area of the FPD

    (A) Interdental space in open margin
    (B) proximal contact of FPD and adjacent natural tooth
    (C) Ridge lap area of Pontic design
    (D) Overcontoured FPD design

Answers:

1. C

    Dental caries is one of the most prevalent disease causing biological failure of the FPD in the form of secondary caries which is not detectable early and in the initial phase of progression(1)

2. B

    Suck- back porosity in casting of FPD is caused by improper pattern position, narrow long sprue, incomplete feeding of molten metal also called Localized shrinkage porosity. (1)

3. B

    Excessive tooth preparation – leaving insufficient tooth structure to resist occlusal forces. (1)

4. A

    Adhesive resin cements are most retentive followed by glass ionomer > polycarboxylate cement > zinc phosphate because of its film thickness and bonding mechanism. (1)

5. B

    Super floss are used for the regular maintenance of mucosal contact area of pontic, having a stiff inserting tip with cushioning pad in between. (1)

Reference:

1. Rosenstiel SF, Land MF, Fjimoto J, eds. Contemporary fixed prosthodontics, 4th ed. St Louis, Mo: Mosby; 2006.

Osseointegration of Dental Implants

Dr. Jitendra Rao, Professor; Dr. Shuchi Tripathi, Associate Professor; Dr.Bhaskar Agarwal Assistant Professor; Department of Prosthodontics and Crown and Bridge

Osseintegration is defined as direct structural and functional connection between living bone and surface living bone and the surface of a load bearing artificial implant typically made of titanium and alloy.

1. Who introduced the concept of Osseointegration?

   (A) Misch
   (B) Branemark
   (C) Atwood
   (D) Weinmann

2. Surface treatment of implant is performed to enhance

   (A) Soft tissue healing
   (B) Bone and implant contact (BIC)
   (C) Stability of implant
   (D) Post-operative healing

3. Types of bone formation during the initial healing of endosseous implants

   (A) Woven bone
   (B) Lamellar bone
   (C) Bundle bone
   (D) Composite bone

4. Classifcation of bone density was defined by

   (A) Misch
   (B) brane mark and Zarb
   (C) Atwood
   (D) Boucher

5. Dense compact bone similar to oak or maple wood is seen in

   (A) D-1
   (B) D-2
   (C) D-3
   (D) D-4

Answers:

1. B

Branemark has introduced the concept of osseointegration [1]

2. B

To enhance the bone implants contact which is 40-60% without surface treatment. [1]

3. A

Type of bone is woven bone in the form primary callus at the initial level of bone healing[1]

4. A

Misc has classified the available bone in the form D1, D2, D3, D4[1]

5. A

D1 bone is very hard one similar to oak or maple wood[1]

Reference:

1. Misch CE. Diagnosis and treatment planning. Contemporary Implant Dentistry. 1st ed. St. Louis: Mosby; 1993.

Single Tooth Implant Rehabilitation

Dr. Jitendra Rao, Professor; Dr.Bhaskar Agarwal Assistant
Professor; Dr. Saumyendra V. Singh, Professor; Department
of Prosthodontics and Crown and Bridge

A 20 year male patient came with fracture of 11 with exposure of pulp, 21 with avulsion of in a road traffic accident. Treatment options can be:

- Endodontic treatment of broken tooth 11, and Fixed partial denture at 11,21 & 22
- Extraction of 11 followed by fabrication removable partial denture at 11,21
- Endodontic treatment of broken tooth 11 and implant retained crown on 21
- Extraction with Immediate implant loading of 11, conventional implant placement on 21 followed by implant retained crown on 11,21

1. What is the ideal inter implant distance?

    (A) 1.0mm
    (B) 1.5mm
    (C) 2.0mm
    (D) 3.0mm

2. While treatment planning of dental implant via radiograph, zone for ideal implant diameter corresponds to the width of the natural tooth is?

    (A) Apical 1/3
    (B) Inter proximal contact
    (C) 2mm below Cementoenamel Junction(CEJ)
    (D) Cement enamel Junction(CEJ)

3. What is the ideal implant abutment distance?

    (A) 1.5mm
    (B) 1mm
    (C) 2.5mm
    (D) 3mm

4. A maxillary central incisor is approximately 10mm at inter proximal contact, 6mm at CEJ, and 4mm at a point below the CEJ. What will be the ideal implant diameter?

    (A) 5,0mm
    (B) 6.0mm
    (C) 10mm
    (D) 4mm

5. While placing implant what should be the minimum distance from vital structre like mental foramen and inferior alveolar nerve?
   (A) 1.0mm
   (B) 1.5mm
   (C) 2.0mm
   (D) 2.5mm

Answers:

1. D

   Interimplant distance is ideally 3mm or greater. This ideal space must have adequate bone in all three dimensions, which should be at least 1mm greater than the diameter of the implant.(1)

2. C

   Tooth has its greatest width at interproximal contacts, is narrower at the CEJ, and is even narrower at the bone contact, which 2mm below the CEJ.(1)

3. A

   This dimension is required to compensate for surgical errors risk and width of the implant or tooth defect which is usually less than 1.4mm.(1)

4. D

   Diameter of an implant can be calculated below the CEJ so ideal diameter will be same as calculated diameter at particular zone.(1)

5. C

   2.0mm of surgical error risk should be maintained between implant and adjacent landmark especially vital structures.(1)

Reference:

1. Misch CE. Diagnosis and treatment planning. Contemporary Implant Dentistry. 1st ed. St. Louis: Mosby; 1993.

Resin Bonded Fixed Partial Dentures

Dr. Saumyendra V. Singh, Professor; Dr. Jitendra Rao, Professor; Dr.Rohan Grover, Junior Resident, Department of Prosthodontics and Crown and Bridge

A 26 year old female patient with high esthetic demands came to a dental clinic seeking replacement of mandibular central incisors which were lost due to trauma 2 years back. The patient was wearing a removable partial denture since one and a half years and wanted fixed prosthetic treatment. The treatment plan decided after investigations, was an implant supported prosthesis with respect to 31 and 41 using a delayed loading protocol. A provisional restoration was required in the interim of implant placement and second stage surgery.

1. The provisional restoration of choice during the healing period would be a
   (A) removable partial denture
   (B) resin bonded fixed partial denture
   (C) fiber reinforced composite restoration
   (D) provisional restoration should not be given

2. What type of resin bonded fixed partial denture is considered ideal for this case?
   (A) Rochette bridge
   (B) Maryland bridge
   (C) Virginia bridge
   (D) Cast mesh fixed partial denture

3. Lost salt technique is employed in which type of resin bonded fixed partial dentures?
   (A) Maryland bridge
   (B) Virginia bridge
   (C) Rochette bridge
   (D) Cast mesh fixed partial denture

4. Most common complication in resin bonded fixed partial dentures is
   (A) Caries of abutment teeth
   (B) Periodontal weaking of abutment teeth
   (C) Debonding
   (D) Fracture of retainers

5. Preferred luting cement for resin bonded fixed partial dentures is
   (A) Glass ionomer cement
   (B) Zinc phosphate
   (C) Zinc polycarboxylate
   (D) Composite resin based cement

Answers:

1. B

   If the edentulous span is short, the resin-bonded fixed partial denture allows tooth replacement with minimal destruction of tooth structure of abutment teeth, and is indicated for short to medium term restorations.[1]

2. A

   The ability to bond cast metal alloys to teeth was first demonstrated clinically by Rochette. Tooth surfaces are etched with acid to provide micromechanical retention for composite resin cement with abutment teeth requiring minimum preparation, thereby making Rochette bridge the ideal resin bonded fixed partial denture in this case.[1]

3. B

   Virginia bridge utilizes particle-roughened retainers by incorporating salt crystals into the retainer patterns to produce roughness on the inner surfaces for added retention.[3]

4. C

   The most common problem associated with resin-bonded fixed partial dentures is debonding of the prosthesis because of the reduced surface area available for bonding of retainers to the abutment teeth.[2]

5. D

   Modified unfilled/filled composite resin with a thin film thickness is commonly used for luting resin-bonded fixed partial dentures due to better mechanical and chemical bonding than the other luting agents.[2]

References:

1. Shillingburg HT, Hobo S, Whitsett L. Resin-bonded fixed partial dentures. Fundamentals of fixed prosthodontics. 3rd ed. Quintessence Publishing Co, Chicago; 1981: 537-63

2. Wassell RW, Walls AWG, Steele JG, Nohl F. A clinical guide to crowns and other extracoronal tooth restorations. Br Dent J 2002;192:135-42

Treatment Planning for Replacing Missing Teeth

Dr. Saumyendra V. Singh, Professor; Dr Shuchi Tripathi,
Associate Professor; Dr. Rohan Grover, Junior Resident,
Department of Prosthodontics and Crown and Bridge

A 46 year old male patient reported to a dental clinic for replacement of missing right mandibular 1st and 2nd premolars lost due to caries 1 year back. The adjacent abutment teeth were healthy having good periodontal support. The patient was a chronic smoker with a history of uncontrolled diabetes for which he was under medication since 5 years.

1. Treatment of choice for replacing missing teeth in this case would be

   (A) Implant supported fixed partial denture
   (B) Removable partial denture
   (C) Fixed partial denture
   (D) Resin bonded fixed partial denture

2. Which of the following are absolute contraindications for implant supported restorations?

   (A) chronic smoking
   (B) uncontrolled diabetes
   (C) old age
   (D) both (a) and (b)

3. The abutments of choice for design of a fixed partial denture in this case would be

   (A) mandibular 1st molar and canine
   (B) mandibular 1st and 2nd molar and canine
   (C) mandibular 1st molar, canine and lateral incisor
   (D) mandibular 1st molar

4. Which of the following are factors in fixed partial denture design

   (A) Root form
   (B) Crown: Root ratio
   (C) Axial inclination of abutment teeth
   (D) Length of lever arm

5. Prolonged sensitivity to heat, cold and pressure after cementation of fixed partial denture is probably related to

   (A) Occlusal trauma
   (B) Improper cementation
   (C) Failure to desensitize abutment teeth
   (D) Caries of abutment teeth

Answers:

1. C

   Uncontrolled diabetic patients are prone to develop infections and vascular complications. Protein metabolism is decreased, hard and soft tissue healing is delayed, nerve regeneration is altered and angiogenesis is impaired. Therefore, implant supported fixed partial denture should not be considered in the present case.[1]

2. D

   The most common immediate postoperative complication after implant surgery is incision line opening. This occurs with greater frequency in smokers because nicotine can contaminate the epithelium and affect blood circulation in the tissues. Also, uncontrolled diabetic patients are prone to develop infections and vascular complications. Therefore, implants are contraindicated in patients having a history of chronic smoking and uncontrolled diabetes.[2]

3. A

   "Ante's Law", as designated by Johnston et al is commonly used for abutment selection. It states that the root surface area of the abutment teeth should be equal to or surpass that of the teeth being replaced with pontics. The combined pericemental area of abutments in all the other options does not meet or exceeds the requirements of Ante's Law.[3]

4. D

   The root form, crown:root ratio, axial inclination of abutment teeth and length of the lever arm are all important factors in fixed partial denture design.[3]

5. A

   After cementation of a fixed partial denture, occlusion should be tested to ensure no premature contacts. There may also be excursive prematurities that may escape detection at try-in. If not corrected, these can cause tooth hypersensitivity, tenderness, and even myofacial disturbances.[4]

References:

1. Misch CE. Diagnosis and treatment planning. Contemporary Implant Dentistry. 1st ed. St. Louis: Mosby; 1993:83-85

2. Misch CE. Complete subperiosteal implants. Contemporary Implant Dentistry. 1st ed. St. Louis: Mosby; 1993:534

3. Shillingburg HT, Hobo S,Whitsett LD. Treatment planning for replacement of missing teeth. Fundamentals of fixed prosthodontics. 3rd ed. Quintessence Publishing Co,Chicago; 1981: 85-103

4. Shillingburg HT, Hobo S, Whitsett LD. Finishing and cementation. Fundamentals of fixed prosthodontics. 3rd ed Quintessence Publishing Co,Chicago; 1981: 385-418

Indications of Fixed Partial Denture

Dr. Saumyendra V. Singh, Professor; Dr Bhaskar Agarwal,
Assistant Professor; Dr. Anusar Gupta, Junior Resident,
Department of Prosthodontics and Crown and Bridge.

A 58-year-old woman requested that her missing upper right back teeth be replaced as she was having difficulty in chewing. She was medically healthy, with no history of parafunctional habits. On clinical examination, maxillary 1st molar and 2nd premolar were found missing. No carious tooth was found and plaque control was satisfactory, with no gingivitis or increase in probing depths.

A fixed partial denture (FPD) was fabricated to replace the missing teeth after clinical and radiographic evaluation.

1. What would be the minimum number of retainers required to fabricate this FPD?
    (A) Four
    (B) Two
    (C) One
    (D) Three

2. The average root surface area of Maxillary First Molar is:
    (A) 433 mm2
    (B) 431 mm2
    (C) 426 mm2
    (D) 220 mm2 .

3. In which of the following situations, fabrication of fixed partial denture is contraindicated?
    (A) Atherosclerosis
    (B) Physically handicapped patients
    (C) Very young patients
    (D) Reduced mouth opening.

4. The optimum crown to root ratio of an abutment should be?
    (A) 2:3
    (B) 3:2
    (C) 1:2
    (D) 1:1

5. Ante's law is concerned with?

   (A) Degree of tipping allowable in an abutment

   (B) Factors concerning retention.

   (C) Crown: Root ratio

   (D) Pericemental root surface area.

Answers:

1. A

   At least two abutment teeth (maxillary right first premolar and second molar) would be required to replace the missing teeth as per Ante's Law (described in key to Q.5). As clinical and radiographic evaluation has been done, it is assumed that conditions were favourable to fabricate an FPD. (1)

2. A.

   Maxillary First Molars have the highest average root surface area of all teeth in the mouth. (1)

3. C

   Fixed Partial Denture is contraindicated in very young patients due to the presence of large pulp chambers which may be exposed during tooth preparation, or cause post preparation sensitivity and pain. (2)

4. A

   Suggested crown to root ratios of abutments for fixed partial denture:
   • Ideal - 1:2
   • Optimum- 2:3
   • Minimum- 1:1 (2)

5. D

   Ante's law in fixed dental prosthodontics, refers to the observation that combined pericemental area of abutment teeth supporting a fixed dental prosthesis should be equal to or greater in pericemental area than tooth or teeth to be replaced. (3)

References:

1. Douglas ED. Treatment Planning. In:Rosenstiel SF, Land MF, Fjimoto J, eds. Contemporary fixed prosthodontics, 4th ed. St Louis,Mo: Mosby; 2006: 82-109.

2. Shillingburg H.T, Hobo S, Whitsett LD, et al, eds. Fundamentals of fixed prosthodontics. 4th ed. Quintessence Publishing Co, Inc: Chicago; 2014: 81-98

3. The Glossary of Prosthodontic Terms. *J Prosthet Dent.*8th ed. 2005; 94(1): 10-92.

Border Molding, its Significance and Materials Used for Border Molding

Dr.Jitendra Rao, Professor, Dr Bhaskar Agarwal, Assistant
Professor, Dr. Himanshi Aggarwal, Senior Resident; Department
of Prosthodontics and Crown and Bridge

A 50 year old patient reported to Prosthodontics department with complaint of unstable upper complete denture, which falls off on mouth opening and jaw movements. He reported that it was made a week ago and he is unable to use it. On clinical examination, denture borders were found to be grossly over-extended, with thick disto-buccal flanges.

1. What is the most likely cause of problem?

   (A) Neuromuscular in-coordination
   (B) Incorrect recording of jaw relations
   (C) Incorrect border molding
   (D) Xerostomia

2. What is the most commonly used material for border molding?

   (A) Tray compound
   (B) Stick modeling compound
   (C) Sticky wax
   (D) Impression plaster

3. Which material is used in single step border molding technique?

   (A) Alginate
   (B) Addition silicone
   (C) Polyether
   (D) Condensation silicone

4. Which material can only be used in sectional border molding technique?

   (A) Polyether
   (B) Addition silicone
   (C) Stick modeling compound
   (D) Condensation silicone

5. What is the amount of flange reduction of custom tray required for border molding?

   (A) 1mm
   (B) 2mm
   (C) 3mm
   (D) 4mm

Answers:

1. C.

As thick disto-buccal flanges and over-extended borders interfere with coronoid process and muscle action. (1)

2. B

Also known as low fusing compound or green stick compound. (1)

3. C

As it meets all requirements of a material that can be used for simultaneous molding of all borders. (1)

4. C

As it is impossible to get the material softened over the full length of the border simultaneously. (1)

5. B (1)

Reference:

1. Davis DM. Developing an analogue/substitute for the maxillary denture-bearing area. In: Zarb GA, Bolender CL, Eckert SE, et al, eds. Prosthodontic Treatment for Edentulous Patients: Complete Dentures and Implant-Supported Prostheses. 12th ed. St Louis, Mo: Mosby; 2004:211-231.

Pontic Designs, Indications and Contraindications

Dr. Saumyendra V. Singh, Professor, Dr. Kopal Goel, Senior
Resident; Dr Rani Ranabhatt, Junior Resident, Department
of Prosthodontics and Crown and Bridge

A 24 year old female patient reported to the department with lateral incisor avulsed due to trauma. Her adjacent central incisor was root canal treated with large access opening and no crown given. Her chief complaint was esthetic concern. She belonged to lower economic strata.

Clinical Treatment:

Pontic design in fixed partial dentures (FPD) should be determined prior to FPD construction. Various pontic designs are ridge lap, modified ridge lap, hygienic, conical and ovate. The patient was given an ovate pontic as it is the most esthetic. Its convex tissue surface resides in a soft tissue depression or hollow which is created in the residual ridge after extraction. This makes a better emergence profile. The pontic design can be easily flossed at the gingival surface.

1. Which pontic design is best indicated in thin ridges in the nonappearance zone?

    (A) Ovate pontic
    (B) Saddle pontic
    (C) Modified ridge lap pontic
    (D) Conical pontic

2. Ovate pontic design is contraindicated in which case?

    (A) Anterior region
    (B) Knife edge ridge
    (C) High smile line
    (D) Posterior region

3. Most unaesthetic pontic design is

    (A) Modified ridge lap
    (B) Ridge lap
    (C) Ovate
    (D) Hygienic

4. To replace a missing canine, the best pontic design is

    (A) Modified ridge lap
    (B) Ridge lap
    (C) Conical
    (D) Hygienic

Answer:

1. D

Ovate and modified ridge lap pontics are used in appearance zone. Saddle pontic is difficult to clean and should not be used. Conical pontics are easily cleansable. (1)

2. B

Ovate pontic can be used in anterior, posterior and high smile line cases. Conical pontic should be used in knife edge ridge. (1)

3. D

Tissue surface of hygienic pontic has to remain clear of the residual ridge by atleast 3mm. (2)

4. A

Modified ridge lap has superior esthetics and is cleansable. (2)

References:

1. Shillingburg H.T, Hobo S, Whitsett LD, et al, eds. Fundamentals of fixed prosthodontics. 3rd ed. Quintessence Publishing Co, Inc: Chicago; 1997: 485-508.

2. Douglas RD. Pontic design. In:Rosenstiel SF, Land MF, Fujimoto J, eds. Contemporary fixed prosthodontics. 4th ed. St Louis, Mo: Mosby; 2006:616-648.

Esthetics in Fixed Partial Denture

Dr. Shuchi Tripathi, Associate Professor; Dr Jitendra Rao,
Professor; Dr Saumyendra V. Singh, Professor, Department
of Prosthodontics and Crown and Bridge

33 year old female patients reported in dental clinic with chief complain of extremely mobile upper left anterior teeth. On examination remained 63 and transposition of 23 at 22 regions was found. In IOPA x-ray, lateral tooth was found to be absent.

1. Most conservative approach with sufficient esthetic would be-

    (A) Extraction of 63, providing FPD for 22, 23 and 24 with conversion of canine as lateral incisor.
    (B) Extraction of 63, orthodontic treatment of 23 at canine region and FPD for 21,22 and 23.
    (C) Extraction of 63, Implant at 23 region and converting 23 as 22.
    (D) Extraction of 63, bodily movement of 23 and implant at22 region.

2. Ideal treatment of this case at around 20 years of age should be-

    (A) Extraction of 63, providing FPD for 22, 23 and 24 with conversion of 23 as 22.
    (B) Extraction of 63, orthodontic treatment of 23 at canine region and FPD for 21,22 and 23.
    (C) Extraction of 63, Implant at 23 and converting 23 as 22.
    (D) Extraction of 63, bodily movement of 23 and implant at22 region

3. Best finish line in this case –

    (A) Chamfer finish line
    (B) Shoulder finish line(900)
    (C) Shoulder finish line(1200)
    (D) Heavy chamfer

4. Tooth considered for cantilever prosthesis-

    (A) Central Incisor
    (B) Canine
    (C) Premolar
    (D) Molar

Answers:

1. A

   Significant esthetics can be seen, provided canine eminence is not very prominent.(1)

2. D

   if age of the patient is favourable, it is better to provide orthodontic treatment and then using implant at lateral incisor as bone width will be sufficient.(2)

3. B

   as in esthetic zone, it is always preferred to use all ceramic restoration.(3)

4. B

   Canines are best suited for cantilever prosthesis due to better bone support.(4)

References:

1. S. F. Rosenstiel, M.F. Land, J. Fujimoto. Contemporary Fixed Prosthodontics, 3rd edition Page no-59-82.

2. S. F. Rosenstiel, M.F. Land, J. Fujimoto. Contemporary Fixed Prosthodontics, 3rd edition Page no-313-353.

3. H.T. Shillingberg, S. Hobo, L.D. Whitsitt et al, Fundamentals of fixed Prosthodontics, 3rd edition, Page no. 151-153.

4. H.T. Shillingberg, S. Hobo, L.D. Whitsitt et al, Fundamentals of fixed Prosthodontics, 3rd edition, Page no. 100-101.

Fixed Partial Denture Failure

Dr. Shuchi Tripathi, Associate Professor; Dr Saumyendra V. Singh, Professor; Dr Bhaskar Agarwal, Assistant Professor, Department of Prosthodontics and Crown and Bridge

A 20 year old female patient came to the department with fractured ceramic from maxillary anterior fixed partial denture in relation to teeth no. 13,12 and 1Patient was quite concerned with her esthetics and wanted to get her confidence back. During clinical examination, Metallic part of FPD was clearly seen. Spacing was noticed between maxillary and mandibular anterior teeth.

1. Best treatment plan for this case is -

   (A) Repair of previous FPD
   (B) Removal of previous FPD and fabricating similar one.
   (C) Removal of previous FPD and fabricating FPD with loop connector.
   (D) Separate crowns on abutments with implant in missing tooth.

2. Best treatment plan for anterior restoration in patient with high lip line-

   (A) All ceramic with equigingival finish lines.
   (B) All ceramic with subgingival finish line
   (C) Metal ceramic with subgingival finish line
   (D) Metal ceramic with equigingival finish line.

3. Best treatment plan for anterior restoration in patient with low lip line-

   (A) All ceramic with equigingival finish lines.
   (B) All ceramic with subgingival finish line
   (C) Metal ceramic with subgingival finish line
   (D) Metal ceramic with equigingival finish line.

4. Best Finish line preparation on facial surface for metal ceramic restoration –

   (A) Chamfer finish line
   (B) Shoulder finish line(900)
   (C) Shoulder finish line(1200)
   (D) Heavy chamfer

5. Best Finish line preparation on lingual/ palatal surface for metal ceramic restoration in anterior teeth –

   (A) Chamfer finish line
   (B) Shoulder finish line(900)
   (C) Shoulder finish line(1200)
   (D) Heavy chamfer

Answers:

1. C

   though best treatment plan for missing tooth is implant, but in given case abutments are already prepared, so it is advisable to maintain. Loop connector is preferred in diastema cases. (1)

2. B

   In high lip line cases gingival portion of anterior teeth is more visible. (2)

3. A

   it s preferable to use supragingival/ equigingival marginal preparation to avoid tissue trauma. (2)

4. C

   Sloped shoulder finish line, minimizes marginal gap width and eliminate unsupported enamel.(3)

5. A

   As it is preferable to use metallic restoration on palatal/lingual surface. (3)

References:

1. Rosenstiel SF, Land MF, Fujimoto J. Contemporary Fixed Prosthodontics, 3rd edition Page no-710.

2. Rosenstiel SF, Land MF, Fujimoto J. Contemporary Fixed Prosthodontics, 3rd edition Page no-59-82.

3. Rosenstiel SF, Land MF, Fujimoto J. Contemporary Fixed Prosthodontics, 3rd edition Page no-216-229.

Restoration of Extensively Damaged Tooth

Dr. Shuchi Tripathi, Associate Professor; Dr Bhaskar Agarwal, Assistant Professor; Dr Jitendra Rao, Professor; Department of Prosthodontics and Crown and Bridge

A 55 year old male patient came with extensively damaged tooth no. 34 with missing 3He reported that he was using removable partial denture for missing tooth and last night tooth next to that got broken while removing the denture. His history revealed previous root canal treatment of first premolar without crown fabrication. On clinical examination, around 2/3rd of crown portion of 34 was missing and palatal part was extensively damaged with only 1.5 mm axial wall left.

1. The minimum ratio of post length to the crown structure is--
   (A) 1:1
   (B) 1:2
   (C) 1:3
   (D) 2:1

2. What should be minimal vertical axial wall covered for crown during P&C fabrication-
   (A) 1mm
   (B) 1.5mm
   (C) 2 mm
   (D) 2.5mm

3. Minimum length of gutta purcha remained at the apex during post preparation in short rooted tooth is-
   (A) 5mm
   (B) 4mm
   (C) 3mm
   (D) 2mm

4. For good prognosis, post diameter should not exceed portion of root cross sectional diameter -
   (A) 1/2
   (B) 1/3
   (C) 1/4
   (D) 1/5

5. Best Choice of dowel selected in this case should be-
    (A) Tapered prefabricated
    (B) Parallel sided prefabricated
    (C) Threaded post
    (D) Custom cast

Answers:

1. A

    minimum ratio of post length to the crown structure is 1:1, while ideally it should be as long as possible without jeopardizing apical seal.(1)

2. A

    vertical axial wall less than 1mm should be extracted as there will be no ferrule effect. (2)

3. C

    Though maintaining at least 4-5 mm of apical seal is recommendable. (1)

4. B

    Increasing beyond 1/3 is not recommendable as it may weaken the root. (1)

5. D

    In elliptical or flared canals, it is better to provide custom cast post and core. (1)

References:

1. S. F. Rosenstiel, M.F. Land, J. Fujimoto. Contemporary Fixed Prosthodontics, 3rd edition Page no-272-312.

2. H.T. Shillingberg, S. Hobo, L.D. Whittsett et al, Fundamentals of fixed Prosthodontics, 3rd edition, Page no. 181-209.

Principles of Tooth Preparation And Finish Lines

Dr Bhaskar Agarwal, Assistant Professor; Dr Jitendra Rao,
Professor; Dr Saumyendra V. Singh, Professor, Department
of Prosthodontics and Crown and Bridge

Principles of tooth preparation are:Preservation of tooth structure, Retention and Resistance form, Structural durability, Marginal integrity and Preservation of periodontisum. Different type of crowns available are Partial veneer crown, Complete cast crown/Metal crown, Porcelain fused to metal crown/PFM or All ceramic crown/ Metal free crown. For all types of crowns, tooth should be prepared to receive the crown under the light of these principles. Featured like grooves, boxes etc. are added in the situation where resistance is compromised and we need extra features to increase resistance. Additionally these act as a guide for placement of crown.

1. If 3 surfaces of a tooth are prepared, what type of crown is to be fabricated

   (A) Partial veneer crown

   (B) Complete cast crown

   (C) Porcelain fused to metal crown

   (D) All ceramic crown

2. Primary purpose of occlusal preparation is

   (A) Preservation of tooth structure

   (B) Structural durability

   (C) Marginal integrity

   (D) Retention and resistance

3. Axial preparation is done for

   (A) Preservation of tooth structure

   (B) Structural durability

   (C) Marginal integrity

   (D) Retention and resistance

4. Seating groove terminates.........from the finish line

   (A) 0.3mm

   (B) 0.4mm

   (C) 0.5mm

   (D) 0.6mm

Answers:

1. B

    complete cast crowns (we always keep the chamfer finish line as it is distinct and easy to capture in an impression, will make a slip joint between the crown margin and the preparation, provides space for an adequate thickness of metal in the margin and also less amount of tooth structure is lost in comparison to shoulder margin) [1]

2. B

    Structural durability(we want to create space for the desired prosthesis so that it may berigid and does not gets fractured) [1]

3. D

    Retention and resistance (so that prosthesis does not get dislodged when forces i.e. against the path of placement, in an apical direction, oblique or horizontal direction are applied) [1]

4. C

    0.5 mm (does not disturbs the finish line, guide the crown into place during cementation and lastly both retention and resistance are enhanced. [1]

Reference:

1. Fundamentals of tooth preparations; Shilingburg H T, Jacobi R and Brackett S E. Quintessence Publishing Co. Inc. Chicago, Illinois. 1987. p13-43, 91-92.

Instrumentation And Partial Veneer Crown

Dr Bhaskar Agarwal, Assistant Professor; Dr. Shuchi Tripathi, Associate Professor, Department of Prosthodontics and Crown and Bridge

A patient comes to the department for replacement of missing Mandibular 1stMolar. History and examination revealed that missing 1st molar was extracted 10 years back and perspective abutment tooth had tipped towards the edentulous space. Treatment was planned keeping in mind the principle that the path of insertion of restoration should be parallel to long axis of the tooth and perpendicular to the plane of occlusion.

1. What can be the treatment option for tilted abutment

    (A) Uprighting tooth orthodontically
    (B) Telescopic crown
    (C) Proximal half-crown
    (D) All of the above

2. 2 The advantages of partial veneer crown

    (A) Preservation of sound tooth structure
    (B) Preservation of periodontism
    (C) Best Retention and Resistance form
    (D) Structural durability

3. which is considered to be a partial veneer crown

    (A) Three quarter crown
    (B) Proximal half-crown
    (C) Seven-eight crown
    (D) All of the above

4. why is a water spray necessary while preparing tooth with a high speed rotary instrument

    (A) To minimize pulpal damage
    (B) Keep the cutting edges clean
    (C) To increase visibility
    (D) All of the above

Answers:

1. D

    All of the above (these all will fulfill the principle that the path of insertion of restoration should be parallel to long axis of the tooth and perpendicular to the plane of occlusion)[1]

2. A

    A and B (at least one or part of the tooth structure is intact mostly the buccal/facial i.e. preservation of tooth structure, the finish line never violets the biological width so preservation of periodontism)[1]

3. D

    All of the above (in all these crown at least one or part of the tooth structure is intact and not cover by the crown)[1]

4. D

    All of the above (prolonged dehydration of freshly cut dentine will damage pulp and water stream directed on the edge of the cutting instrument will clean it and displace the debris allowing good visibility and cleanliness)[1]

Reference:

1. Fundamentals of tooth preparations; Shilingburg H T, Jacobi R and Brackett S E. Quintessence Publishing Co. Inc. Chicago, Illinois. 1987. P61-62, 95-96, 115-119, 189-190.

Periodontium And Full Veneer Crown

Dr Bhaskar Agarwal, Assistant Professor; Dr. Shuchi Tripathi, Associate Professor; Dr Jitendra Rao, Professor, Department of Prosthodontics and Crown and Bridge

A 45 year old auto driver reported with fractured restoration in mandibular 1st molar. History and radiographic examination revealed that tooth was root canal treated three years back and he did not get the crown after root canal treatment. Finish line (in any preparation) should be planned keeping in mind, marginal integrity with the restoration, respect of biologic width and ease of cleaning the margin by the patient. For preservation of periodontium, biologic width should never be violated.

1. what can be the treatment options?

    (A) All ceramic crown
    (B) Complete cast crown
    (C) Porcelain fused to metal crown
    (D) All of the above

2. what should be the angle of convergence of the prepared tooth for best retention and resistance form?

    (A) 3
    (B) 4
    (C) 6
    (D) 12

3. In general, what kind of finish line is preferred for marginal integrity of a complete cast crown?

    (A) Shoulder
    (B) Chamfer
    (C) Shoulder with bevel
    (D) Knife edge

4. Width of connective tissue attachment in relation to biologic width is

    (A) 1.07mm
    (B) 1.00mm
    (C) 0.97mm
    (D) 2.04mm

Answers:

1. D

   All of the above (the case does not tell us for destruction of Buccal surface so partial veneer can be planned, If facial surface is involved and comes in esthetic zone then Porcelain fused to metal and if not in esthetic zone then complete cast crown.[1]

2. C

   6 (the acceptable taper for adequate retention is 3 degree so the angle of convergence formed will be 3+3=6)[1]

3. B

   Chamfer (will make a slip joint between the crown margin and the preparation, provides space for an adequate thickness of metal in the margin and thus gives a better marginal integrity)[1]

4. A

   1.07mm (Biologic width i.e. 2.04mm, is the combined width of epithelial tissue attachment i.e. 0.97mm and connective tissue attachment i.e. 1.07mm)[2]

References:

1. Fundamentals of tooth preparations; Shilingburg H T, Jacobi R and Brackett S E. Quintessence Publishing Co. Inc. Chicago, Illinois. 1987. p18, 45-56, 87.

2. Carranza's Clinical periodontology; 10th ed. Newman MG, Takei HH, Klikkevol PR and Carranza FA. Elsevier Inc. p 1044.

Chapter - 9

Public Health Dentistry

Dental Fluorosis

Dr Vinay Kumar Gupta, Assistant Professor,
Department of Public Health Dentistry

A dental checkup campaign was organized in a village at Kanpur road, Lucknow. A 15 year old male child came with complaint of brownish staining of tooth. He noticed staining since he was 12 yr. old, these became darker with time. He spent 6 years of early life at Unnao district, drinking hand pumpground water. His father had similar stains. On clinical examination, corroded appearance of upper anterior with attrition of canine and pitting in lower molars was seen.

1. What would be the clinical diagnosis?

   (A) Fluorosis stain
   (B) Tetracycline stain
   (C) Tobacco stain
   (D) Tea stain

2. If the diagnosis was fluorosis, what category would it be?

   (A) Mild
   (B) Moderate
   (C) Severe
   (D) Very mild

3. The teeth that would be mostly affected with fluorosis

   (A) all primary teeth
   (B) all permanent teeth except third molars
   (C) incisors, canines, premolar and third molars
   (D) only molars

4. Confirmation of fluorosis is based on

   (A) Family History
   (B) Type of drinking water
   (C) Early Residence
   (D) All the above

5. Treatment of this case includes all except

   (A) Bleaching
   (B) Crown
   (C) Micro/ macro abrasion
   (D) Laminates & veneering

Answers:

1. A

   Consumption of water containing high level of fluoride by infant /child during first 6 yr. of life.

2. C

   Corroded appearance is the featured of severe fluorosis.

3. B

   As the child resided in the affected area till 6 years, third molars will not be involved because their calcification begins after 8 years.

4. D

   Diagnosis of dental fluorosis should be made from familial history, place of residence and quality of drinking water.

5. A

   The treatment options for fluorosis are varied depending upon individual cases. In severe fluorosis, bleaching is not done.

References:

1. Hiremath SS. Textbook of Preventive and Community Dentistry. 2nd ed. India: Elsevier, 2011.394-396.

2. I Anand Sherwood. Fluorosis varied treatment options.J Conserv Dent. 2010; 13: 47–53.

Pit and fissure sealants

Dr. Vinay Kumar Gupta, Assistant Professor,
Department of Public Health Dentistry

A dental checkup campaign was organizedin a school. A mother of 7 year old girl child came with the complaint that her daughter had pain in lower left posterior region and blackening of teeth. Clinical examination revealed all deciduous molar were carious, possibly with no pulp involvement and all permanent newly erupted 1st molars present had deep pits and fissures, further history revealed that the child had daily intake of over 10 candies.

1. What preventive measure can be adapted for the permanent molars

    (A) Apply pit & fissure sealant to molars
    (B) Amalgam filling to molars
    (C) Fluoride application to molars
    (D) Not to do anything

2. Occlusal sealants are retained on enamel surface chiefly by

    (A) Mechanical retention in deep pits and fissures
    (B) Chemical bonding between sealant and enamel
    (C) Direct adhesiveness of sealant
    (D) Mechanical retention by sealant penetration into the etched enamel

3. Pit and fissure sealant should be placed in all conditionsexcept

    (A) Presence of deep occlusal pit and fissures in newly erupted molars
    (B) Presence of incipient lesions in pit and fissure systems
    (C) Children with medical- physical impairment with high risk caries
    (D) Presence of shallow pit and fissures of molars

4. Which of following factors will reduce the retention of occlusal sealant?

    (A) Saliva contamination of etched enamel
    (B) Moisture contamination during sealant polymerization
    (C) Presence of prism-less enamel surface
    (D) All of the above

5. What are the preventive measures to be undertaken in this case?

    (A) Topical fluoride application
    (B) Pit and fissure sealants of newly erupted molars
    (C) Dietary restriction of sticky foods
    (D) All of above

Answers:

1. A

   Child shows sign of high caries activity, so to save newly erupted molars apply pit & fissure sealant.

2. D

   Occlusal sealants are retained on enamel surface chiefly by mechanical retention with etched enamel (by formation of resin tags).

3. D

   All are indications of pit & fissure sealants except d.

4. D

   Adequate isolation is the most critical aspect of sealant application. Prism less enamel (c), seems to be relatively resistant to etching.

5. D

   Child shows sign of high caries activity. All preventive measure should be taken to save tooth from further involvement.

References:

1. Hiremath SS. Textbook of Preventive and Community Dentistry. 2nd ed. Indian: Elsevier, 2011: 432-434.

2. Burrow MF, Burrow JF, Makinson OF. Pits and fissures: etch resistance in prism less enamel walls. Australian Dental Journal 2001;46:(4):258-262.

Nursing Bottle Caries

Dr. Seema Malhotra, Reader, Department of Pedodontics,
Saraswati Dental College, Lucknow and Dr. Vinay Kumar Gupta,
Assistant Professor, Department of Public Health Dentistry

A mother & children oral health education program was organized in a pre-school of Lucknow. A 5 year old girl child reported with pain in left lower posterior region. Her mother reported bottle feeding at night. Clinical examination revealed upper front teeth and lower left primary molars were grossly decayed. Lower right primary molar was also carious, and lower incisors unaffected.

1. What is the diagnosis of this child?

    (A) Nursing bottle caries

    (B) Rampant caries

    (C) Both of above

    (D) None

2. The most possible cause of above condition

    (A) Not cleaning mouth after intake of food

    (B) Prolongedbottle feeding

    (C) Not brushing properly

    (D) Spoon feeding

3. The first teeth that become involved in nursing bottle caries usually are

    (A) Mandibular canine

    (B) Maxillary anterior

    (C) Mandibular anterior

    (D) Maxillary and mandibular anterior

4. What will the dentist do in the first appointment of a nursing bottle caries patient?

    (A) Start endodontic treatment of poorly decayed teeth

    (B) Excavation of decayed portion and restoration

    (C) Start pulpotomy

    (D) Extraction

5. Best possible preventive strategy to be undertaken by pre-school mothers is

    (A) Cleaning of tooth with gauze after bottle feeding at night

    (B) Stop chocolates

    (C) Avoid sugar addition to drinks

    (D) Avoid sharing spoon with the child

Answers:

1. A

This is aunique pattern of dental decay in young children due to prolonged nursinghabit and involves upper anteriorand lower molars but not lower anterior.

2. B

Nursing bottle caries is caused by prolongedbottle feeding, especially before sleeping without mouth rinsing/ cleaning.

3. B

There is a unique pattern of involvement of teeth; maxillary incisors followed by molars

4. B

On the 1st appointment all lesions should be excavatedand restored.

5. A

Parents should be instructed to clean the child's teeth after every feed in this manner.

References:

1. Tandon S. Textbook of Pedodontics. 2nd ed., India: Paras Medical Publisher 2009: 217-221.

Oral Submucous Fibrosis (OSMF)

Dr. Vinay Kumar Gupta, Assistant Professor,
Department of Public Health Dentistry

A 23 year old male presented with limited mouth opening in acamp organized in a slum area. On taking history, the patient told about difficulty in opening of mouth, burning sensation when consuming spicy food and tobaccochewing since last 6-7 years. Clinical examination revealed poor oral hygiene with staining of teeth, marble like appearance of mucosa, fibrotic cheek tissue andmouth opening of two fingers. The clinical presentation of the patient is displayed below.

1. What is the most probable diagnosis of this case?
    (A) Trismus
    (B) OSMF
    (C) Ankylosis of TMJ
    (D) Fibrosis due to irradiation/ burn

2. Pathogenesis of OSMF:
    (A) Increased collagen phagocytosis by fibroblasts
    (B) Stimulation of fibroblast proliferation and collagen synthesis
    (C) Increase secretion of collagenase
    (D) Decrease in collagencross linkage

3. What are the possible management options of thepatient?
    (A) Elimination of Habit
    (B) Elimination of Habit and surgical release at retro molar area
    (C) Elimination of Habit, muscle extension exercises, placental extract injections
    (D) Antibiotics

4. Histological finding at affectedsite would be
    (A) Non-keratinised mucosa with fibrosis of connective tissue which is acellular
    (B) Atrophic and parakeratinised mucosa with acellular fibrosis
    (C) Keratinized mucosa with cellular fibrosis of connective tissue
    (D) Parakeratinised mucosa with no fibrosis of connective tissue

5. Rate ofmalignant transformation in OSMF is
    (A) 10%
    (B) 1%
    (C) 20%
    (D) 25%

Answers:

1. B

   Complaint of limited mouth opening, leathery appearance of mucosa, burning sensation of oral mucosa and history oftobacco chewing lead to a probable diagnosis of oral submucous fibrosis.

2. B

   Pathogenesis of OSMF has been suggested as stimulation of fibroblast proliferation and collagen synthesis, decreased secretion of collagenase, deficiency in collagen phagocytosis by fibroblasts and increase in collagen cross linkage by fibroblasts.

3. C

   Management of OSMF includeselimination of habit, nutritional support (high protein, Vitamin B etc), immune modulatory drugs (local & systemic application of glucocorticoids and placental extracts) & physiotherapy (forceful mouth opening and heat therapy)

4. B

   Histologically epithelial changes in OSMF are hyperplasia (early) and atrophy (advanced). Lesions of the palate show predominantlyorthokeratosis and those of buccal mucosa, parakeratosis.

5. A

   Oral submucous fibrosis has malignant transformation of 7-13%.

References:

1. Rajendran R, Sivapathasundaram B, editors. Shafer'sTextbook of oral pathology, 7th ed.India: Elsevier 2012: 98-101.

2. Peter S. Essential of Public Health Dentistry, 5th ed. India: Arya Medi Publishing, 2013: 329.

Atraumatic Restorative Treatment (ART)

Dr. Vinay Kumar Gupta, Assistant Professor,
Department of Public Health Dentistry

In a village of 2000 occupants, there is no electricity or water supply. Inhabitants have poor living standards and unavailability of resources. The only way to reach there is by two wheelers. The nearest primary health center is 20 km away, with no facility for dental treatment. One primary school is present. Only unqualified dentists are available for treatment. On examination most people had dental decay without involving pulp.

1. What restorative approach should be used to treat the carious teeth

    (A) Amalgam restoration approach
    (B) Composite restoration approach
    (C) ART approach
    (D) None of the above

2. Principle of ART is

    (A) Removing carious tooth tissue using hand instrument only
    (B) Removing carious tooth tissue using rotary instrument only
    (C) Restore the cavity with adhesive cement
    (D) Removing carious tissue using hand instrument only & restoring cavity with adhesive cement

3. Indication of ART is

    (A) Exposure of pulp
    (B) Painful teeth with chronic inflammation of pulp
    (C) Presence of swelling or fistula near the carious tooth
    (D) Carious tooth without pulpal involvement

4. Reason to use Glass Ionomer Cement (GIC) for ART are all except

    (A) Fluoride release
    (B) Chemical bonding
    (C) Mechanical bonding
    (D) Biocompatibility

5. What type of GIC do we use in ART

    (A) Type II
    (B) Type IV
    (C) Type IX
    (D) Type V

Answers:

1. C

   ART procedure was originally developed for deprived communities, not able to obtain dental care.

2. D

   Principle of ART is removing carious tooth tissue using hand instrument only & restore the cavity with adhesive cement.

3. D

   Choice d is indication of ART and all others are contraindications.

4. C

   GIC chemically bonds to enamel & dentine. Fluoride release from restoration prevents & arrest caries. GIC is biocompatible.

5. C

   Glass Ionomer type IX cement is used for ART.

References:

1. Hiremath SS. Textbook of Preventive and Community Dentistry. 2nd ed. Indian:Elsevier, 2011: 440-441.

2. Lopez N, Rafalin SS, Berthold P. Atraumatic Restorative Treatment for Prevention and Treatment of Caries in an Underserved Community. American Journal of Public Health August 2005, Vol 95, No. 8; 1338-1339.

Biostatistics

Dr. Vinay Kumar Gupta, Assistant Professor,
Department of Public Health Dentistry

The fasting blood sugar of 9 individuals was as follows 90, 95, 101, 98, 99, 95, 102, 87, 115.

1. What is the arithmetic mean of blood sugar of these 9 individuals?

    (A) 98
    (B) 99
    (C) 100
    (D) 102

2. What is the arithmetic median of blood sugar of these 9 individuals?

    (A) 98
    (B) 99
    (C) 100
    (D) 102

3. What is the arithmetic mode of blood sugar of these 9 individuals?

    (A) 95
    (B) 98
    (C) 90
    (D) 100

4. The range of fasting blood sugar of these 9 individuals was

    (A) 90-110
    (B) 80-115
    (C) 87-115
    (D) 95-115

5. The standard deviation in fasting blood sugar range of above individuals was

    (A) 8
    (B) 9.6
    (C) 9.2
    (D) 8.6

Answers:

1. A

    Arithmetic meanis calculated by first adding individual observation and then dividing this no. of observations.

2. A

    To obtain median, the Data is first arranged in an ascending or descending order and then value of the middle observation is considered the median. If there were 10 values instead of 9, the median would be calculated by taking the average of two middle values.

3. A

    It is the most commonly occurring value in a distribution of data.

4. C

    Range is the simplest measure of dispersion. It is defined as the difference between the highest and lowest figure in a given sample.

5. C

    Standard deviation (SD) is the most frequently used measure of deviation.

    Steps involve in calculating SD are:
    a) First of all, take the deviation of each value from the arithmetic mean,$(x-x)$
    b) Then square each deviation-$(x-x)^2$
    c) Add up the squared deviations-$\sum(x-x)^2$
    d) Divide the result by the number of observations n [or (n-1) in case the sample size is less than 30]
    e) Then take the square root, which gives the standard deviation.

x	(x-x)	(x-x)^2
90	-8	64
95	-3	9
101	3	9
98	0	0
99	1	1
95	-3	9
102	4	16
87	-11	121
115	17	289
		518

S.D = $\sqrt{\sum(x-x)^2 / n-1}$ = $\sqrt{518/9-1}$ = $\sqrt{518/8}$ = $\sqrt{64.75}$ = 8.047 (1)

References:

1. K. park. Park's textbook of preventive and social medicine. 18th ed. India: Banarsidas bhanot publishers, 2005: 646-647.

Oral Cancer

Dr Vinay Kumar Gupta, Assistant Professor,
Department of Public Health Dentistry

A 48 year old male patient came with a complaint of chronic non healing ulcer on left side of tongue since 2 months, rapidly increasing in size. The lesion had a 10mm diameter with irregular margins. The patient gave history of heavy tobacco chewing since approximately 15 years.

1. The most probable diagnosis is

    (A) Oral cancer
    (B) Apthous ulcer
    (C) Ranula
    (D) Fibroma

2. Confirmatory diagnosis of this case can be done by

    (A) Screening
    (B) Toluidine blue staining
    (C) Biopsy
    (D) Ultrasound

3. Commonest cancer of oral cavity is

    (A) Tongue
    (B) Floor of mouth
    (C) Lip
    (D) Gingiva

4. The best possible way to prevent oral cancer at community level is

    (A) Education about basic factors causing it
    (B) Ban on tobacco products
    (C) Proper nutrition
    (D) Periodic visit to dentist

5. Key to early detection of cancer at community level

    (A) X-ray
    (B) Screening
    (C) Biopsy
    (D) Blood examination

Answers:

1. A

   Any ulcer of mucosa which fails to heal within 2 weeks of appropriate therapy, with features as presented in the case, should raise suspicions of oral cancer.

2. C

   Biopsy is a procedure in which tissue sample is excised from site for examination and evaluated under microscope.

3. A

   Commonest cancer of oral cavity worldwide is that of the tongue.

4. A

   Best way to prevent oral cancer at community level is health education about factors associated with oral cancer.

5. B

   Screening for oral cancer is key to early detection at community level.

References:

1. Hiremath SS. Textbook of Preventive and Community Dentistry. 2nd ed. India: Elsevier, 2011: 162-166.

Epidemiology (Case Control study)

Dr Vinay Kumar Gupta, Assistant Professor,
Department of Public Health Dentistry

In a case control study, the distribution of gutka and non gutka chewers in case (oral cancer patients) and control (no oral cancer subjects) subjects in a study sample was as given below:

	Case (Oral cancer)	Control (without oral cancer)
Gutka chewers	20 (a)	15 (b)
Non Gutka chewers	15 (c)	20 (d)

The case group was found to be consuming gutka more frequently than control and difference was statistically significant (p<0.05).

1. This indicates:

   (A) Gutka is the cause of disease
   (B) Incidence of disease was more in those consuming gutka
   (C) The disease can be cured if gutka is stopped
   (D) An association exists between gutka and oral cancer

2. Odds ratio (OR) of getting oral cancer in gutka chewers is:

   (A) 0.44
   (B) 1.0
   (C) 1.7
   (D) 2.5

3. Exposure rate of cases a/a+c

   (A) 50%
   (B) 57%
   (C) 67%
   (D) 70%

4. Case control study is also called

   (A) Retrospective
   (B) Prospective
   (C) Prevalence
   (D) Incidence

5. All of the following are advantages of case control studies except:
    (A) Useful in rare disease
    (B) Incidence can be calculated
    (C) Odds ratio can be calculated
    (D) Cost-effective and inexpensive

Answers:

1. D

    Case control study assess the statistical association between exposure and occurrence of disease. Incidence is measured by cohort study.

2. C

    Odds ratio=a x d/b x c=20 x 20/15 x 15=1.7

3. B

    Exposure rate of cases a/a+c =20/35=57%.

4. A

    Case control study is also called Retrospective study.

5. B

    Incidence can only be determined by a cohort study.

Reference:

1. K. Park. Park's textbook of preventive and social medicine. 18th ed. India: Banarsidas bhanot publishers, 2005: 65-68.

Acute Fluoride Toxicity

Dr. Vinay Kumar Gupta, Assistant Professor,
Department of Public Health Dentistry

A male child aged 4 years weighing around 9 Kg from a well off family, ingested 50mg of adult toothpaste due to craving for mint flavor. The parents found the child vomiting and crying with abdominal pain. The child complained of tingling sensation of the extremities.

1. What is the most probable diagnosis?

   (A) Acute fluoride toxicity
   (B) Chronic fluoride toxicity
   (C) Allergic reaction
   (D) None

2. Main gastro intestinal site of absorption for fluoride is

   (A) Stomach
   (B) Small and large Intestine
   (C) Large intestine
   (D) Oral cavity

3. In this case home remedy we can use

   (A) Vinegar
   (B) Water
   (C) Milk
   (D) NaHCO3

4. Nausea, the most frequently encountered symptom in acute fluoride toxicity, is due to

   (A) Formation of hydrogen peroxide
   (B) Formation hydrofluoric acid
   (C) Formation hydrochloric acid
   (D) Formation of bicarbonates

5. In acute fluoride toxicity, chances are of

   (A) Hypocalcaemia
   (B) Hypercalcaemia
   (C) Hyponatrimia
   (D) Hypernatrimia

Answers:

1. A

   Nausea, vomiting, abdominal pain, tingling sensation of the extremities indicate acute fluoride toxicity.

2. A

   Absorption of fluoride is mainly from the Stomach.

3. C

   Calcium rich preparation (milk) can relieve gastrointestinal symptoms.

4. B

   Most frequently encountered symptoms in acute fluoride toxicity is nausea. This is caused by fluoride combining with hydrogen in the gastric juice to form hydrofluoric acid, a stomach irritant.

5. A

   In acute fluoride poising hypocalcaemia may be detected.

References:

1. Hiremath SS. Textbook of Preventive and Community Dentistry. 2nd ed. India: Elsevier, 2011: 395.

2. Peter S. Essential of Public Health Dentistry, 5th ed. India: Arya Medi Publishing, 2013: 521-557.

Oral Health Survey

Dr Vinay Kumar Gupta, Assistant Professor, Department of Public Health Dentistry

Population of India is approximately 1.25 billion and previous scattered studyreportsshows poor oral conditions. A well implemented oral health policy is required to improve this. To form anoral health policy, policy makers should have proper data. Ministry of health and family welfarehave directed the dental council of India (DCI) to collect proper data.

1. What approach should DCI use to collect information about oral health of a community?
   (A) WHO 1997 performa
   (B) WHO 1986 performa
   (C) Proforma using DMFT index
   (D) Proforma using CPITN

2. Which one is the first step to conduct a survey?
   (A) Select the sample
   (B) Designing the investigation
   (C) Establish the objective
   (D) Analyze the data

3. Index ages for oral health survey are
   (A) 5,15,25,35 and 65-70 years
   (B) 5,10,15,30 and 60-70 years
   (C) 5, 12, 15, 35-44 and 65-74 years
   (D) 5-10, 15-35 and 40-65 years

4. To conduct pilot survey in a population, usualindex ageselected is
   (A) 2 years
   (B) 15 years
   (C) 35-44 years
   (D) 65-74 years

5. Which age has been chosen globally for monitoring caries for international comparison?
   (A) 5 years
   (B) 12 years
   (C) 15 years
   (D) 35-44 years

Answers:

1. A

    There are several approaches to collecting information about oral health of a community. WHO oral health surveymeasures the prevalence and nature of oral diseases in a community and describes the community's oral health needs. WHO provides a systematicapproach to collection and reporting of data on oral disease and conditions in the WHO 1997 Proforma.

2. C

    First step to conduct a survey is to establish the objective.

3. C

    Index ages for oral health survey are 5, 12, 15, 35-44 and 65-74 years.

4. A

    A pilot survey is one that includes only the most important subgroup in the population-usually 12 years.

5. B

    12 yrs. has been chosen globally for monitoring caries for international comparison and monitoring of disease trend.

Reference:

1. Hiremath SS. Textbook of Preventive and Community Dentistry. 2nd ed. Indian: Elsevier, 2011: 190-194.

Printed in the United States
by Bookmasters

Printed in the United States
By Bookmasters